Respiratory
Pharmacology and
Pharmacotherapy

Series Editors:

Dr. David Raeburn
Discovery Biology
Rhône-Poulenc Rorer Ltd
Dagenham Research Centre
Dagenham
Essex RM10 7XS
England

Dr. Mark A. Giembycz
Department of Thoracic Medicine
National Heart and Lung Institute
Imperial College of Science, Technology and Medicine
London SW3 6LY
England

Asthma: Epidemiology, Anti-Inflammatory Therapy and Future Trends

Edited by
M. A. Giembycz
B. J. O'Connor

Springer Basel AG

Editors:

Dr. Mark A. Giembycz
Department of Thoracic Medicine
National Heart and Lung Institute
Imperial College of Science,
Technology and Medicine
London SW3 6LY
England

Dr. Brian J. O'Connor
Clinical Studies Unit
The Royal Brompton National Heart
and Lung Hospital
Sydney Street
London SW3 6NP
England

A CIP catalogue record for this book is available from the library of Congress, Washington D.C., USA

Deutsche Bibliothek Cataloging-in-Publication Data

Asthma: epidemiology, anti-inflammatory therapy and future trends / ed. by Mark A. Giembycz ; Brian J. O'Connor. – Basel ; Boston ; Berlin : Birkhäuser, 2000
(Respiratory pharmacology and pharmacotherapy)
ISBN 978-3-0348-9585-9   ISBN 978-3-0348-8480-8 (eBook)
DOI 10.1007/978-3-0348-8480-8

The publisher and editor cannot assume any legal responsibility for information on drug dosage and adminis-tration contained in this publication. The respective user must check its accuracy by consulting other sources of reference in each individual case.

The use of registered names, trademarks, etc. in this publication, even if not identified as such, does not imply that they are exempt from the relevant protective laws and regulations or free for general use.

ISBN 978-3-0348-9585-9

© 2000 Springer Basel AG
Originally published by Birkhäuser Verlag in 2000
Softcover reprint of the hardcover 1st edition 2000

Printed on acid-free paper produced from chlorine-free pulp. TCF ∞

Cover design: Markus Etterich

ISBN 978-3-0348-9585-9

9 8 7 6 5 4 3 2 1

Contents

List of Contributors

C. Richard W. Beasley, Wellington Asthma Research Group, Department of Medicine, Wellington School of Medicine, P.O. Box 7343, Wellington South, New Zealand; e-mail: Beasley@wnmeds.ac.nz

John R. Britton, Division of Respiratory Medicine, University of Nottingham, City Hospital, Hucknall Road, Nottingham NG5 1PB, UK

K. Fan Chung, National Heart and Lung Institute, Imperial College School of Medicine, Dovehouse St., London SW3 6LY, UK; e-mail: f.chung@ic.ac.uk

John Costello, Department of Respiratory Medicine and Allergy, Guy's, King's & St. Thomas' School of Medicine, King's College London, Bessemer Road, London SE5, UK

Julian Crane, Wellington Asthma Research Group, Department of Medicine, Wellington School of Medicine, P.O. Box 7343, Wellington South, New Zealand; e-mail: Crane@wnmeds.ac.nz

David J. Evans, Respiratory Medicine, Royal Brompton Hospital, Sydney Street, London SW3 6NP, UK

Duncan M. Geddes, Respiratory Medicine, Royal Brompton Hospital, Sydney Street, London SW3 6NP, UK

Freddy E. Hargreave, Asthma Research Group, St. Joseph's Hospital, McMaster University, Hamilton, Ontario, Canada L8N 4A6; e-mail: hargreav@fhs.mcmaster.ca

Peter König, Department of Child Health, University of Missouri, N708 Health Sciences Center, 1 Hospital Drive, Columbia, MO 65212, USA

Sarah A. Lewis, Division of Respiratory Medicine, University of Nottingham, City Hospital, Hucknall Road, Nottingham NG5 1PB, UK

Paul M. O'Byrne, Asthma Research Group and Department of Medicine, McMaster University, Hamilton, Ontario, Canada L8N 3Z5

Clive P. Page, Sackler Institute of Pulmonary Pharmacology, Division of Pharmacology and Therapeutics, Guy's, King's & St. Thomas', School of Biomedical Sciences, 5th Floor, Hodgkin Building, Guy's Campus, London SE1 9RT, UK; e-mail: clive.page@kcl.ac.uk

K. Parameswaran, Asthma Research Group, St. Joseph's Hospital, McMaster University, Hamilton, Ontario, Canada L8N 4A6

Neil E. Pearce, Wellington Asthma Research Group, Department of Medicine, Wellington School of Medicine, P.O. Box 7343, Wellington South, New Zealand; e-mail: Pearce@wnmeds.ac.nz

Søren Pedersen, University of Odense, DK-5000 Odense, Denmark

Malcolm R. Sears, Firestone Regional Chest and Allergy Unit, St. Joseph's Hospital, McMaster University, Hamilton, Ontario, Canada L8N 4A6; e-mail: searsm@fhs.csu.mcmaster.ca

D. Robin Taylor, Department of Medicine, Dunedin School of Medicine, University of Otago, P.O. Box 913, Dunedin, New Zealand; e-mail: robin.taylor@stonebow.otago.ac.nz

Asthma: Epidemiology, Anti-Inflammatory Therapy and Future Trends
ed. by M. A. Giembycz and B. J. O'Connor
© 2000 Birkhäuser Verlag/Switzerland

CHAPTER 1
Epidemiology of Asthma Mortality

C. Richard W. Beasley, Neil E. Pearce and Julian Crane

Wellington Asthma Research Group, Department of Medicine, Wellington School of Medicine, Wellington South, New Zealand

1. Introduction

The epidemiology of asthma mortality has been controversial since Osler stated in the *Principles and Practice of Medicine*, published in 1901, that the "the asthmatic pants into old age" [1]. Certainly asthma deaths were rare in the first half of this century, although since this time, the patterns of asthma mortality have become considerably more complex. There have been epidemics of asthma deaths in six Western countries in the 1960s, and again in New Zealand in the 1970s. Another feature observed in many countries has been a more gradual increase in asthma mortality, which commenced in the 1940s and has been particularly marked in the 1970s and 1980s. During the 1990s, mortality has declined in some, but not in other countries. In this chapter, we commence by briefly considering issues relevant to the interpretation of long-term time trends in asthma mortality. We then discuss the international trends in asthma mortality throughout the 20th century, focusing primarily on the possible causes for the mortality epidemics and the gradual rise in asthma mortality which has occurred over recent decades. Finally, we review markers of an increased risk of asthma mortality, the characteristics of patients experiencing a fatal or near fatal attack of asthma, and factors that can provoke such episodes.

2. Long-Term Time Trends

2.1. Validity of Mortality Data

International time trends in asthma mortality are inherently difficult to interpret due to the many different factors that may change in different countries over this time. It is crucial that the mortality data is valid, and in this respect a number of key issues need to be considered including the accuracy of death certificates, changes in disease classification, and changes in diagnostic fashion [2].

Almost all comparative studies of asthma mortality have been confined to the 5 to 34 years age group, because the diagnosis of asthma mortality is more firmly established in this group [3]. By eliminating younger children in whom the diagnosis may be confused with other conditions such as bronchiolitis, and older patients in whom it may not be possible to differentiate the diagnosis of asthma from chronic bronchitis and emphysema, routine death certificates have been shown to be reasonably accurate. For example, Sears et al. [4] observed that in patients aged 5 to 34 years, the recorded information was considered accurate in 98% of all certified deaths, and in 100% of deaths coded as asthma in national mortality data (Fig. 1). The accuracy declined with increasing age and was less than 70% in those aged 65 years or more. Most studies of this type have only examined the possibility of false positive reporting (i.e. deaths from other causes being falsely attributed to asthma). However, in one study in which false negative reporting was examined (i.e. asthma deaths being falsely assigned to other categories), it appeared to be very rare [5].

Changes in disease classification are also of concern, as the International Classification of Diseases has gone through several major changes in coding practices for asthma deaths since the early 1900s [6]. These largely involved changes in the coding of deaths due to "Asthma and bronchitis" which were assigned to bronchitis during some periods and to asthma during others (Tab. 1). However, these changes have primarily affected the data for the older age-groups, and they appear to have had little effect on the key trends in the 5–34 age group [2]. For example, the most important revision occurred with the change from ICD-4 to ICD-5, when the method of coding the underlying cause of death was changed, but no major changes in mortality rates occurred [2]. A further significant change occurred with the change from ICD-8 to ICD-9; however, bridge coding exercises found that the maximum possible increase that could be attributed to the change was approximately 5% [7, 8].

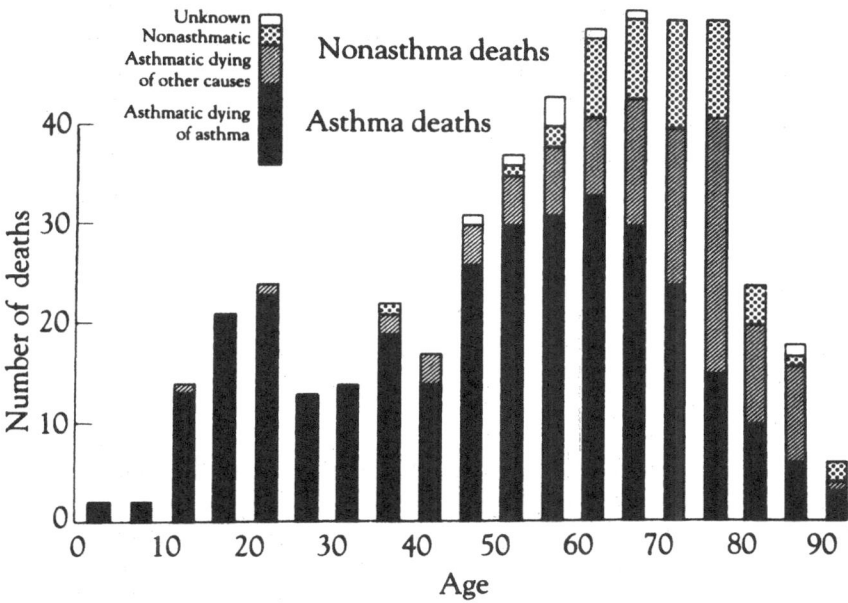

Figure 1. Accuracy of certification of asthma deaths as judged by a review panel of physicians, of 492 cases with asthma in Part 1 of the death certificate or on the coroner's report of cause of death. (Source: adapted from ref. [4].)

Table 1. Changes to coding of asthma deaths during this century

Classification	Years	Comments
Bertillon	1908–1922	"Asthma and bronchitis" coded according to which was judged to be underlying cause of death.
ICD 3	1923–1929	"Asthma and bronchitis" coded according to which was judged to be underlying cause of death.
ICD 4	1930–1939	"Asthma and bronchitis" coded according to which was judged to be underlying cause of death.
ICD 5	1940–1949	"Asthma and bronchitis" coded as bronchitis "Asthmatic bronchitis" coded as asthma.
ICD 6	1950–1958	"Asthma and bronchitis" coded as asthma.
ICD 7	1959–1967	"Asthma and bronchitis" coded as bronchitis, unless the asthma was specified as allergic.
ICD 8	1968–1978	"Asthma and bronchitis" coded as bronchitis.
ICD 9	1979–1988	"Asthma due to bronchitis" coded as bronchitis. "Bronchitis due to asthma" coded as asthma.
ICD 10	1989–	"Asthma due to bronchitis" coded as bronchitis. "Bronchitis due to asthma" coded as asthma.

The effects of changes in diagnostic fashion over time are more difficult to assess, although several attempts have been made by simultaneously examining time trends in other respiratory diseases which could be confused with asthma [2, 6]. In general, these exercises have found that changes in diagnostic fashion could not account for the most striking time trends (such as the 1960s mortality epidemics), but it is not possible to exclude changes in diagnostic fashion as a partial explanation for the more gradual changes in asthma mortality.

It is with these considerations in mind that the different patterns of asthma mortality that have been observed in different countries during this century are discussed.

2.2.   1900 to 1960

Those western countries in which the relevant data has been published indicate that asthma mortality was uniformly low and relatively stable between 1900 and 1940 (Fig. 2) [6, 9–11]. The death rate began to increase gradually in the 1940s in a number of countries including New Zealand and Australia, in which a three-fold increase over a 15-year period was observed. Mortality declined again in the late 1950s in New Zealand, England and Wales, but not in Australia. In contrast, little change in asthma mortality rates was observed in the USA during this period.

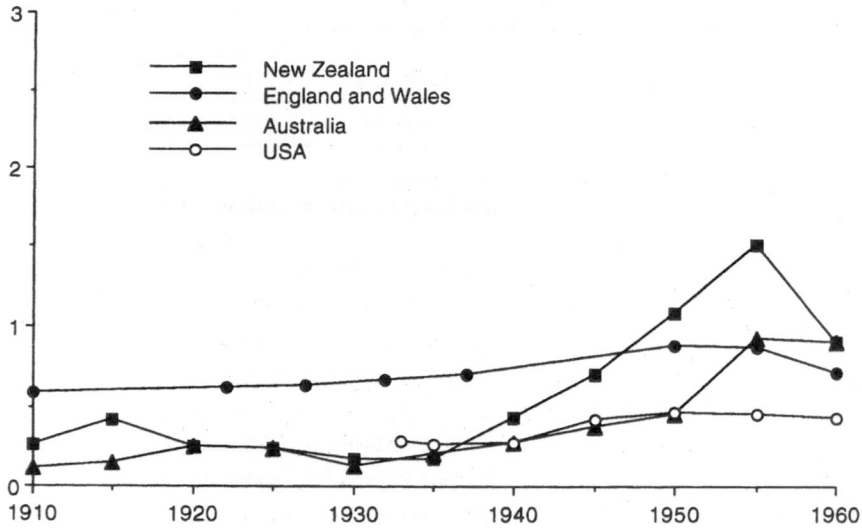

Figure 2. Asthma mortality (per 100 000) in persons aged 5–34 years in New Zealand, Australia, England and Wales, and the USA 1910–1960. (Source: adapted from refs. [6, 9–11])

Although the interpretation of death rates over such an extended period is difficult, the historical data is likely to be of acceptable accuracy in this age group and the patterns observed did not appear to be due to changes in coding or diagnostic fashion. Possible factors include an increase in asthma prevalence due to changes in environmental risk factors such as aeroallergens, diet, smoking, occupational exposures, or the incidence of environmental protective factors such as respiratory infections, as has been recently postulated [12]. Alternatively, the gradual changes in mortality could have been due to changes in the management of asthma. In this respect, interest has focused primarily on the introduction of isoprenaline as an atomiser spray during the 1940s when mortality began to increase, and the introduction of corticosteroids in the 1950s when mortality declined. It is difficult to investigate these hypotheses, because of the gradual nature of the changes and the lack of precise data on the many different putative factors during this period.

2.3. 1960s Epidemics (Fig. 3)

In the mid 1960s, asthma mortality increased dramatically in at least six western countries; England and Wales, Scotland, Ireland, New Zealand, Australia and Norway [13]. In these countries, the mortality rates increased two- to 10-fold within a 2- to 5-year period (Tab. 2). Other countries such as the United

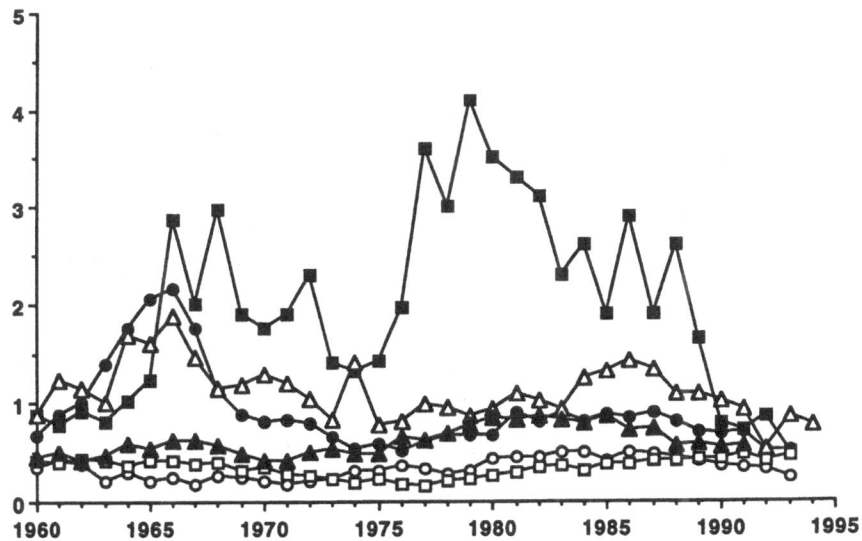

Figure 3. International patterns of asthma mortality in persons aged 5–34 years, 1960–1994, showing the different trends. (■—■) New Zealand; (●—●) England and Wales; (△—△) Australia; (▲—▲) West Germany; (○—○) Canada; (□—□) United States. (Source: adapted from refs. [2, 29, 36])

Table 2. Mortality from asthma at ages 5 to 34 years in 14 countries

	1959	1960	1961	1962	1963	1964	1965	1966	1967	1968
England & Wales	0.66	0.68	0.89	1.00	1.40	1.76	2.05	2.18	1.76	1.13
Scotland	0.82	1.08	0.79	0.70	1.23	1.63	1.32	2.59	1.77	1.22
Rep. Of Ireland	0.90	0.45	0.71	0.55	0.47	1.18	1.42	1.06	1.36	0.66
Australia	1.06	0.89	1.23	1.15	1.03	1.70	1.60	1.88	1.44	-
New Zealand	0.81	0.88	0.78	0.92	0.82	1.03	1.24	2.87	1.99	-
Sweden	-	-	0.64	0.48	0.51	0.76	0.31	0.62	0.55	-
Denmark	0.15	0.15	0.24	0.19	0.34	0.24	0.28	0.66	0.42	-
FR Germany	0.39	0.41	0.53	0.42	0.45	0.59	0.54	0.63	0.56	-
Netherlands	0.42	0.68	0.35	0.42	0.52	0.42	0.55	0.51	0.59	0.38
Belgium	0.24	0.42	0.24	0.36	0.46	0.38	0.65	0.37	-	-
United States	0.37	0.41	0.40	0.43	0.41	0.36	0.42	0.41	0.38	-
Japan	0.71	0.86	0.84	0.89	0.99	1.03	1.00	1.01	1.01	-
Norway	0.13	0.13	0.00	0.26	0.51	0.76	1.26	1.00	0.68	0.49
Canada	0.30	0.34	0.41	0.37	0.24	0.33	0.32	0.31	0.26	0.35

Note: Dash indicates that data were not available
(From Stolley PD (1972) *Am Rev Respir Dis* 105: 883. With permission)

States, Denmark, Sweden, Canada, Germany and The Netherlands did not experience epidemics, although in some countries such as Japan, significant increases in asthma mortality were noted within more narrowly defined age groups [14]. The initial detailed examination of mortality trends in England and Wales concluded that the epidemic was real and was not due to changes in death certification, disease classification or diagnostic practice [15]. The most likely explanation was an increase in case fatality, possibly due to new methods of treatment. Interest focused initially on the possible role of pressurised metered dose beta agonist aerosols which had been introduced in the early 1960s, however it was soon apparent that while this may explain the observed trends in some countries such as England and Wales (Fig. 4) [16], it could not explain the international patterns.

Subsequent examination of international time trend data suggested that the epidemics were related to the use of a high-dose beta agonist aerosol isopre-

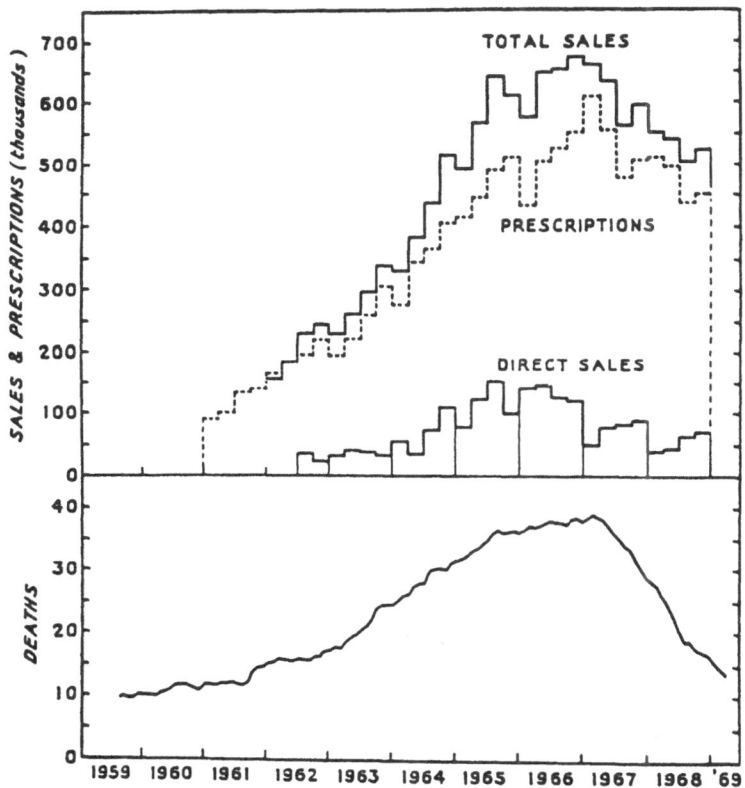

Figure 4. Asthma mortality (per 100 000) in persons aged 5–34 years, compared with sales and prescriptions of β-agonist preparations in England and Wales for 1959–1968. (Reproduced with permission from ref. [16])

Table 3. Cross-classification of countries by presence or absence of an epidemic of asthma mortality and presence or absence of sales of isoprenaline forte aerosols

Epidemic of asthma mortality in the 1960s	Isoprenaline forte Aerosols		
	Available	Not available	Total
Present	6	0	6
Absent	2	6	8
TOTAL	8	6	14

naline forte, which contained a concentration of isoprenaline two to eight times greater than the standard isoprenaline MDI available in other countries [13]. Epidemics occurred only in countries where the high-dose preparation of isoprenaline was available, and in the two countries which marketed the high-dose preparation and had no increase in mortality, it was introduced late into their markets and *per capita* sales were low (Tab. 3). Countries such as the United States, Denmark, Canada, Sweden and Germany that did not market the high-dose preparation of isoprenaline did not experience an epidemic. In countries experiencing epidemics, case series identified that many of the patients who died from asthma had used excessive amounts of this drug in the situation of severe asthma [17]. Unfortunately, formal analytical epidemiological studies were not undertaken because the epidemic declined before there was time to conduct them. Nevertheless the weight of evidence suggested that the use of the isoprenaline forte inhaler was the major, although probably not the only, cause of the epidemics of asthma mortality.

Although this isoprenaline forte hypothesis was subsequently disputed in many texts and reviews, this reinterpretation was not based on any new substantial evidence, and in fact the further analyses that were undertaken strengthened the original conclusions [18]. Alternative hypotheses concerning under-treatment with oral or inhaled corticosteroids are implausible, since such problems of under-treatment applied to most countries, irrespective of whether they experienced epidemics, over a long period prior to, rather than during the epidemics. The mortality rate declined following warnings from regulatory bodies, a marked reduction in the sales of isoprenaline forte, and other changes in medical practice.

2.4. The Second New Zealand Epidemic (Fig. 3)

A second asthma mortality epidemic began in New Zealand in the mid-1970s. Jackson et al. [5] investigated the epidemic and concluded that it was real and could not be explained by changes in the classification of asthma deaths, inaccuracies in death certification or changes in diagnostic fashion, or changes in the incidence or prevalence of asthma. The most likely explanation, as for the

Table 4. Prescribed inhaled β-agonist and the relative risk of dying from asthma: results from published epidemiological studies

Specific β-agonist	Relative risk*					
	1st NZ Study	2nd NZ Study	3rd NZ Study	Saskatchewan Study (1)	Saskatchewan Study (2)	Japanese Study[#]
Salbutamol	0.7	0.7	0.6	0.9	1.1	1.0
Fenoterol	1.6	2.0	2.1	5.3	11.8	5.0
Reference:	[19]	[20]	[21]	[24]	[25]	[28]

* Relative risk of death, unadjusted odds ratios
During the period of these studies salbutamol and fenoterol were available in preparations dispensing 100 μg/puff and 200 μg/puff respectively
Saskatchewan Study: (1) case-control (2) cohort
[#] Based on market share; this study did not include a formal control group

1960s epidemics, appeared to be an increased case fatality rate related to changes in the management of asthma in New Zealand.

These initial investigations led to the formal examination of prescribed drug therapy and asthma mortality in New Zealand. In a series of three case-control studies, which employed different methods and incorporated different data sources, at different time periods throughout the epidemic, an increased risk of asthma death was found in patients prescribed the beta agonist fenoterol but not other asthma medications (Tab. 4) [19–21]. The association between fenoterol and asthma deaths was particularly strong in subgroups with more severe asthma, a pattern which essentially rules out the possibility that the findings were due to confounding by severity [22], an interpretation that was supported by more detailed analyses [23].

A subsequent case-control study from Saskatchewan, Canada also found that the prescription of the high-dose preparation of fenoterol was associated with an increased risk of death when compared with the more commonly prescribed beta agonist, salbutamol (Tab. 4) [24, 25]. Although the authors raised the possibility of a general beta agonist class effect, their subsequent analyses indicated that these particular findings may largely be due to confounding by severity [26].

Studies from two other countries have examined the issue of specific beta agonist use and asthma mortality. A cohort study based in Germany found that in older patients with chronic obstructive respiratory disease (CORD), the prescription of fenoterol was associated with a 10-fold increased risk of mortality when compared with salbutamol [27]. More recently, an epidemiological study in Japan has found a five-fold increased risk of mortality with fenoterol in children [28].

By their nature, epidemiological studies such as those discussed are unable to identify the underlying mechanisms by which the high-dose preparations of

isoprenaline forte and fenoterol led to asthma mortality epidemics in the populations in which they were widely used. There are two potential groups of
mechanisms that have been proposed [29–32]: those relating to the regular use
leading to worsening asthma control, and those relating to their over-use in the
situation of a life-threatening attack of asthma, in which the cardiac side-
effects are likely to be particularly harmful in the presence of severe hypoxia.
It is likely that both these groups of mechanisms are relevant to the increased
mortality associated with the use of fenoterol and isoprenaline, which are relatively non-selective potent full beta agonists, and which have been shown to
have both greater adverse chronic and acute side-effects when compared with
other beta agonist drugs [29, 31, 33, 34].

Similar to the New Zealand experience with isoprenaline forte, the asthma
mortality rate fell dramatically with initial warnings and subsequent restriction
of fenoterol in New Zealand (Fig. 5). The time trend data were inconsistent
with other hypotheses that have been proposed including a class effect of beta
agonist drugs, under-prescribing of inhaled corticosteroids (during the epidemic New Zealand had the highest *per capita* use of inhaled corticosteroids),
or socio-economic factors [35]. Thus the epidemiological evidence suggests
that fenoterol was the major, although not the only, cause of the second New
Zealand asthma mortality epidemic, similar to the role of isoprenaline forte
during the first New Zealand asthma mortality epidemic.

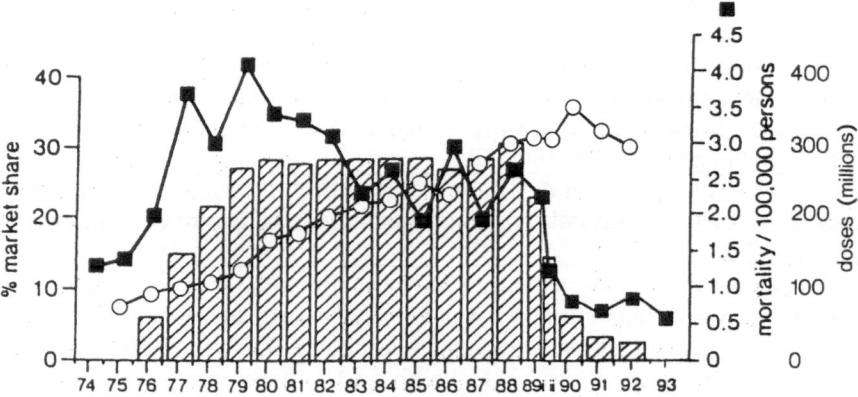

Figure 5. Asthma mortality (per 100 000) in persons aged 5–34 years (■), market share of fenoterol
(□) and overall β-agonist use by metered dose inhaler (○) in New Zealand. The data for 1989 are
divided into two periods due to the initial regulatory restrictions with fenoterol in mid-1989. (Source:
adapted from ref. [35].)

2.5. Gradual Increase in Asthma Mortality

Although no other countries have apparently experienced epidemics, a more gradual increase in asthma deaths has occurred in many countries during the 1970s and 1980s. This background increase has occurred not only in countries which experienced the first epidemic of deaths in the 1960s, but also in other countries unaffected by previous increases in mortality. It has been difficult to determine the causes of this trend, as death from asthma is a complex phenomenon and many factors relevant to the causation of asthma mortality have changed to differing degrees in different countries during this period. Despite this complexity, a number of observations can be made.

2.5.1. Magnitude: In a number of countries the magnitude of this "gradual" increase has been substantial. For example, between the mid-1970s and mid-1980s, the mortality rate increased by more than 40% in many countries throughout the world (Tab. 5) [7, 29, 36]. In many of these countries, the marked increases in mortality occurred after a period of previously stable asthma mortality rates.

2.5.2. Variation: There is both a wide variation in the reported asthma mortality rates in some countries with similar lifestyles and comparable approaches to the management of asthma (e.g. Australia, England and Canada), and conversely, similar asthma mortality rates in other countries with different lifestyles and approaches to the management of asthma (e.g. Japan, Sweden

Table 5. Asthma mortality (per 100 000) in persons aged 5–34 years in 15 countries between the mid-1970s and mid-1980s

	1975–1977	1985–1987	Percentage Increase
Australia	0.86	1.42	65
Canada	0.33	0.47	42
Denmark	0.14	0.36	157
England & Wales	0.57	0.90	58
Finland	0.29	0.21	−28
France	0.24	0.51	113
Italy	0.05	0.17	240
Japan	0.44	0.59	34
Netherlands	0.20	0.22	10
Singapore	0.75	0.88	17
Sweden	0.37	0.54	46
Switzerland	0.31	0.45	45
USA	0.19	0.40	111
West Germany	0.59	0.78	32

and the United States). There appears to be no unifying hypothesis that explains this international variation.

2.5.3. Prevalence: The gradual increase in mortality rates has occurred during the same period in which the prevalence of asthma has also increased. Asthma prevalence studies which have been repeated during this period using standardised methods in the same population group, have observed a consistent increase in the prevalence of asthma symptoms [37, 38]. This increase has been observed in a wide range of countries with differing lifestyles and in some countries has been of considerable magnitude.

In addition, available data suggest an increase in the prevalence of severe asthma, as indicated by the international trends of increasing hospital admissions for asthma in children. This increase, which began in the 1960s has been most pronounced in the younger age groups (Fig. 6) [39]. Detailed studies of

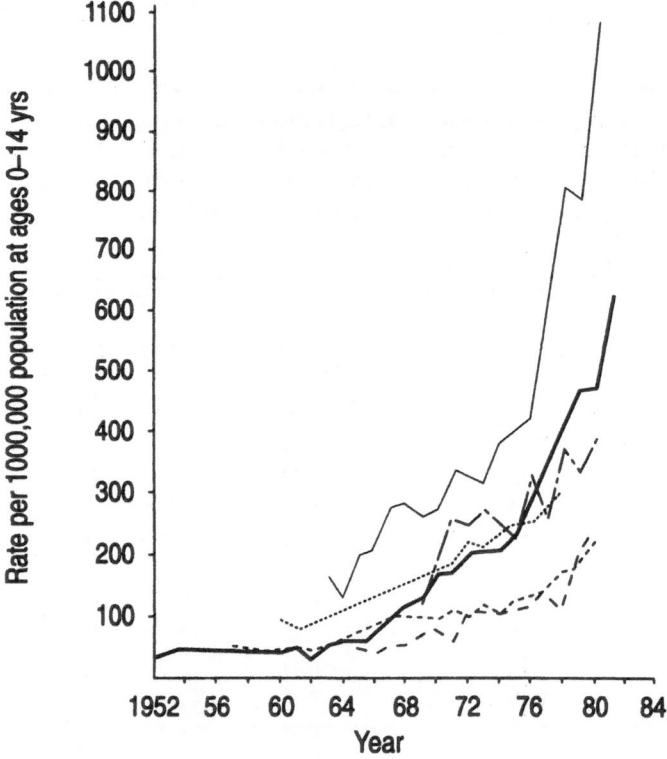

Figure 6. Admissions to hospital with asthma (per 100 000) in 0–14 year olds in a number of different countries since the 1950s. (Reproduced with permission from ref. [39]). (———) Queensland, Australia; (— · —) Tasmania, Australia; (━━━) New Zealand; (··········) Canada; (-----·) England and Wales; (– – –) USA.

the circumstances of the hospital admissions have established that these trends cannot be completely explained by an increase in readmissions, diagnostic transfer from related disease categories, or changes in medical practice such as the threshold for admission, but are likely to reflect an increase in the prevalence of severe asthma [40]. Indeed, limited data suggest that the severity of children hospitalised due to asthma may have actually increased during the 1980s [41, 42]. During the 1990s, the hospital admission rates have stabilised or decreased in several countries including the United Kingdom [40] and New Zealand [43].

2.5.4. Case Fatality Rates: It is evident from these considerations that when making international comparisons of asthma mortality, it is necessary to also consider the asthma prevalence rates in the countries being compared. This is now possible with the standardised international asthma prevalence data published from the European Community Respiratory Health Survey (ECHRS) [43] and the International Study of Asthma and Allergies in Childhood (ISAAC) [44]. These data have allowed an assessment of national case fatality rates which provides a different perspective of the international differences in asthma mortality rates (Tab. 6). This specific analysis based on the ISAAC data [45] indicates that amongst Western countries, a five-fold difference may exist in the case fatality rates, defined by the ratio of the asthma mortality rates to the prevalence rates of severe asthma within each country. This suggests that while the prevalence of severe asthma is one determinant of asthma mortality rates, other factors unrelated to the occurrence of severe disease may also play

Table 6. Comparison of asthma mortality rates with prevalence rates of severe asthma in 12 countries

	Asthma mortality rate	Prevalence of severe asthma*	Ratio
Australia	0.86	8.3	0.10
Canada	0.25	8.0	0.03
England & Wales	0.52	8.7	0.06
Finland	0.21	3.1	0.07
France	0.40	2.8	0.14
Italy	0.23	2.0	0.12
Japan	0.73	2.1	0.35
New Zealand	0.50	8.0	0.06
Sweden	0.12	2.0	0.06
USA	0.47	10.0	0.05
West Germany	0.44	5.7	0.08

Asthma mortality rate (per 100 000) in persons aged 5–34 years in 1993
* Asthma prevalence rates defined as self-reported episodes of wheezing sufficient to limit speech in previous 12 months, in 13–14 year old children, 1993–1995 (Source: adapted from ref. [45].)
NB: Mortality and prevalence data are not available in the same age group

a major role. This approach also identifies countries such as Japan in which the asthma mortality rates are disproportionately high in relation to the prevalence of severe asthma. Investigations into the reasons for such variations have the potential to identify the major risk factors for some of these international mortality patterns.

2.5.5. Relationships Between Time Trends: When presented individually, the trends in asthma prevalence, morbidity and mortality all suggest increases over recent decades. When reviewed together, it is evident that there are differences in these trends in terms of both the time-courses and the magnitude of the changes [11]. This would suggest that a single explanation for the causes of these trends is unlikely, and that there are significant differences in the relative importance of the different risk factors contributing to such trends.

2.5.6. Population Groups: Analysis of trends in asthma mortality rates within countries often reveals differences between specific population groups [46–49]. This is illustrated by studies from the USA, in which the asthma mortality rates are greater in disadvantaged populations such as the Blacks and Hispanics [46, 47], those who are poorly educated, live in large cities, or are poor [11, 46, 47, 50]. It is likely that through the investigation of such high risk populations, our understanding of the risk factors that contribute to asthma mortality will be improved.

2.5.7. Environmental Exposures: One feature which is not evident from national mortality data is the occurrence of epidemics in discrete locations, associated with environmental exposures. Probably the best studied example is that of the epidemics of life-threatening attacks of asthma (and fatal asthma) in Barcelona in the 1980s, associated with environmental exposure to airborne soybean dust [51, 52]. While the causative agent may be difficult to identify with general environmental exposure, a wide range of sensitising agents have been implicated in the occupational setting as causes of severe asthma [53]. These studies suggest that repeated environmental exposure to a single organic aeroallergen can lead to recurrent episodes of life-threatening attacks of asthma in a community whenever exposure reaches a sufficient level.

2.5.8. Seasonal Trends: Seasonal trends in asthma mortality have been observed in a number of countries including the United Kingdom (Fig. 7) [54], France [55] and the USA [56]. In each of these countries, asthma mortality in the 5 to 34 year age group is highest in the summer months, in contrast to the older age groups, in which the peak occurs in the winter. It is likely that this trend may relate to reduced access to or availability of medical care during the summer holidays, in view of the associated reduction in hospital admissions during this period [54, 56].

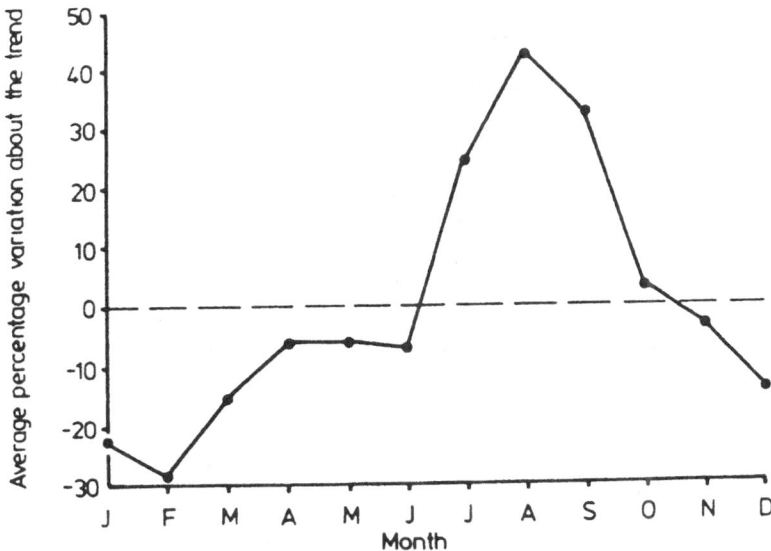

Figure 7. Average monthly variation in deaths from asthma in 5–34 year age group in England and Wales 1960–82. (Reproduced with permission from ref. [54])

2.6. Most Recent Trends

There has been a gradual fall in asthma mortality since the late 1980s in some but not all countries in which accurate mortality statistics are kept (Fig. 3). Countries in which such reductions have been observed include Australia, Canada, Denmark, West Germany, Sweden, England and Wales. It is possible that this reduction may relate to changes in management, in particular the greater use of inhaled corticosteroid therapy. In support of this view are the studies which have shown improved clinical outcome with inhaled corticosteroid therapy [57], and their protective effects against mortality [58]. However, the time trend evidence is not conclusive in this regard, particularly as some countries such as the United States and Japan have experienced increases in mortality during this period, despite similar marked increases in the use of inhaled corticosteroid therapy. It is likely that other (unknown) factors may well account for a significant component of the recent mortality decline in those countries in which this trend has been observed.

3. Studies of Other Risk Factors for Asthma Mortality

Although most analytical epidemiological studies of asthma deaths have focused on pharmacological risk factors, several case-control studies have examined other risk factors for asthma deaths. These risk factors can be categorised as involving characteristics of the disease (asthma severity) and characteristics of the patient (such as psychosocial factors). These factors are relevant both to clinicians who wish to identify patients who are at increased risk of death and to epidemiologists who wish to control for asthma severity in studies of asthma mortality.

3.1. Asthma Severity

A number of markers of asthma severity have been associated with an increased risk of asthma death as listed in Table 7 [24, 59–61]. Amongst these markers, a hospital admission for asthma in the previous 12 months, and the occurrence of multiple hospital admissions for asthma in the previous 12 months are the most reliable and easily ascertained, and carry a greatly increased risk of asthma death. However, they may be present in only about one-half of cases dying from asthma, and so their absence does not necessarily mean that a patient is not "at risk". With respect to the use of "prescribed oral corticosteroids" as a marker, the evidence is equivocal, probably because this class of drugs may be beneficial in the severe group of patients to whom it is prescribed; thus it may identify a high-risk group of patients, whose risk is in turn lowered by use of oral corticosteroids.

Amongst patients with a recent hospital admission for asthma, the marker associated with the highest risk of death is a previous intensive care unit admission for asthma [60], and in particular the requirement for mechanical ventilation, which has a 5-year mortality rate of about 20% [61]. The use of other markers of acute asthma severity is difficult due to the poor quality and paucity of available data. However, if available they contribute to the overall assessment of risk, with a $PaCO_2$ of 45 mmHg or more being associated with an up to four-fold risk of subsequent death, and a PEF of less than 100 l/min being associated with an approximately two-fold risk of subsequent death [59, 61].

3.2. Characteristics of the Asthmatic

Several studies have examined characteristics of the asthmatic which may be associated with an increased risk of death. In particular, it has been observed that in addition to the underlying asthma severity, the risk of asthma death is also associated with psychiatric disease, psychosocial problems, and other psychological characteristics of the patient. These problems have been studied in depth by Strunk et al. [63], who reported that children were at an increased risk of asthma death if there were conflicts between the patient's parents and medical staff regarding management, depressive symptoms, or a disregard of asthma symptoms. Other characteristics which have been identified in "at risk"

Table 7. Case-control studies of markers of asthma severity and subsequent risk of death

Study base	Rea et al. [60] Asthmatics		Ryan et al. [61] Asthmatics with recent hospital admission		Crane et al. [59] Asthmatics with recent hospital admission		Spitzer et al. [24] Asthmatics with 10+ prescriptions in 1978–1987		Joseph et al. [67] Asthmatics with 10+ prescriptions in 1978–1987	
	OR	(95%CI)	OR	(95%CI)	OR	(95%CI)	OR	(95%CI)	OR	(95%CI)
Chronic severity markers:										
Three or more categories of asthma drugs	3.0	(1.0–11)			1.7	(0.9–3.3)		-		
Oral steroids	-		2.3	(1.6–3.3)	1.3	(0.6–2.8)	3.1	(1.5–6.5)		
Admission within 12 months	16.0	(2.5–666)			3.5	(1.8–6.9)		-		
5+ admissions within 12 months	-				8.8	(1.2–56)		-		
A&E visit within 12 months	8.5	(2.0–76)				-		-		
Acute severity markers:										
Previous life-threatening attack	∞	(13.0–∞)								
$PaCO_2 \geq 45$ mmHg	-		1.9	(1.1–3.1)	4.0	(0.9–21)		-		
$PaO_2 < 60$ mmHg	-		1.2	(0.7–1.9)		-		-		
$FEV_1 < 1.0$ litres	-		0.8#	(0.3–1.9)	1.5	(0.1–34)		-		
FVC <40% pred	-		1.6	(0.8–3.0)		-		-		
PEF <100 l/min	-				1.9	(0.7–5.4)		-		
$K^+ < 3.5$ mmol/l	-				0.4	(0.1–1.5)		-		
Patient characteristics:										
Psychosocial problems (psychotropic medications)	3.5	(1.0–13.7)	1.7	(1.2–2.5)	3.7	(1.3–10.8)			3.2	(1.4–7.5)
Discontinuity of medical care	20.1	(4.0–100)								
Non-compliance	∞	(5.2–∞)								

* Cases and controls who were prescribed fenoterol were excluded,
\# $FEV_1 < 40\%$ predicted

patients include discontinuity of general practice care, poor compliance with therapy, family dysfunction, poor social support, and risk-taking behaviour [60, 64–66].

One practical marker which can be used by clinicians or epidemiologists to identify the existence of psychosocial problems is the prescription of psychotropic drugs, such as antipsychotics and sedatives, the use of which are associated with an increased risk of death [59, 61, 67]. The observation that the past use of antipsychotics with recent discontinuation (as against continuous use) is associated with a particularly high risk of death suggests that antipsychotic use is a "marker" of a patient at high risk of mortality, rather than directly increasing the risk fatality through a pharmacological effect such as depression of the central nervous system or impaired respiratory drive [67].

3.3. Circumstances of Fatal Episode

Information concerning the circumstances associated with death from asthma has been obtained from national or regional descriptive asthma mortality surveys, in which close relatives or friends of the deceased, and general practitioners have been interviewed and the medical records have been reviewed when available. From such studies, undertaken in a number of Western countries over the last 30 years, similar management problems have been consistently identified in association with the fatal outcome [17, 49, 68–75]. These can be broadly grouped into those relating to the long-term care and those relating to the treatment of the life-threatening attack (Tab. 8).

Problems associated with long-term management include lack of appreciation by both the patient and their doctor, of the patient's chronic asthma severity and risk of serious morbidity or mortality. This was often compounded by a discontinuity of general practice care and psychosocial problems. As a result, there was commonly inadequate use of, and poor compliance with preventive therapy and an over-reliance on bronchodilator drugs.

Table 8. Management problems associated with fatal outcome in asthma

---

Long term:

    Lack of appreciation of chronic asthma severity and risk of death
    Poor compliance with management
    Discontinuity of medical care
    Under-utilisation of inhaled corticosteroids

Fatal attack:

    Delay in seeking medical help
    Inability to recognise the severity of the attack
    Over-reliance on bronchodilator therapy
    Insufficient systemic steroid use
    Lack of written guidelines for management

Similar problems have been identified with the treatment of the severe attack that led to death. In particular, in the majority of cases, there was a lack of recognition by the patient, family or doctor of the severity of the fatal attack, in part due to the infrequent use of objective measures of asthma severity such as lung function measurements. This results in delay in seeking emergency medical services, despite the development of a life-threatening attack of asthma. Linked with this delay is the excessive self-administration of bronchodilator and the lack of an agreed management plan detailing instructions on when to seek medical care and what treatment to take in this situation.

3.4. Life-Threatening Attacks

Consideration of the circumstances relating to life-threatening attacks of asthma is relevant to asthma mortality, on the assumption that the pathophysiological mechanisms and precipitating factors involved in these clinical situations are likely to be similar. While there are reasons to be cautious in the use of information on near fatal attacks in this way, there are some practical advantages, in particular that detailed information of the circumstances of the severe attack can often be obtained, when such information is not usually available in fatal asthma [76].

Case series of life-threatening attacks of asthma have revealed three main patterns of presentation [77–79]. The first presentation is that of a sudden precipitate attack in which the asthmatic patient may develop a life-threatening attack of asthma within minutes or hours of the onset of the first symptoms. The second type of presentation is characterised by a gradual worsening, evolving over several days to weeks, leading to progressively more severe asthma and the gradual development of respiratory failure. A third pattern is that of a severe attack which occurs quickly after a few days of unstable asthma. Clinical features, including the time-course of the response to treatment, suggest that bronchospasm may play the primary role in the pathogenesis of precipitate asthma, whereas worsening airways inflammation would cause mucous plugging which may be the predominant pathophysiological process involved in the more gradual presentations.

Information concerning the different precipitating factors that have been identified as the cause of life-threatening attacks of asthma are also relevant to the causation of fatal asthma (Tab. 8). The most common cause of a severe attack of asthma is a viral respiratory tract infection, accounting for up to 80% of episodes in children, and up to 30% in adults [80, 81]. Although many different viruses may precipitate an attack of asthma, the most common are rhinoviruses and coronaviruses, which are responsible for the "common cold" [80, 81], and *Chlamydia pneumoniae* infection which has recently been implicated in the pathogenesis of recurrent severe attacks of asthma [82].

One of the common causes of a precipitate life-threatening attack is allergen exposure in a sensitised individual [77, 78, 83]. The particular allergen

Table 9. Precipitating factors contributing to a life-threatening attack

---

- Viral respiratory tract infections
- Allergen exposure
- Weather changes
- Drugs -NSAIDs
- Emotional stress
- Foods, including preservatives
- Air pollution

---

responsible will often vary in different populations and individuals, however it is not uncommon for outbreaks of severe asthma to occur in a community due to one specific allergen, as occurred in the soybean-induced epidemics of severe asthma in Barcelona, [51, 52] and in seasonal-related episodes of life-threatening asthma relating to *Alternaria* exposure in the United States [84]. A further feature is that there may be a number of related factors which interact in the development of life-threatening attacks. For example, thunderstorms have been shown to cause the release of allergen containing starch granules, following the osmotic rupture of rye-grass pollen grains by rainwater, thereby provoking attacks of severe asthma in sensitised individuals [85]. The importance of atopy in the underlying pathogenesis of life-threatening attacks of asthma is also illustrated by the findings that severe "brittle" asthmatics with frequent near fatal attacks of asthma are more atopic than asthmatics with less severe forms of asthma [86].

Aspirin and other non-steroidal anti-inflammatory drugs taken as medications or naturally present in foodstuffs may also be a common provoking factor in near-fatal asthma. In one series of asthmatic patients requiring mechanical ventilation, aspirin sensitivity was recognised in about 25% of the cases [62]; in other series sensitivity to aspirin has been considered to be the cause of the life-threatening attack in about 10% of patients [78, 86]. Allergic reactions to foodstuffs such as nuts and peanuts may also precipitate fatal or near fatal attacks of asthma, particularly if features of anaphylaxis are present [87, 88]. Patients with known anaphylactic food sensitivity appear to be at high risk of death from severe asthma [88] and conversely both adults and children with a pre-existing diagnosis of asthma are at increased risk of fatal or near fatal anaphylaxis [89].

4. Summary

In considering the epidemiology of asthma mortality, it is important to distinguish between asthma mortality epidemics and asthma deaths during non-epidemic periods. There is convincing evidence that the major cause of the epidemics of asthma deaths was the use of the high-dose preparations of isoprenaline forte and fenoterol. In contrast, there are many different factors that may have contributed to asthma deaths in individual patients during non-epidemic periods. These include increases in asthma prevalence and severity, characteristics of the disease and its management, characteristics of the patient, and exposure to precipitating factors that can provoke life-threatening asthma attacks. However, it is currently unclear to what extent these various factors may explain international patterns of asthma mortality. Thus, there is a continuing need to monitor international patterns and time trends in asthma mortality, and to conduct further studies into the causes of asthma deaths in both populations and in individuals.

Acknowledgements

The Wellington Asthma Research Group is supported by Programmes Grants from the New Zealand Health Research Council and the Guardian Trust (Trustee of the David and Cassie Anderson Medical Charitable Trust).

References

1 Osler W (1901) *The principles and practice of medicine*. (4th ed.) Pentland, Edinburgh
2 Jackson R (1993) A century of asthma mortality. *In*: R Beasley, NE Pearce (eds): *The role of beta agonist therapy in asthma mortality*. CRC Press, New York, 29–47
3 British Thoracic Association BTAResearch Committee (1984) Accuracy of death certificates in bronchial asthma. *Thorax* 39: 505–9
4 Sears MR, Rea HH, de Boer G, Beaglehole R, Gillies AJ, Holst PE, O'Donnell TV, Rothwell AP (1986) Accuracy of certification of deaths due to asthma: a national study. *Am J Epidemiol* 124: 1004–11
5 Jackson RT, Beaglehole R, Rea HH, Sutherland DC (1982) Mortality from asthma: a new epidemic in New Zealand. *Br Med J* 285: 771–4
6 Beasley R, Smith K, Pearce N, Crane J, Burgess C, Culling C (1990) Trends in asthma mortality in New Zealand, 1908–1986. *Med J Australia* 152: 570–3
7 Jackson R, Sears MR, Beaglehole R, Rea HH (1988) International trends in asthma mortality: 1970 to 1985. *Chest* 94: 914–8
8 Lambert PM (1981) Oral theophylline and fatal asthma. *Lancet* ii: 200–1 (letter)
9 Speizer FE, Doll R (1968. A century of asthma deaths in young people. *Br Med J* 3: 245–6
10 Baumann A, Lee S Trends in asthma mortality in Australia, 1911–1986 (1990) *Med J Australia* 153: 366 (letter)
11 Weiss KB, Gergen PJ, Wagener DK (1993) Breathing better or wheezing worse? The changing epidemiology of asthma morbidity and mortality. *Annu Rev Public Health* 14: 491–513
12 Becklake MR, Ernst P (1997) Environmental factors. *Lancet* 350(SII): 10–13
13 Stolley PD (1972) Why the United States was spared an epidemic of deaths due to asthma. *Am Rev Respir Dis* 105: 883–90
14 Mitsui S (1986) Death from bronchial asthma in Japan. *Sino-Jpn J Allergol Immunol, Soshiran* 3: 249–57
15 Speizer FE, Doll R, Heaf P (1968) Observations on recent increases in mortality from asthma. *Br Med J* 3359
16 Inman MHW, Adelstein AM (1969) Rise and fall of asthma mortality in England and Wales in relation to use of pressurised aerosols. *Lancet* 2: 279–85
17 Fraser PM, Speizer FE, Waters SD, Doll R, Mann NM (1971) The circumstances preceding death from asthma in young people in 1968 to 1969. *Br J Dis Chest* 65: 71–84
18 Stolley PD, Schinnar R (1978) Association between asthma mortality and isoproterenol aerosols: a review. *Prev Med* 7: 319–38

19 Crane J, Pearce N, Flatt A, Burgess C, Jackson R, Kwong T, Ball M, Beasley R (1989) Prescribed fenoterol and death from asthma in New Zealand, 1981–83: case-control study. *Lancet* 1: 917–22

20 Pearce N, Grainger J, Atkinson M, Crane J, Burgess C, Culling C, Windom H, Beasley R (1990) Case-control study of prescribed fenoterol and death from asthma in New Zealand, 1977–1981. *Thorax* 45: 170–5

21 Grainger J, Woodman K, Pearce N, Crane J, Burgess C, Keane A, Beasley R (1991) Prescribed fenoterol and death from asthma in New Zealand, 1981–1987: a further case-control study. *Thorax* 46: 105–11

22 Beasley R, Burgess C, Pearce N, Grainger J, Crane J (1994) Confounding by severity does not explain the association between fenoterol and asthma death. *Clin Exp Allergy* 24: 660–8

23 Sackett DL, Shannon HS, Browman GW (1990) Fenoterol and fatal asthma. *Lancet* 46 (letter)

24 Spitzer WD, Suissa S, Ernst P, Horwitz RI, Habbick B, Cockcroft D, Bovin JF, McNutt M, Buist AS, Rebuck A (1992) The use of beta agonists and the risk of death and near death from asthma. *N Engl J Med* 326: 501–6

25 Suissa S, Ernst P, Boivin J-F, Horwitz RI, Cockroft D, Blais L, McNutt M, Buist AS, Spitzer WO (1994) A cohort analysis of excess mortality in asthma and the use of inhaled beta agonists. *Am J Respir Crit Care Med* 149: 604–10

26 Suissa S (1995) The case-time-control design. *Epidemiology* 6: 248–53

27 Criée C-P, Quast CH, Ludtke R, Laier-Groeneveld G, Huttemann U (1993) Use of beta agonists and mortality in patients with stable COPD. *Eur Respir J* 6: 426S (abstract)

28 Matsui T (1996). Asthma deaths and β_2-agonists. current advances in paediatric allergy and clinical epidemiology. K Shimomiya (ed): Selected proceedings from the 32nd annual meeting of the Japanese Society of Paediatric Allergy and Clinical Immunology. Churchill Livingstone, Tokyo, 161–4

29 Sears MR, Taylor DR (1994) The β_2-agonist controversy: observations, explanations and relationship to epidemiology. *Drug Safety* 11(4): 259–83

30 Taylor DR, Sears MR (1994) Regular adrenergic agonists: evidence, not reassurance, is what is needed. *Chest* 106: 552–9

31 Beasley R, Pearce N, Crane J, Windom H, Burgess C (1991) Asthma mortality and inhaled beta agonist therapy. *Aust NZ J Med* 21: 753–63

32 Collins JM, McDevitt DG, Shanks RG, Swanton JG (1969) The cardiotoxicity of isoprenaline during hypoxia. *Br J Pharmacol* 36: 35–45

33 Trembath PW, Greenacre JK, Anderson M, Dimmock S, Mansfield L, Wadsworth J, Green M (1979) Comparison of four weeks treatment with fenoterol and terbutaline aerosols in adult asthmatics. *J Allerg Clin Immunol* 63: 395–400

34 Bremner P, Siebers R, Crane J, Pearce N, Beasley R, Burgess C (1996) Partial *versus* full beta receptor agonism—a clinical study of inhaled albuterol and fenoterol. *Chest* 109(4): 957–62

35 Pearce N, Beasley R, Crane J, Burgess C, Jackson R (1995) End of the New Zealand asthma mortality epidemic. *Lancet* 345: 41–4

36 Sears MR (1991) Worldwide trends in asthma mortality. *Bull Int Union Tubercul Lung Dis* 66: 79–83

37 Peat JK, van den Berg RH, Green WF, Mellis CM, Leeder SR, Woolcock AJ (1994) Changing prevalence of asthma in Australian children. *BMJ* 308: 1591–6

38 National Institutes of Health National Heart Lung Blood Institute World Health Organisation Workshop Report (1995) Chapter 2, Epidemiology. *In: Global initiative for asthma: Global strategy for asthma management and prevention*, 10–24

39 Mitchell EA (1985) International trends in hospital admission rates for asthma. *Arch Dis Child* 60: 376–8

40 Lung and Asthma Information Agency. Trends in hospital admissions for asthma: Factsheet 95/1. Dept Public Health Sciences, St George's Hospital Medical School, London

41 Gergen PJ, Weiss KB (1990) Changing patterns of asthma hospitalization among children: 1979 to 1987. *JAMA* 264: 1688–92

42 Williams MH (1989) Increasing severity of asthma from 1960 to 1987. *N Engl J Med* 320: 1015–6

43 Burney PGJ, Luczynska C, Chinn S, Jarvis D (1994) The European Community Respiratory Health Survey. *Eur Respir J* 7: 954–60

44 Asher MI, Keil U, Anderson HR, Beasley R, Crane J, Martinez F, Mitchell EA, Pearce N, Sibbald

B, Stewart AW et al (1995) International Study of Asthma and Allergies in Childhood (ISAAC): rationale and methods. *Eur Respir J* 8: 483–91

45 Asher MI, Anderson HR, Stewart AW, Crane J, Anabwani G, Beasley R, Björkstén B, Burr M, Keil U, Lai C et al World-wide variations in the prevalence of asthma symptoms: International Study of Asthma and Allergies in Childhood (ISAAC). *Eur Respir J*; *in press*

46 Weiss KB, Wagener DK (1990) Changing patterns of asthma mortality: identifying populations at high risk. *JAMA* 264: 1683–7

47 Sly MR (1988) Mortality from asthma, 1979–1984. *J Allerg Clin Immunol* 82: 705–17

48 Ehrlich RI, Bourne DE (1994) Asthma deaths among coloured and white South Africans: 1962 to 1988. *Respir Med* 88: 195–202

49 Sears MR, Rea HH, Beaglehole R, Gillies AJD, Holst PE, O'Donnell TV, Rothwell RPG, Sutherland DC (1985) Asthma mortality in New Zealand: a two-year national study. *N Z Med J* 98: 271–5

50 McFadden ERJr Warren EL (1997) Observations on asthma mortality. *Ann Intern Med* 127: 142–47

51 Anto JM, Sunyer J (1986) Asthma Collaborative Group of Barcelona. A point source asthma outbreak. *Lancet* 1: 900–3

52 Anto JM, Sunyer J, Rodriguez-Roisin R, Suarez-Cervera M, Vazquez L (1989) Toxicoepidemiological Committee. Community outbreaks of asthma associated with inhalation of soybean dust. *N Engl J Med* 320: 1097–102

53 Chan-Yeung M, Lam S (1986) Occupational asthma. *Am Rev Respir Dis* 133: 686–703

54 Khot A, Burn R (1984) Seasonal variation and time trends of deaths from asthma in England and Wales 1960–82. *BMJ* 289: 233–4

55 Cadet B, Robine JM, Leibovici D (1994) Dynamic of asthma mortality in France: Seasonal variation and peaking of mortality in 1985–87. *Rev Epidemiol Santé Publ* 42: 103–18

56 Weiss KB (1990) Seasonal trends in US asthma hospitalizations and mortality. *JAMA* 263: 2323–8

57 Toogood JH, Jennings BH, Baskerville JC, Lefcoe NM (1993) Aerosol corticosteroids. *In*: EB Weis, M Stein (eds): *Bronchial asthma: mechanisms and therapeutics*, 3rd edition. Little, Brown and Co, Boston, 818–41

58 Ernst P, Spitzer WO, Suissa S, Cockroft D, Habbick B, Horwitz RI, Boivin JF, McNutt M, Buist AS (1992) Risk of fatal and near-fatal asthma in relation to inhaled corticosteroid use. *JAMA* 268: 3462–4

59 Crane J, Pearce NE, Burgess C, Woodman K, Robson B, Beasley R (1992) Markers of risk of asthma death or readmission in the 12 months following a hospital admission for asthma. *Int J Epidemiol* 21: 737–44

60 Rea HH, Scragg R, Jackson R, Beaglehole R, Fenwick J, Sutherland DC (1986) A case-control study of deaths from asthma. *Thorax* 41: 833–9

61 Ryan G, Musk AW, Perera DM, Stock H, Knight JL, Hobbs MS (1991) Risk factors for death in patients admitted to hospital with asthma: a follow-up study. *Aust NZ J Med* 21: 681–5

62 Marquette CH, Saulnier F, Leroy O, Wallaert B, Chopin C, Demarcq JM, Durocher A, Tonnel AB (1992) Long-term prognosis of near-fatal asthma. *Am Rev Respir Dis* 146: 76–81

63 Strunk RC, Mrazek DA, Fuhrmann GS, LaBrecque JF (1985) Physiologic and psychological characteristics associated with deaths due to asthma in childhood: a case-controlled study. *JAMA* 254: 1193–8

64 Joseph KS (1977) Asthma mortality and antipsychotic or sedative use. What is the link? *Drug Safety* 16: 351–4

65 Campbell DA, Yellowlees PM, McLennan G, Coates JR, Frith PA, Gluyas PA, Latimer KM, Luke CG, Martin AJ, Ruffin RE (1995) Psychiatric and medical features of near fatal asthma. *Thorax* 50: 254–9

66 Miller TP, Greenberger PA, Patterson R (1992) The diagnosis of potentially fatal asthma in hospitalized adults: patient characteristics and increased severity of asthma. *Chest* 102: 515–8

67 Joseph KS, Blais L, Ernst P, Suissa S (1996) Increased morbidity and mortality related to asthma among asthmatic patients who use major tranquillisers. *Br Med J* 312: 79–83

68 MacDonald JB, MacDonald ET, Seaton A, Williams DA (1976) Asthma deaths in Cardiff 1963–74: 53 deaths in hospital. *BMJ* 2: 721–3

69 Ormerod LP, Stableforth DE (1980) Asthma mortality in Birmingham 1975–7: 53 deaths. *BMJ* 280: 687–90

70 British Thoracic Association (1982) Death from asthma in two regions of England. *BMJ* 285: 1251–5

71 Johnson AJ, Nunn AJ, Somner AR, Stableforth DE, Stewart CJ (1984) Circumstances of death from asthma. *BMJ* 288: 1870–2

72 Manning P, Murphy E, Clancy L, Callaghan B (1987) Asthma mortality in the Republic of Ireland 1970–84 and an analysis of hospital deaths in a single year. *BMJ* 80: 406–9

73 Rea HH, Sears MR, Beaglehole R, Fenwick J, Jackson RT, Gillies AJ, O'Donnell TV, Holst PE, Rothwell RP (1987) Lessons from the national asthma mortality study: circumstances surrounding death. *N Z Med J* 100: 10–3

74 Robertson CF, Rubinfeld AR, Bowes G (1990) Deaths from asthma in Victoria: a 12-month study. *Med J Australia* 152: 511–7

75 Fletcher HJ, Ibrahim SA, Speight N (1990) Survey of asthma deaths in the Northern region 1970–85. *Arch Dis Child* 65: 163–7

76 Beasley R, Pearce N, Crane J (1993) Use of near fatal asthma for investigating asthma deaths. *Thorax* 48: 1093–4

77 Wasserfallen J-B, Schaller M-D, Feihl F, Perret CH (1990) Sudden asphyxic asthma: a distinct entity? *Am Rev Respir Dis* 142: 108–11

78 Ruffin RE, Latimer K, Schembri DA (1991) Longitudinal study of near fatal asthma. *Chest* 99: 77–83

79 Arnold AG, Lane DJ, Zapata E (1982) The speed of onset and severity of acute severe asthma. *Br J Dis Chest* 76: 157–63

80 Pattemore PK, Johnston SL, Bardin PG (1992) Viruses as precipitants of asthma symptoms: epidemiology. *Clin Exp Allergy* 22: 325–36

81 Johnston SL, Sanderson G, Pattemore PK, Smith S, Bardin PG, Bruce CB, Lambden PR, Tyrrell DA, Holgate ST (1993) Use of polymerase chain reaction for diagnosis of picornavirus infection in subjects with and without respiratory symptoms. *J Clin Microbiol* 31: 111–7

82 Magee J (1998) Could *Chlamydia pneumoniae* be asthma villain? *Lancet* 351: 344

83 Molfino NA, Slutsky AS (1994) Near-fatal asthma. *Eur Respir J* 7: 981–90

84 O'Hollaren MT, Yunginger JW, Offord KP, Somers MJ, O'Connell EJ, Ballard DJ, Sachs MI (1991) Exposure to aeroallergen as a possible precipitating factor in respiratory arrest in young patients with asthma. *N Engl J Med* 324: 359–63

85 Knox RB (1993) Grass pollen, thunderstorms and asthma. *Clin Exp Allergy* 23: 354–9

86 Miles J, Cayton R, Ayres J (1995. Atopic status in patients with brittle and non-brittle asthma: a case-control study. *Clin Exp Allergy* 25: 1074–82

87 Sampson HA, Mendelson L, Rosen JP (1992) Fatal and near-fatal anaphylactic reactions to food in children and adolescents. *N Engl J Med* 327: 380–4

88 Bock SA, Atkins FM (1989) The natural history of peanut allergy. *J Allerg Clin Immunol* 83: 900–4

89 Yunginger JW, Sweeney KG, Sturner WQ, Giannandrea LA, Teigland JD, Bray M, Benson PA, York JA, Biedrzycki L, Squillace DL et al (1988) Fatal food-induced anaphylaxis. *JAMA* 260: 1450–2

Asthma: Epidemiology, Anti-Inflammatory Therapy and Future Trends
ed. by M. A. Giembycz and B. J. O'Connor
© 2000 Birkhäuser Verlag/Switzerland

CHAPTER 2
Epidemiology of Childhood Asthma

John R. Britton and Sarah A. Lewis

Division of Respiratory Medicine, University of Nottingham, City Hospital, Hucknall Road, Nottingham, NG5 1PB, UK

1. Definitions

1.1. Definition of Asthma in Children

Over recent years, wheezing illness in children of the Western world has become synonymous with asthma, but as in adults there remains no universally accepted epidemiological definition of the condition. Existing definitions of asthma in adults are more descriptive than definitive, focussing on the clinical characteristics of reversible airways obstruction, chronic airway inflammation, and increased bronchial responsiveness to a variety of stimuli. The definition of asthma in children is even more difficult however, partly because of practical contraints on the objective measures of airflow in young children, and also because of the particular susceptibility of infants and younger children to wheeze in response to viral respiratory tract infection. Although the term wheezy bronchitis was used to describe this condition, the emergence of evidence in the 1970s that children with either a diagnosis of bronchitis or of asthma differed from healthy controls with respect to family and personal history of allergic disease and personal atopy [1], that some children with the diagnosis of wheezy bronchitis responded positively to asthmatic therapy [2], and that children were more likely to be treated appropriately if their condition acquired the label asthma [3], lead to an increased tendency to diagnose asthma in these children. The nature of the condition now labelled childhood asthma may therefore be at least as diverse as diagnosed asthma in adults, and probably reflects contributions from virtually any process resulting in the production of the symptom of wheeze. It is therefore extremely difficult to identify and define unique wheezing conditions in children, and the working definitions adopted in practice inevitably reflect a substantial degree of compromise.

1.2. Working Epidemiological Definitions of Asthma in Children

Measurements of asthma prevalence in children have tended to rely on parental reporting of asthma diagnoses and associated symptoms. Doctor-diagnosed asthma is one of the more commonly used terms in epidemiological surveys to identify asthma cases, yet there are considerable objections raised to it. In the first 6 years of life, wheezing is itself a very common symptom and the proportion of children with wheeze who acquire a doctor given diagnosis of asthma is related to age, frequency of wheezing episodes and the association of wheeze with shortness of breath [4], suggesting that a diagnosis of asthma is heavily dependent on the duration and severity of symptoms, but not to any specific definition. More importantly, in view of the variations in diagnostic labelling of childhood wheezing which have taken place over recent years [5] and between populations, doctor-diagnosed asthma is clearly an unreliable measure with which to establish temporal or spatial differences in asthma prevalence.

For epidemiological purposes, parentally-reported symptoms have served as a widely used alternative. Symptom-based measurements have the advantage of simplicity, relative independence from diagnostic trends, and the capacity to detect intermittent disease. Parental responses to questions on current wheeze have been shown to be highly repeatable at a 4–6 month interval [6, 7] and in relation to a respiratory physician diagnosis of asthma as gold standard, to have a high level of sensitivity [8]. However, wheeze is not a symptom specific to diagnosed asthma, there is no agreed way of grading the severity of wheezing symptoms and the word wheeze is not readily translatable into some languages. Also, by comparison with general practice medical records, parental recall of respiratory symptoms may be biased in relation to the severity and persistence of symptoms [9].

General Practitioner (GP) medical records have provided a further source of information on wheezing illness, but these too are potentially biassed by the impact that symptom severity and general health awareness have on GP consultation. Thus, parentally-completed symptom-based questionnaires have become the main source of information on childhood asthma prevalence and, for all its potential faults, parentally-reported wheeze in the past 12 months has evolved as the most widely used measure of the prevalence of asthma in children. Problems associated with comprehension and with poor response have been reduced by using video presentations of clinical signs and symptoms and interviews with appropriately trained interviewers rather than self-administered questionnaires [10]. In the last few years the International Study of Asthma and Allergies in Childhood (ISAAC) initiative has generated a standardised questionnaire with an accompanying video and this has been used across a number of international centres [11], to begin to provide comparable estimates of childhood asthma prevalence using standardised methodologies.

2. Natural History of "Wheezing" in Children

Wheezing in early childhood is very common, and prevalence estimates for wheeze during the first 5 years of life of up to 32% have been reported in UK studies [6, 12, 13]. These observations are consistent with a finding based on GP records that 25% of parents consulted as a result of their child's wheezing before the age of 5 years of whom approximately half did so in the first 12 months [9]. However, there is now increasing recognition that, in the first year of life, wheezing illness is common but the vast majority is episodic and confined to episodes of lower respiratory tract infection [14].

Many children who wheeze in the first few years of life experience a resolution of their symptoms before school age. Martinez et al. and Brooke et al. have followed children with pre-school wheezing to show that only about 40% of these children were still wheezing in the early school years [15, 16], whilst children who wheeze only in the first 12 months of life have been shown to have no greater risk of subsequent asthma than children with no history of wheezing [17].

After age 5, the incidence of wheezing for the remainder of childhood is relatively low, estimated from the 1958 British birth cohort at 1% per year for children aged 8–11 and 0.7% from age 12–16 [18]. However wheezing in this age group may be associated with a poorer prognosis through childhood into adulthood, particularly if symptoms are more severe or persistent. Two Australian cohort studies have provided valuable information on the natural history of childhood wheezing, and from the first of these studies it has emerged that, of children who wheezed at age 7, only 23% had no respiratory symptoms at age 14 [19]. The second cohort, which was enriched with children with more severe asthma, tended to show a less favourable prognosis, with 80% of children with persistent symptoms at age 7 continuing to wheeze into adolescence, and over 90% of those with persistent wheezing at age 14 continuing to experience symptoms at age 21 [20].

The two distinct patterns of natural history thus described for childhood wheezing have lead to the suggestion that there are two distinct subgroups of wheezing in early childhood. According to this hypothesis, most childhood wheezing occurs in the first years of life, is associated with viral infection, and has a favourable prognosis, whilst in a minority, wheezing in infancy is an early manifestation of wheezing which will persist through childhood into adulthood. Wheezing that persists is probably more likely in children who are atopic and have other allergic diseases [16, 21–25]. In contrast, infants with a family history of allergic disease or a personal history of allergic symptoms do not show an increased predisposition to wheezing within the first year of life [26–28]. Data from the Children's Respiratory Study in Tuscon, Arizona, which was the first prospective study initiated at birth and with measurements of airway function, serum IgE levels, allergic sensitisation, and wheezing illness collected through early childhood, confirmed this association in that, whilst children who wheezed in the first 3 years of life and persisted in wheezing to age 6 were more likely than never wheezers to have mothers with a history of asthma and to have elevated serum IgE levels at birth and age 6, children with transient wheezing before age 3 only did not differ from never wheezers in either of these respects [15]. However, children with transient early wheezing also differed from persistent wheezers with respect to lung function measured in the first months of life, confirming that wheezing lower respiratory tract illness is associated with lower levels of airway function [28–31]. Initially, it was not possible to ascertain whether this relationship was the result of airway damage caused by the respiratory tract illness or if the same factors determined the risk of respiratory tract illness and lung function. However, the Tucson study is now one of two studies demonstrating that diminished airway function exists in children who wheeze in infancy prior to the onset of the first wheezing respiratory tract illness [31, 32], and suggesting that pre-existing abnormalities in airway function predispose to wheezing in response to viral infections in infancy.

It therefore appears that the two types of early wheezers, distinguished initially by the natural history of their illness, also differ with respect to the pathology of the condition, such that early transient wheezing is attributable to lower airway calibre and a consequent increased risk of wheezing in episodes of viral infection whilst persistent wheezing is associated with an allergic predisposition. Recent work on the 1970 British birth cohort has suggested that the two types of wheezing also have distinct aetiologies [33].

Interestingly, longer term cohort data suggest that the favourable prognosis which has been described for wheezing in association with viral infection in infancy, may not be sustained throughout adult life. Baker and colleagues have demonstrated that respiratory tract infection in infancy may be associated with reduced airway function and with an increased risk of COPD in later life [34, 35]. Early wheezing may therefore still represent a marker of susceptibility to significant airflow obstruction in later life, but it would appear that this is an effect distinct from what is perceived to be asthma.

3. Temporal Changes in the Prevalence of Childhood Asthma and Allergic Disease

3.1. Temporal Changes in Hospital Asthma Admission Rates

Changes in hospital admission rates for asthma in children provided one of the earliest indications that the prevalence or severity of the condition might be increasing. In England and Wales, from 1958 to 1985, hospital admissions for childhood asthma increased 14-fold in the 0–4 age group and seven-fold in the 5–14 age group [36]. It is likely that this was at least in part due to changes in medical care and in particular to the introduction of nebuliser therapy [37] which was initially a hospital-based treatment and may therefore have contributed to increased parent expectations and preference for hospital care and to an increase in self-referral to hospital casualty departments [36, 38, 39]. However, there does not seem to have been a corresponding change in the severity of hospital admissions [36], suggesting either that there was a real increase in the prevalence of asthma over this time span or an increase in the proportion of asthmatic children having severe attacks, or that there was an increase in presentation of previously untreated disease.

3.2. Temporal Changes in the Prevalence of Asthma and Wheezing in Children

There is relatively little information other than that based on hospital admissions with which to establish temporal changes in the prevalence of wheezing in pre-school children. However, serial surveys from the UK [5, 40–42], Australia [43, 44] and the USA [45], using several different methodologies, from parental questionnaires and interviews through to GP records, have shown an increase in the prevalence of diagnosed asthma in pre-adolescent children over the past few decades. Asthma histories obtained from medical records on army conscripts have provided inconsistent evidence of a larger increase in the adolescent age group; a 600% increase was observed between 1966 and 1989 in Finland [46]. Several studies in pre-adolescence have also shown a substantial increase in the labelling of current wheezing as asthma [5, 40, 41], suggesting that some of the increase in asthma prevalence which took place over these years was due to an increased use of asthma as a diagnostic label. Nevertheless, these studies were also consistent in finding evidence for a smaller, though significant increase in the reported occurrence of current wheezing in these countries during the 1970s and 80s; wheezing in the past 12 months increased from 9.8% to 15.2% over 15 years in 12 year olds in Wales [40], from 11.5% to 12.8% over 3 years in 5–11 year olds in England [5], from 10.4% to 27.6% over 10 years in 8–10 year olds of Australia [44], and wheezing in the past 3 years from 10.4% to 19.8% over 25 years in 8–13 year olds in Scotland [41]. The Welsh and Australian studies alone had objective measures of wheezing illness, comprising bronchial responsiveness to exercise and histamine respectively, and both demonstrated increases over the same time scales in the prevalence of bronchial hyperresponsiveness. However, the increase in exercise-induced bronchoconstriction observed in the Welsh study was modest, at just 15%, in relation to the magnitude of the increase in prevalence of symptoms.

There is relatively little information on whether the severity of asthma in affected children has changed, but most of the available studies indicate an increase in morbidity in addition to an increase in prevalence. The Welsh study cited above found a relatively greater increase in the prevalence of severe grades of exercise-induced hyperreactivity than that of milder response to exercise between the two studies [40]. Burney et al. showed a trend towards an increased prevalence of wheeze on most days and nights and persistent wheeze in successive annual British cohorts born between 1961 and 1973 [47]. Comparisons of the latest two British birth cohorts originating in 1958 and 1970 revealed a three-fold increase in the prevalence of more frequent attacks of wheezing in 16 year olds [48]. These data contrast however with the findings of a UK survey of 8-year-old children which encorporated more detailed

Table 1. Prevalence studies of childhood wheezing in the UK since 1980

Year	Ref	Age of Subjects	No. of Subjects	Method	Prevalence of wheeze	
					Ever	Last 12 months
1984	[51]	5–13	5287	PQ	15%	
1985	[9]	5	369	MR	25%	
1985	[5]	5–11	3675	PQ	17.7%	11.5%
1986	[7]	7	1275	PQ	19.4%	12.0%
1986	[7]	11	1218	PQ	18.3%	12.3%
1988	[40]	12	965	PQ	22.3%	15.2%
1989	[5]	5–11	13 544	PQ	16.4%	12.8%
1989	[41]	8–13	3403	PQ	19.8 (last 3 years)	
1991	[38]	7–8	3070	PQ	12.3%	
1993	[6]	4–5	385	PQ	17%	

Data collection methods:
PQ: Parental Questionnaire,
MR: Medical Records

measures of the severity of wheezing and found little change in the prevalence of frequent attacks of wheezing, speech limiting attacks or school absence due to wheezing between 1978 and 1991 [49].

Nevertheless, the most recent prevalence surveys from Britain have shown little evidence of a continuing increase in childhood wheezing illness. The prevalence of wheezing in primary school age children has been estimated in a number of separate surveys during the late 1980s and 1990s, and despite differences in targeted age groups, geographical locations, size and type of sample and survey methodology, findings since 1980 have consistently provided estimates of between 11.5 and 15.2% for the 12-month period prevalence of wheezing in the 5–13 years age group (Tab. 1). Hospital admission rates for asthma may also have stabilised in some areas [50].

3.3. Evidence for an Increase in Atopy and Atopic Disease

Since wheezing that is associated with atopy may represent part of the more severe spectrum of wheezing in children [52], the limited evidence of an increase in morbidity in asthmatic children suggests an increase in expression of an allergic disease. A comparison of the prevalence of atopic dermatitis in the three British national birth cohorts, originating in 1946, 1958 and 1970 provided some of the first evidence that the prevalence of allergic disease might be increasing, for the proportion of children with a parentally-reported history of eczema by age 5–7 increased from 5.1% in the earliest cohort, to 12.2% in the most recent cohort [53]. The Scottish and Welsh surveys of asthma prevalence [40, 41] additionally asked parents about hayfever and eczema in their children. These two studies were consistent in showing a doubling in the parentally-reported prevalence of eczema since the 1970s, from 5.3% to 12% in Scotland and from 5% to 16% in Wales, and substantial increases in the prevalence of hayfever, the magnitude of the increase being greater over the 25 year time span of the Scottish study (from 3.2% to 11.9%) than over the shorter period of the Welsh study (from 9% to 15%). These findings are consistent with the increase in prevalence of hayfever and eczema at age 16 reported between the 1958 and 1970 British birth cohorts [54], and with British general practice morbidity statistics which show a doubling in the consultation rates for both conditions between 1970 and 1980 [42]. The increase in the prevalence of eczema and hayfever thus appears to have been at least as great as the increase in self-reported childhood wheezing.

Temporal changes in the self-reported prevalence of hayfever and eczema are subject to similar diagnostic and health care related trends as described for asthma [55]. There have been relatively few comparable cross-sectional population studies using objective measures of atopy. In a representative sample of adults in South West London the proportion of subjects with at least one positive skin prick test reaction increased significantly from 23% in 1974 to 46% in 1988, which supports a doubling in the prevalence of atopy over this time period [56]. A similar study in Tucson, USA, showed a slightly smaller increase over 8 years from 39% to 50% [57], but the increase in sensitisation to local aeroallergens between 1982 and 1992 in Australian children was smaller and non-significant [44]. The limited number of available objective serial measurements tend, therefore, to support an increase in the prevalence of atopy during the 1970s which may not have continued into the late 1980s and 90s.

3.4. An Increase in Wheezing as an Expression of Atopy?

Since the increase in asthma prevalence seems to have occurred simultaneously with an increase in the prevalence of atopy and of other atopic disease in developed societies, it is plausible that the increase in wheezing has occurred as a result of a general rise in the underlying prevalence of allergic sensitisation. However, Peat et al. have described a doubling in the prevalence of asthma in Australia between 1982 and 1992, which was concurrent with a much smaller and non-significant increase in atopy but with evidence of an increase in airway hyperreactivity in atopic children [44]. A similar pattern indicative of an increased tendency to wheeze in those with other expressions of allergic disease emerged from our own comparison of the 1958 and 1970 British birth cohorts [48], so that, in some environments at least, wheezing may also have become a more common expression of atopy.

4. Spatial Differences in the Prevalence of Wheeze and Atopy

Comparisons of wheeze and atopy prevalence between populations and countries can provide insight into the contribution of the environment in the development of these conditions and into those environmental factors which are likely to be the more important. However, differences in methodology, diagnostic criteria and age range between appropriate studies have limited the extent to which this is possible. Table 2 shows the results of recent studies focused to address this issue, and it is evident that, even allowing for differences in methodology and cultural differences in the interpretation of questions, there seems to be considerable international variation in the prevalence of childhood wheezing illness. These data suggest that childhood asthma is more common in Australasia, which is consistent with the geographical pattern of asthma mortality, admissions, and therapeutic drug use [58–60]. These studies also suggest that the prevalence of respiratory symptoms is two to three times lower in the more recently developed or developing countries of China, Malaysia and Hong Kong than in Western populations, and similarly very low prevalence rates have been described in areas of Africa [61, 62]. Racial differences in genetic susceptibility could explain some of the geographical differences in prevalence of childhood wheezing illness, but that this does not fully explain the observed spatial differences is confirmed by studies of children of

Table 2. International comparisons of the prevalence of childhood wheezing

Ref.	Year	Country	Method and criteria	Age group	Prevalence
[67]	1991	Australia (Adelaide)	Self-reported wheeze in the past year (ISAAC questionnaire/video)	12–15	29%/37%
		Australia (Sydney)			30%/40%
		England			29%/30%
		Germany			20%/27%
		New Zealand			28%/36%
[68]	1994	Hong Kong	Parentally-reported wheeze in the past 12 months	11–20	4%
		Malaysia			5%
		China			1%
[69]	1994	Hong Kong	Parentally reported wheeze in the past 12 months	12	5%
		Melbourne			22%
		Switzerland			6%
		Chile			21%
		Fiji			21%
[70]	1994	New Zealand	Parentally-reported wheeze in the past 12 months	12	18%
		Wales			15%
		South Africa			18%
		Sweden			9%

similar genetic origin living in different environments. The reunification of East and West Germany has provided a unique opportunity to compare the development of childhood respiratory and allergic conditions in ethnically similar populations who have lived in different environments for a number of years. Surveys using identical methods in the two areas have shown an increased prevalence of cough and wheezing in East Germany, in particular that labelled bronchitis and associated with a cold, in comparison with the West, but reduced rates of asthma [63]. One interpretation of this study is that asthma is more common in children exposed to a Western lifestyle and perhaps the more convincing evidence for this supposition comes from comparisons of rural and urban communities of less developed countries, the latter being relatively recently exposed to Western influences. Van Niekerk et al. showed in 1979 that asthma was more prevalent in an urban than in a rural Xhosa community [61], Keeley et al. showed in 1991 that the prevalence of "reversible airways obstruction" measured as exercise reactivity was greater in urban than in rural Zimbabwe [64], and more recently, we have shown a higher prevalence of wheeze and diagnosed asthma in urban relative to rural Ethiopia [62]. The perception in these countries is that the increase in asthma prevalence is related to the adoption of a more Western lifestyle.

International comparisons of positivity to skin prick tests reveal that there are also wide variations in levels of atopy and specific IgE sensitivity (Tab. 3).

Table 3. Between country and area comparisons of atopy levels in children

Ref	Year	Country	Age group	Criteria for +vty	Atopy prevalence ≥ 1 +ve skin test		Mite	Pollen
[68]	1994	Malaysia	11–20	≥3 mm	64%	60%	17%	
		Hong Kong			58%	55%	6%	
		China			49%	43%	6%	
[71]	1989	New Zealand	5–15	≥3 mm	46%	30%	33%	
[72]	1994	Fiji	9–10	≥3 mm	36%	25% *	<10% *	
[44]	1994	Australia						
		Belmont (humid)	8–10	≥3 mm	29%	21%	12%	
		Wagga Wagga (dry)			35%	15%	22%	
[73]	1996	UK	8–11	≥1 mm	35%	not given	not given	
[74]	1994	West Germany	9–11	≥3 mm	37%	10%	21% (grass)	
		East Germany			18%	4%	8% (grass)	
[75]	1994	Sweden (rural)	10–12	≥3 mm	24%	2%	19%	
		Sweden (urban)			35%	2%	27%	
		Poland (urban)			14%	0.3%	10%	
[76]	1994	Sweden (north rural)	7–9	≥3 mm	27%	5%	16%	
		Sweden (south urban)			14%	4%	10%	
[62]	1997	Ethiopia (urban)	10–19	≥3 mm	5.9%	2.8%	3.3% (mixed threshings)	

* estimated from graphical representation

Specific IgE levels are clearly associated with the level of exposure to specific allergens, such that sensitisation to the housedust mite seems to predominate in the more humid countries, whilst sensitivity to pollens is more common in drier climates. Nevertheless, it is also clear that the prevalence of atopy, defined in terms of positivity by skin prick test to at least one local aeroallergen, across Westernised countries is reasonably consistent at 30–40%, Australia and New Zealand having the higher levels, comparatively low in Poland and East Germany, and relatively uncommon in the developing society of Jimma, Ethiopia [62]. The geographical pattern of the prevalence of atopy and allergic disease is similar to the described pattern of asthma prevalence, and our own findings that in urban Ethiopia as in the Western world, atopy was by far the strongest risk factor for asthma [62], is consistent with the suggestion that the spatial distribution of atopy largely explains that of allergic wheezing illness.

5. Migrant Studies of Wheeze and Atopy

Perhaps the most persuasive evidence that the prevalence of asthma and of atopy vary with the geographical environment rather than simply genetic background comes from studies of first generation migrants. Individuals who move from areas of relatively low to relatively high asthma or atopy prevalence seem to be more likely to develop these conditions than children remaining in the country of origin. South African children living in urban Cape Town were more likely to be asthmatic than their non-migrant counterparts living in the rural Transkei area [61], and migrant Tokelauan children living in New Zealand had a significantly increased risk of the development of asthma, eczema or rhinitis defined by self-reported history and medical examination than those remaining in Tokelau [65]. Interestingly the most marked increase in the latter study occurred in the under 4 years age group who were more likely to be born in, or to have lived in New Zealand early in life. That the development of asthma, in particular, may be closely associated with the geographical environment of infancy is suggested by the studies of Smith et al., who have shown a lower prevalence of asthma in migrant children to the UK born in India or Pakistan than in children of similar origin born in the UK, and Reid et al., who have shown that British migrants to the USA had a higher prevalence of respiratory illness than Norwegian migrants [66].

6. Aetiology of Wheezing Illness in Children

6.1. Evidence for the Importance of the Environment in the Development of Asthma and Atopy in Childhood

Although genetic factors are known to be important in the development of atopy, and probably also in the expression of asthma, the data on the spatial and secular distribution of asthma outlined above demonstrates that the development and progression of atopic disease is largely explained by environmental factors. The spatial distribution of disease and relatively greater increase in prevalence in developing societies suggest that factors relating to the Westernisation of a society may be important, and may also help to explain the increase in the Western world. The fact that atopic disease is usually first expressed in the first few years of life, and that the origins of respiratory disease, even that occurring in later life [77], is related to the geographical region of early childhood, suggest that environmental exposures occurring very early in life may be of especial significance. To date, however, the exposures involved have not been identified, and untangling the aetiology of asthma in children is complicated by the fact that more than one aetiologically distinct disease entity may be involved. To date a wide range of environmental factors have been linked with the development of asthma and wheezing illness in children, including maternal smoking, low birth weight, pre-term birth, low birth order, maternal age, breast feeding, month of birth, levels of housedust mite exposure, keeping pets in the home, damp housing, indoor and outdoor pollution, diet, respiratory infections and exposure to other childhood illnesses and/or vaccinations.

6.2. Maternal Smoking

There have been extensive investigations into the effects of parental smoking upon children's lung health, and the evidence is consistent that, after adjustment for relevant social class factors, maternal smoking is associated with about a 1.5 fold increase in the risk of wheezing and lower respiratory illness in the first few years of life [78–83]. Where the smoking habits of both parents have been considered, maternal smoking has been the more important in almost all studies [79, 81], and whilst this could reflect the more prolonged post-natal exposure to maternal smoking, there is also evidence that pre-natal exposure is particularly important [80].

There is strong evidence from cross-sectional data that parental smoke exposure is associated with diminished airway function in children [79, 84–86]. Whilst many of the early studies suggested that the respiratory illness in early life to which the children of smoking mothers were disposed was the antecedent cause of the lowered levels of function that were observed [87–91], subsequent evidence has shown significantly reduced pulmonary function soon after birth in children of mothers who smoke in pregnancy [29, 92, 93], suggesting that *in utero* exposure to cigarette smoke impairs airway development, and support for this theory has been provided through animal models [94].

The relationship between pre- or post-natal parental smoking and respiratory symptoms in children over the age of two is less clear. Some authors have found no significant effect of maternal smoke exposure in school age children, but interestingly most have found an odds ratio for this effect which is larger than one [95–97]. Others have shown a significant increase in risk of respiratory symptoms in relation to parental smoking, though the size of the effect has generally been smaller than that seen in relation to wheezing in infancy, with estimates of 1.23 (95% CI 1.05–1.37) in relation to wheezing in the last year in 6- to 9-year-old children [98], and 1.35 (1.01–1.81) in relation to current wheezing in children from age 6 to 12 [99]. As in the case of early wheezing, the larger effects have generally arisen in relation to maternal, rather than paternal smoking [98], but again it has proved difficult to separate the effects of current and *in utero* exposure to maternal cigarette smoke. In support of a detrimental effect of postnatal as well as prenatal smoke exposure, however, some authors have described a significant dose response relationship with the number of smokers in the home [98, 100], and an increase in relation to paternal smoking in homes where the mother did not smoke [101]. Moreover, certain children, and in particular those with diagnosed asthma, may be more susceptible to the effects of passive smoke exposure and may experience more severe or frequent symptoms as a consequence [102–104].

Active smoking is associated with an increase in total serum immunoglobulin E (IgE) [105–107], and possibly with an elevated risk of allergic sensitisation to some occupational allergens [108], leading to speculation that passive smoke exposure might increase the risk of allergic sensitisation in children. However, the available evidence in relation to allergic symptoms and atopy tends not to support this suggestion, and indeed three large studies have now shown negative associations between parental smoke exposure and atopy [109–111]. It therefore seems unlikely that parental smoking, either before or after birth increases the risk of allergic sensitisation in childhood.

6.3. Low Birth Weight and Prematurity

Low birth weight and prematurity have been associated with an increased risk of respiratory symptoms in infancy [112–115], and also with an increased risk of asthma in older children [116, 117]. Some authors have speculated that mechanical ventilation used in the management of preterm children may itself induce lung damage, but others have shown that the effects of low birth weight or premature birth seem to be independent of neonatal respiratory illness or mechanical ventilation after birth [118]. A further possibility is that maternal asthma predisposes to premature labour [116], but children born prematurely or of low birth weight do not appear to be at increased risk of the development of atopy. Premature and low birth weight children do however appear to have a lower mean level of airway function measured soon after birth [119, 120], and it seems more likely that persistent wheezing in such children is a condition attributable to poor airway calibre, rather than IgE mediated disease. Barker et al. have shown an interesting link between birth weight and lung function in adults [35], suggesting either that the effect of low birth weight on pulmonary function is irrecoverable or that there is some programming effect by which birth weight effects the subsequent growth of the lung.

Birth weight and gestation are clearly strongly correlated, yet they may be differentially measures of fetal growth and fetal maturity [121, 122]. Only two studies to date have attempted to separate the relative effects of each upon lung function and respiratory symptoms. The results of the first were inconsistent in demonstrating that lung function was independently related only to low birthweight, whilst respiratory symptoms were independently related only to prematurity [112], and the more recent study of new born infants has demonstrated a reduced airway size in relation to small birthweight in premature babies, but no reduction in pulmonary function in relation to prematurity *per se* [120]. The evidence so far therefore suggests that the effects of low birth weight and prematurity are explained by some factor of the *in utero* environment which leads to retardation in infant weight gain; fetal undernutrition is a possible explanation.

Nevertheless, it is also recognised that exposure to maternal smoking *in utero* is an important cause of low birth weight [123, 124], and a probable cause of pre-term birth [125, 126]. A study set in Shanghai, where smoking by women in pregnancy is rare, suggested that in the absence of maternal and other passive smoke exposure there may be no increased risk in relation to low birth weight, but that the detrimental effect of passive smoke exposure might be increased in children of low birth weight [115]. Thus the complex relationship between the effects of *in utero* and passive smoking, birth weight and gestation in relation to the risk of respiratory symptoms and the development of asthma in children has yet to be fully elucidated.

6.4. Maternal Age

There is some consistency in the observation that wheezing illness in infancy [114, 127] as well as in later childhood [33, 128] may be increased in relation to young maternal age, yet the occurrence of hayfever seems to be more rather than less likely with increasing maternal age [129, 130]. In some countries smoking is now commonest in young women, and is therefore a potential confounder of this relationship, though the increase in risk of wheezing in the children of young mothers is reported to be independent of the effect of smoking [127]. The interpretation which has been put on this finding is that children of young mothers experience adverse circumstances *in utero* or in childhood leading to suboptimal respiratory growth or function, and one possibility is that in the teenage years, nutritional requirements for the mother's own growth may compete with the needs of the fetus [131].

6.5. Birth Order

Strachan et al. have shown in two British datasets that atopy and the occurrence of hayfever in adolescence are strongly inversely related to the number of siblings [109, 129, 130, 132], and a similar association has now been shown in children of East and West Germany [110]. Since the association in the British data was stronger in relation to the number of older than to the number of younger siblings, it has been speculated that earlier or increased exposure to viral infections early in life may be involved in this association, as discussed below.

6.6. Month of Birth

Bjorksten et al. have demonstrated an increased risk of pollen allergy in children born in Finland in March and April, about 3 months before the period of highest exposure to pollen [133], and also that children born between February and April were at maximum risk of sensitisation to birch pollen, and those born between April and May were at maximum risk of mugwort allergy [134]. The maximum risk of sensitisation appeared to occur in those born 2–3 months before the period of maximum environmental exposure. These data indicate that there may be a relatively greater risk of sensitisation upon exposure to allergens in early life. This suggestion has since been supported by studies showing an increased risk of sensitisation to housedust mite and cat in those born in the autumn [135], but also disputed on the basis of several studies showing no such association [136] and the likely publication bias in reporting of random associations with month of birth. Collectively, however, these findings have led to the suggestion that there is a "window of opportunity" in very early childhood during which time genetically predisposed children may be at a relative greater risk of sensitisation to the allergens to which they are exposed, and that allergen avoidance during this period might reduce the risk of allergic disease. In conflict with this suggestion, studies which have looked at the effect of month of birth on the prevalence of allergic symptoms have produced largely inconsistent results, and one possibility is that the month of birth simply alters the allergen to which an individual becomes sensitised rather than the risk of sensitisation *per se*. Evidence from intervention studies is limited. In one major study, Arshad et al. showed that avoidance of food allergen and housedust mite in the first year produced a six fold reduction in the occurrence of atopic disease at 1 year in high-risk children [137]. In relation to allergic sensitisation but not to asthma, the effect was sustained to age 4 [138], and interestingly, lower rates of sensitisation were observed to a number of different aeroallergens, not simply housedust mite antigen. Nevertheless, evidence on the development of sensitivity to occupational allergens, which has provided an analogous model within which to look at the relationship between timing of exposure and onset of symptoms, suggests that sensitisation can occur in adults upon exposure to a new allergen [139]. A population based study in Tuscon, Arizona, showing that within 6 years migrants into the area had an increased level of sensation to local aeroallergens to a similar level to that seen in the native population, provided further support for this suggestion [57]. It therefore seems likely that avoidance of environmental allergens in early life may simply postpone rather than prevent sensitisation to a specific allergen, or result in sensitisation to an alternative allergen.

6.7. Housedust Mite Exposure

In the UK, the majority of children with asthma are sensitised to the housedust mite; as many as 94% have skin sensitivity to this allergen in relation to 30% in those without asthma [140]. As a result, much debate has centred around the extent to which the increase in asthma prevalence can be attributed to an increase in exposure and sensitisation to the housedust mite allergen, with speculation that modern, centrally heated, well-insulated housing has caused increases in housedust mite levels, and that earlier and increased exposure has caused an increased likelihood of sensitisation and more frequent or severe symptoms. Consistent with this hypothesis, there was a dramatic increase in allergic disease following modernisation of housing design in Japan [141] and there is evidence from some Western countries including Australia of increases in the prevalence of housedust mite exposure [44]. Some studies have also shown a relationship between the risk and degree of sensitisation and the level of housedust mite exposure [140, 142], and some, but not all, have demonstrated that current asthma symptoms, severity of symptoms, hospital admissions in asthmatic children, and airway reactivity are associated with levels of housedust mite exposure [143–145]. On the other side of this argument however the evidence from studies of lung function and symptoms in asthmatic children after reduction in housedust mite levels in the home suggest that any effect is modest [146], and the fact that asthma has increased in areas of the world where the housedust mite does not flourish and in which sensitisation to other allergens are more important risk factors for asthma also suggest that increased exposure to the housedust mite is not the sole explanation for the described rise in allergic disease.

6.8. Pets

Sixty-eight percent of asthmatic children are sensitised to cat allergen [147], and some studies have suggested that keeping furry pets is a risk factor for current symptoms [148, 149], if only in children sensitised to the relevant allergen [150]. Whilst some cross-sectional studies have not demonstrated an association between the presence of pets in the home or the levels of animal danders and increased respiratory symptoms [7, 151], Brunekreef et al., in showing that the highest prevalence of pet allergy was in homes where pets were no longer present but owned at some stage in the past, have suggested that these negative findings are erroneous and caused by the selective removal of pets from the homes of sensitised children [151]. Nevertheless, a lower risk of atopy in children from homes with a pig living in the house in a recent study in Guinea Bissau appears to be inconsistent with an important effect of animal exposure [152].

6.9. Damp and Mould in the Home

Dampness and mould in the home has been associated with an increased prevalence of respiratory symptoms in children [150, 153–156]. However, many of the studies showing this association have relied on parental reporting both of respiratory symptoms and of dampness and it is likely that a public perception that damp housing must be detrimental to respiratory health may be partly responsible for these findings [97, 157]. Alternatively, sensitivity to the housedust mite, which thrive in damp homes, or to the airbourne spores of fungal moulds, are possible mechanisms for a causal link between damp conditions and asthma. One carefully conducted case control study, which used observer and parentally reported measures of damp and mould, has shown that, whilst parents of asthmatic children were slightly more likely to report damp in the home, there was a significant relationship between reported dampness and mould and respiratory symptoms or asthma, that this was related to an increased sensitivity to mould and housedust mite in children living in damp housing, and that damp housing was only associated with increased respiratory symptoms in children sensitised to one of these allergens [157]. A remaining question however is whether the effect of damp housing is truly independent of the effect of parental smoke exposure, since a number of these studies provide limited data on the effect of adjustment for this likely confounder.

6.10. Breast Feeding

The question of whether or not breast feeding protects against the development of atopic diseases in general, and asthma in particular, is a source of persistent controversy. Some studies have shown breast feeding to be highly protective [158–161], whilst others have shown no effect [162, 163], or even a positive association between breast feeding and atopic disease [129, 130, 164]. On the grounds that when children at high risk of allergy are followed prospectively from birth some initially show an allergic response to food allergens only [165,

166], and that eczema is the main disease manifestation of food allergy, notably to cow's milk, it would seem plausible that early avoidance of food antigens might prevent or delay the onset of childhood eczema. This hypothesis is supported by at least one randomised trial showing that within breast fed children at high risk of allergic disease, manipulation of maternal diet to avoid specific food antigens such as milk and eggs which are known to be transmitted through breast milk, reduces the risk of atopic eczema [167]. However, it is also recognised that allergic reactions to food peak in infancy and that the prevalence of food allergy reduces with age, and what is not clear is whether avoidance of food or other allergens in infancy has any sustained impact on the likelihood of allergic disease, or whether it simply delays onset.

That breast feeding may also have a protective role in wheezing in the first few years of life [168], perhaps in non-atopic children only [169, 170], is also plausible, since there is substantial evidence that prolonged breast feeding protects against early childhood infections, including respiratory tract infections [171, 172]. This effect has not been satisfactorily separated from confounding by maternal smoking, but if true, breast feeding might conversely predispose an individual to the subsequent development of allergic disease, if the hypothesis that early infections are protective (see below) has any foundation. Two large cross-sectional studies showing an increased incidence of hayfever by adolescence or early adulthood in those breastfed as infants would appear to support this proposition [129, 130]

6.11. Outdoor Pollution

The rise in asthma prevalence over recent decades has occurred at a time of increasing appreciation of environmental issues, and this in conjunction with the recognition that acute pollution episodes such as the London smog of 1952 caused excess deaths from respiratory conditions, have led to widespread speculation that air pollution was responsible for the increases and high levels of asthma prevalence in children. As a result of these concerns in the UK, the Committee on the Medical Effects of Air Pollutants was formed to examine the evidence to date on the effects on respiratory health and the development of allergic disease of current pollution levels [173]. Some of the most persuasive evidence related to the fact that levels of sulphur dioxide and black smoke have actually substantially reduced over the same time span as the increase in asthma prevalence in the UK, and that levels of ozone and nitrogen dioxide have changed very little in polluted areas. Furthermore, population-based studies of genetically similar children exposed long term to very different pollution levels, such as those of the American six cities study, children of East and West Germany, and children of Sweden and Poland, show little association between traditional pollutants such as black smoke and sulphur dioxide and asthma prevalence. Indeed, in areas of East Germany and Poland, where the levels of sulphur dioxide and particulates were highest, the prevalence of asthma, bronchial hyperresponsiveness, atopic sensitivity, hayfever and rhinitis, were lower than in the less polluted areas of West Germany and Sweden [63, 75]. These findings provoked the alternative suggestion that some aspect of the new types and distribution of pollutant levels in West Germany or Sweden, perhaps relating to car vehicle emissions, was responsible. There is very limited evidence in support of a relation between the risk of atopy and exposure to high traffic density, restricted to one study showing an increased prevalence of cedar pollen allergy in areas of high traffic volume [174], but to date, four published studies have shown a consistent, though modest, association between exposure to traffic and asthma prevalence in children [175–178]. Chamber and panel studies have demonstrated that at current outdoor ambient levels, ozone is the only measurable new pollutant to show any effect on respiratory symptoms [179–182] or response to allergen [183]. Short-term daily variations in ozone are associated with temporary reductions in lung function in children [184–186], which, superimposed on the deteriorating lung function of asthmatic children, might provoke symptoms which would otherwise not have occurred. This effect is however, small, and unlikely to be important at a population level. However, that constituents of traffic pollution are involved in the initiation of asthma is difficult to reconcile with the apparent lack of an urban/rural variation in the prevalence of asthma in the UK [187–189] or elsewhere in the developed world. Overall, the current evidence and the finding of the Committee on the Medical Effects of Air Pollution is that, while increased levels of certain pollutants might incite attacks of asthma in a small number of asthmatics particularly susceptible to the effects of air pollution, there is little support for air pollution as an initiator of asthma, or as the cause of the increased prevalence of asthma over recent decades.

6.12. Indoor Pollution

With the possible exception of exposure to environmental tobacco smoke, there is relatively little evidence on the impact of exposure to indoor air pollutants such as those emanating from gas stoves, wood stoves, and fireplaces, despite the fact that these are likely to have greater relevance than outdoor pollutant levels, since children spend over 80% of their time indoors. Indoor pollution is likely to have increased over recent years as a result of better insulation of houses, and in the presence of unvented gas appliances, levels of the nitrogen oxides are considerably higher indoors than outdoors. There is evidence, from some but not all studies, that children who live in homes with gas stoves have reduced lung function [98, 190] and experience more respiratory symptoms, particularly in the first few years of life, than those who live in homes that use other fuels for cooking [190–193]. Though the reported effects are fairly small, nevertheless the importance of this exposure lies in the fact that 30–60% of the population in most European and American countries use gas appliances for cooking or heating.

Smoke that emanates from wood stoves and fireplaces is a potential source of several indoor pollutants. Wood burning, in addition to producing hydro-carbons and respirable particules, is a significant source of carbon monoxide. Interestingly, whilst coal and wood combustion have been reported to increase the risk of upper and lower respiratory tract infection, Von Mutius et al. have shown an inverse relationship between homes using open coal or wood burn-ing fires and the development of atopy and allergic disease [194]. This finding was thus consistent with the possibility that respiratory tract infections have a protective role in the development of atopy. It also suggests however that this particular source of indoor pollution is unlikely to form an important cause of allergic disease.

6.13. Diet

More recently, dietary intake has received much attention as a possible expla-nation for the world-wide variations, trends in prevalence, and association with Westernisation [195], particularly because the western diet has changed dra-matically over the last 20–30 years with an increase in processed foods, and a decrease in fresh fruits, vegetables and fish [196]. Moreover, there is now sub-stantial evidence that in adults dietary factors may be involved in the aetiolo-gy of asthma. The hypothesis that the high and increasing sodium content of Western diets may contribute to a higher prevalence of asthma has received particular attention, and has been supported by some cross-sectional epidemi-ological studies [197–199] and experimental clinical trials [200–202], though not in all cases [203, 204]. Our own work has suggested that some of the inconsistency in these findings may be explained by inverse correlation between sodium and magnesium intakes, since a high magnesium intake seems to be associated with reduced airway hyperreactivity and higher lung function in the general population [205]. Other nutrients implicated in the aeti-ology of asthma include the antioxidant vitamins C and E [198, 206], which may protect the lung against the oxidant damage caused by exposure to ciga-rette smoke and other air pollutants, and eicosapentaenoic acid found in fish oil, which may have a role in preventing or reducing inflammation in the air-way [207–209]. Whilst these findings have mainly arisen from studies of adults, a recent Australian study has shown a reduced prevalence of asthma and airway responsiveness in children with a high intake of fish oil [210], Demissie et al. have shown an increase in bronchial responsiveness but not asthma with increasing salt intake [211], Powell et al. have shown that children with asthma have a lower antioxidant status than healthy controls [212], and less specifically, Carey et al. have recently shown that Asian children living in Britain who ate a traditional Indian diet were at a reduced risk of asthma rela-tive to those eating a British diet [73]. There is thus increasing evidence that dietary factors may be involved in determining respiratory health in children as well as adults. It has been speculated that such changes may also have acted to increase the risk of allergic sensitisation, and that these changes might thus have contributed to the increase in all allergic diseases over recent years [195]. However, an alternative hypothesis is that the influence of dietary trends has operated through changes in maternal diet in pregnancy, and indirect evidence that this may be influential has arisen from an apparent association between large head circumference at birth and adult IgE levels [213]. The argument that follows is that head size could be a marker of disproportionate growth, and that this in turn is a marker of fetal undernutrition in late gestation which itself results in slower maturation of the immune system. However, there is currently little direct evidence for the effect of maternal nutrient levels on the subsequent development of atopy or allergic disease in the child.

6.14. Viral and Other Infections

Older data has suggested that viral infection occurring during early life could be a risk factor for the development of asthma, because children who wheezed in response to viral infection in early childhood seemed to be more likely to develop subsequent asthma [88, 214–218]. It was suggested that viral infections could alter the lung and immune system, leading to reduced airway calibre, increased allergic sensitisation and persistent bronchial reactivity. More recently, it has been recognised that wheezing in children may not be a homogeneous condition and that most children who wheeze in response to viral infection do so in the first few years of life with an early resolution of symptoms. Martinez et al. have found that such children do not seem to be at increased risk of the subsequent development of atopy [15], suggesting that viral infections do not increase the risk of the development of allergic disease, and that in these children, reduced lung function pre-existed the viral infection [32]. That viral infection might conversely protect a child from the development of atopy is a hypothesis which has emerged from a number of recent findings. Martinez et al. have shown that children who had non-wheezing, but not wheezing, lower respiratory tract illness before age 3 years had lower IgE levels at 6 years, and those with more than one non-wheezing LRI before age 3 were less likely to be atopic at age 6 [219]. A low prevalence of asthma is reported in New Guinea in which there is a very high rate of respiratory infection [220], and an increased rate of respiratory infection but reduced rate of atopy has been found in East relative to West Germany [63]. A hypothesis that early infection might direct the development of the developing immune system against allergic sensitisation would also explain the strong inverse relationship between the prevalence of atopy and atopic disease and the number of siblings in the household. Recent studies showing a reduced risk of atopy in West African children who contracted measles infection [152], in Italian military students seropositive to hepatitis A [221], and in Japanese children with delayed hypersensitivity to mycobacterium tuberculosis [222] have provided further support for the suggestion that early respiratory or non-respiratory infections may act to inhibit the development of allergic disease. Helminth parasites may have a similar action, and indeed the allergic response which is now responsible for so many unwanted allergic symptoms may once have conferred biological advantage in immunity against parasitic infections [223].

7. Conclusion—What Has Caused the Increase?

There seems to be little doubt that childhood asthma is a condition which has increased in prevalence in the developed world over the last 30 years, whilst remaining relatively rare in a number of developing societies. The picture that has emerged of childhood asthma is however of a heterogeneous condition, in terms of its natural history, pathogenesis and its aetiology, in that there may be a subset of children who wheeze early in life, with a condition associated with small airways, and partly attributable to maternal smoking or low birth weight, but whose symptoms have a good prognosis after infancy. A smaller group have a more persistent condition, more closely associated with an allergic predisposition, and since the increase in childhood asthma has occurred simultaneously with an increase in other allergic disease phenotypes and with the underlying prevalence of atopy, it seems most likely that it is an increase in allergic asthma which has occurred over recent years. Whilst atopy is partly genetically determined, there are substantial reasons for believing that environmental factors must underlie the increase in atopy over such a short time span, and the pattern of prevalence and increase in both asthma and atopy is consistent with there being an aspect or aspects of a Western lifestyle which are responsible. However, there remains no satisfactory explanation for the increase. Changes in air pollution, increased smoking by women in pregnancy, a tendency to bottle feed rather than breast feed and from an earlier age and increased exposure to environmental allergens have all been implicated but the direction and magnitude of the effects of each are inconsistent with an important contribution from any one of these factors. Our own analyses of the two most recent British birth cohorts found that temporal changes in all of maternal smoking, birth weight, infant feeding practices, maternal age, and occupational social class had a minimal contribution to the increase in prevalence of allergic disease between the two cohorts [48, 54]. Moreover, whilst the development of hayfever and eczema were strongly related to birth order in both sets of children, our analyses provided little evidence that the small reductions in family size which have occurred over the past decades could explain much of the increase in these diseases.

One factor which is linked to a western lifestyle and which has changed in a direction which would appear to be generally deleterious is diet, and this remains a contender as a contributor to the increase in childhood asthma. Additionally, however, recent advances in our comprehension of the immunological processes involved in the development of allergic disease, have provided a potential mechanism by which exposure to infections, and also to pathogens, in early life might protect against the development of atopy [220]. It may therefore be improved health care, the introduction of immunisation programs against certain common infectious diseases of childhood, a direct effect of a specific immunisation itself, or the more hygienic environment in which we now live which holds the key to the increase in allergic disease. One further factor which has consistently emerged as a strong and independent determinant of the occurrence of allergic disease in older children and adults is high socioeconomic status, and though the factors underlying this association have yet to be determined, nevertheless, there is no doubt that in many developed societies, individuals are relatively more affluent and enjoy a considerably better standard of living now than 20 or 30 years ago. Whatever the factors involved, the rise in prevalence of allergic disease seen across the developed world over recent decades may therefore finally emerge as a necessary and obligatory consequence of a Western lifestyle.

References

1 Williams H, McNicol KN (1969) Prevalence, natural history, and relationship of wheezy bronchitis and asthma in children. An epidemiological study. *Br Med J* 4: 321–325
2 Speight ANP (1983) Underdiagnosis and undertreatment of asthma in childhood. *Br Med J* 286: 1253–1256
3 Anderson HR, Bailey PA, Cooper JS, Palmer JC, West S (1983) Medical care of asthma and wheezing illness in children: a community survey. *J Epidemiol Community Health* 37: 180–186
4 Luyt DK, Burton P, Brooke aM, Simpson H (1994) Wheeze in preschool children and its relation with doctor diagnosed asthma. *Arch Dis Child* 71: 24–30
5 Hill R, Williams J, Tattersfield A, Britton J (1989) Change in use of asthma as a diagnostic label for wheezing illness in schoolchildren. *Br Med J* 299: 898
6 Luyt DK, Burton PR, Simpson H (1993) Epidemiological study of wheeze, doctor diagnosed asthma, and cough in preschool children in Leicestershire. *Br Med J* 306: 1386–1390
7 Clifford RD, Radford M, Howell JB, Holgate ST (1989) Prevalence of respiratory symptoms among 7 and 11 year old schoolchildren and association with asthma. *Arch Dis Child* 64: 1118–1125
8 Jenkins MA, Clarke JR, Carlin JB, Robertson CF, Hopper JL, Dalton MF et al (1996) Validation of questionnaire and bronchial hyperresponsiveness against respiratory physician assessment in the diagnosis of asthma. *Int J Epidemiol* 25: (3)609–616
9 Strachan DP (1985) The prevalence and natural history of wheezing in early childhood. *J Roy Coll Gen Prac* 35: 182–184
10 Shaw RA, Crane JA, Pearce N (1992) Comparison of a video questionnaire with the IUATLD written questionnaire for measuring asthma prevalence. *Clin Exp Allergy* 22: 509–510
11 Asher MI, Keil U, Anderson HR, Beasley R, Crane J, Martinez F et al (1995) International study of asthma and allergies in childhood (ISAAC): Rationale and methods. *Eur Resp J* 8: 483–491
12 Park ES, Golding J, Carswell F, Stewart-Brown S (1986) Preschool wheezing and prognosis at 10. *Arch Dis Child* 61: 642–646
13 Ogston SA, Florey cd Walker CHM (1985) The Tayside infant morbidity and mortality study: effect on health and using gas for cooking. *Br Med J* 290: 957–960
14 Wright AL, Taussig LM, Ray CG (1989) The Tucson children's respiratory study. II Lower respiratory tract illness in the first year of life. *Am J Epidemiol* 129: 1232–1246
15 Martinez FD, Wright AL, Taussig LM, Holberg CJ, Halonen M, Morgan WJ et al (1995) Asthma and wheezing in the first six years of life. *N Engl J Med* 332: 133–138
16 Brooke AM, Lambert PC, Burton PR, Clarke C, Luyt DK, Simpson H (1995) The natural history of respiratory symptoms in preschool children. *Am J Respir Crit Care Med* 152: (6)1872–1878

17 Dodge R, Martinez FD, Cline MG, Lebowitz MD, Burrows B (1996) Early childhood respiratory symptoms and the subsequent diagnosis of asthma. *J Allerg Clin Immunol* 98 (1): 48–54

18 Anderson HR, Pottier AC, Strachan DP (1992) Asthma from birth to age 23: incidence and relation to prior and concurrent atopic disease. *Thorax* 47: 537–542

19 Giles GG, Gibson HB, Lickiss N, Shaw K (1984) Respiratory symptoms in Tasmanian adolescents: a follow up of the 1961 birth cohort. *Aust NZ J Med* 14: 631–637

20 Martin AJ, McLennan LA, Landau LI, Phelan PD (1980) The natural history of childhood asthma to adult life. *Br Med J* 280: 1397–1400

21 Jenkins MA, Hopper JL, Bowes G, Carlin JB, Flander LB, Giles GG (1994) Factors in childhood as predictors of asthma in adult life. *Br Med J* 309: 90–93

22 Kokkonen J, Linna O (1993) The state of childhood asthma in young adulthood. *Eur Resp J* 6: 657–661

23 Roorda RJ, Gerritsen J, Vanaalderen WMC, Knol K (1993) Skin reactivity and eosinophil count in relation to the outcome of childhood asthma. *Eur Resp J* 6: 509–516

24 Ross S, Godden DJ, Abdalla M, McMurray D, Douglas A, Oldman D et al (1995) Outcome of wheeze in childhood: The influence of atopy. *Eur Resp J* 8: (12)2081–2087

25 Peat JK, Salome CM, Woolcock AJ (1990) Longitudinal changes in atopy during a 4-year period: relation to bronchial hyperresponsiveness and respiratory symptoms in a population sample of Australian schoolchildren. *J Allerg Clin Immunol* 85: 65–74

26 Sims DG, Gardner PS, Weightman D, Turner MW, Soothill JF (1981) Atopy does not predispose to RSV bronchiolitis or postbronchiolitic wheezing. *Br Med J* 282: 2086–2088

27 Cogswell J, Halliday DF, Alexander JR (1982) Respiratory infections in the first year of life in children at risk of developing atopy. *Br Med J* 284: 1011–1013

28 Young S, Okeeffe PT, Arnott J, Landau LI (1995) Lung function, airway responsiveness, and respiratory symptoms before and after bronchiolitis. *Arch Dis Child* 72: 16–24

29 Tager IB, Hanrahan JP, Tosteson TD, Castile RG, Brown RW, Weiss ST et al (1993) Lung function, pre- and post-natal smoke exposure, and wheezing in the first year of life. *Am Rev Respir Dis* 147: 811–817

30 Clarke JR, Reese A, Silverman M (1992) Bronchial responsiveness and lung function in infants with lower respiratory tract illness over the first six months of life. *Arch Dis Child* 67: 1454–1458

31 Stick SM, Arnott J, Turner DJ, Young S, Landau LI (1991) Bronchial responsiveness and lung function in recurrently wheezy infants. *Am Rev Respir Dis* 144: 1012–1015

32 Martinez FD, Morgan WJ, Wright AL, Holberg CJ, Taussig LM (1988) Diminished lung function as a predisposing factor for wheezing respiratory illness in infants. *N Engl J Med* 319: 1112–1117

33 Lewis S, Richards D, Bynner J, Butler N, Britton J (1995) Prospective study of risk factors for early and persistent wheezing in childhood. *Eur Resp J* 8: 349–356

34 Barker DJP, Osmond C (1986) Childhood respiratory infection and adult chronic bronchitis in England and Wales. *Br Med J* 293: 1271–1275

35 Barker DJP, Godfrey KM, Fall C, Osmond C, Winter PD, Shaheen SO (1991) Relation of birth weight and childhood respiratory infection to adult lung function and death from chronic obstructive airways disease. *Br Med J* 303: 671–675

36 Anderson HR (1970) Increase in hospital admissions for childhood asthma: trends in referral, severity, and readmissions from to 1985 in a health region of the United Kingdom. *Thorax* 1989; 44: 614–619

37 Anderson HR (1990) Trends and district variations in the hospital care of childhood asthma: results of a regional study 1970–85. *Thorax* 45: 431–437

38 Strachan DP, Anderson HR (1992) Trends in hospital admission rates for asthma in children. *Br Med J* 304: 819–820

39 Storr J, Barrell E, Lenney W (1988) Rising asthma admissions and self referral. *Arch Dis Child* 63: 774–779

40 Burr ML, Butland BK, King S, Vaughan-Williams E (1989) Changes in asthma prevalence: two surveys 15 years apart. *Arch Dis Child* 64: 1452–1456

41 Ninan TK, Russell G (1992) Respiratory symptoms and atopy in Aberdeen schoolchildren: evidence from two surveys 25 years apart. *Br Med J* 304: 873–875

42 Fleming DM, Crombie DL (1987) Prevalence of asthma and hay fever in England and Wales. *Br Med J* 294: 279–283

43   Robertson CF, Heycock E, Bishop J, Nolan T, Olinsky A, Phelan PD (1991) Prevalence of asthma in Melbourne schoolchildren: changes over 26 years. *Br Med J* 302: 1116–1118
44   Peat JK, van den Berg RH, Green WF, Mellis CM, Leeder SR, Woolcock AJ (1994) Changing prevalence of asthma in Australian children. *Br Med J* 308: 1591–1596
45   Gergen PJ, Mullally DI, Evans R (1976) National survey of prevalence of asthma among children in the United States, to 1980. *Pediatrics* 1988; 81: 1–7
46   Haahtela T, Lindholm H, Bjorksten F, Koskenvuo K, Laitinen LA (1990) Prevalence of asthma in Finnish young men. *Br Med J* 301: 266–268
47   Burney PGJ, Chinn S, Rona RJ (1990) Has the prevalence of asthma increased in children? Evidence from the national study of health and growth 1973–86. *Br Med J* 300: 1306–1310
48   Lewis S, Butland B, Strachan D, Bynner J, Richards D, Butler N et al (1996) Study of the aetiology of wheezing illness at age 16 in two national British birth cohorts. *Thorax* 51: (7) 670–676
49   Anderson HR, Butland BK, Strachan DP (1994) Trends in prevalence and severity of childhood asthma. *Br Med J* 308: 1600–1604
50   Hyndman SJ, Williams DRR, Merrill SL, Lipscombe JM, Palmer CR (1994) Rates of admission to hospital for asthma. *Br Med J* 308: 1596–1600
51   Johnston IDA, Bland JM, Anderson HR (1987) Ethnic variation in respiratory morbidity and lung function in childhood. *Thorax* 42: 542–548
52   Burrows B, Sears MR, Flannery EM, Herbison GP, Holdaway MD, Silva PA (1995) Relation of the course of bronchial responsiveness from age 9 to age 15 to allergy. *Am J Respir Crit Care Med* 152: 1302–1308
53   Taylor B, Wadsworth J, Wadsworth M, Peckham C (1984) Changes in the reported prevalence of childhood eczema since the 1939–45 war. *Lancet* ii: 1255–1257
54   Butland BK, Strachan DP, Lewis S, Bynner J, Butler N, Britton J (1997) An investigation of the increase in hay fever and eczema at age 16 observed between the 1958 and 1970 British birth cohorts. *Br Med J* 315: 717–721
55   Williams HC (1992) Is the prevalence of atopic dermatitis increasing? *Clin Exp Dermatol* 17: 385–391
56   Sibbald B, Rink E, D'Souza M (1990) Is the prevalence of atopy increasing? *Br J Pharmacol* 40: 338–340
57   Barbee RA, Kalterborn W, Lebowitz MD (1987) Longitudinal changes in allergen skin test reactivity in a community population sample. *J Allergy Clin Immunol* 79: 16–24
58   Jackson RT, Beaglehole R, Rea HH, Sutherland DC (1982) Mortality from asthma: a new epidemic in New Zealand. *Br Med J* 285: 771–774
59   Keating G, Mitchell EA, Jackson R, Beaglehole R, Rea H (1984) Trends in sales of drugs for asthma in New Zealand, Australia, and the United Kingdom, 1975–81. *Br Med J* 289: 348–351
60   Mitchell EA (1985) International trends in hospital admission rate for asthma. *Arch Dis Child* 60: 376–378
61   Van Niekerk CH, Weinberg EG, Shore SC, Heese HD, Van Shalkwyk DJ (1979) Prevalence of asthma: a comparitive study of urban and rural Xhosa children. *Clin Allergy* 9: 319–324
62   Yemaneberhan H, Bekele Z, Venn A, Lewis S, Parry E, Britton J (1997) Low prevalence of wheeze and asthma, and the disassociation of their relation with atopy in urban and rural areas of Ethiopia. *Lancet* 350: 85–90
63   von Mutius E, Fritzsch C, Weiland SK, Roll G, Magnussen H (1992) Prevalence of asthma and allergic disorders among children in united Germany: a descriptive comparison. *Br Med J* 305: 1395–1399
64   Keeley DJ, Neill P, Gallivan S (1991) Comparison of the prevalence of reversible airways obstruction in rural and urban Zimbabwean children. *Thorax* 46: 549–553
65   Waite DA, Eyles EF, Tonkin SL, O'Donnell TV (1980) Asthma prevalence in Tokelauan children in two environments. *Clin Allergy* 10: 71–75
66   Reid DD, Fletcher CM (1971) International studies in chronic respiratory disease. *Br Med Bull* 27: 59–64
67   Pearce N, Weiland S, Keil U, Langridge P, Anderson HR, Strachan D et al (1993) Self-reported prevalence of asthma symptoms in children in Australia, England, Germany and New Zealand: an international comparison using the ISAAC protocol. *Eur Respir J* 6: 1455–1461
68   Leung R, Ho P (1994) Asthma, allergy, and atopy in three south-east Asian populations. *Thorax* 49: 1205–1210

69 Leung R, Bishop J, Robertson CF (1994) Prevalence of asthma and wheeze in Hong Kong schoolchildren: An international comparative study. *Eur Resp J* 7: 2046–2049

70 Burr ML, Limb ES, Andrae S, Barry DMJ, Nagel F (1994) Childhood asthma in four countries: A comparative survey. *Int J Epidemiol* 23: 341–347

71 Crane J, O'Donnell TV, Prior IA, Waite DA (1989) The relationships between atopy, bronchial hyperresponsiveness, and a family history of asthma: A cross-sectional study of migrant Tokelauan children in New Zealand. *J Allergy Clin Immunol* 84: 768–772

72 Flynn MGL (1994) Respiratory symptoms, bronchial responsiveness, and atopy in Fijian and Indian children. *Am J Respir Crit Care Med* 150: 415–420

73 Carey OJ, Cookson JB, Britton J, Tattersfield AE (1996) The effect of lifestyle on wheeze, atopy, and bronchial hyperreactivity in Asian and White children. *Am J Respir Crit Care Med* 154: 537–540

74 Burney PGJ, Luczynska C, Chinn S, Jarvis D, Vermeire P, Dahl R et al (1994) The European Community Respiratory Health Survey. *Eur Resp J* 7: 954–960

75 Braback L, Breborowicz A, Dreborg S, Knutsson A, Pieklik H, Bjorksten B (1994) Atopic sensitization and respiratory symptoms among Polish and Swedish school children. *Clin Experiment Allergy* 24: 826–835

76 Aberg N, Hesselmar B, Aberg B, Eriksson B (1995) Increase of asthma, allergic rhinitis and eczema in Swedish schoolchildren between 1979 and 1991. *Clin Experiment Allergy* 25: 815–819

77 Osmond C, Barker DJP, Slattery JM (1990) Risk of death from cardiovascular disease and chronic bronchitis determined by place of birth in England and Wales. *J Epidemiol Community Health* 44: 139–141

78 Schenker MB, Samet JM, Speizer FE (1983) Risk factors for childhood respiratory disease. *Am Rev Respir Dis* 128: 1038–1043

79 Ferris BG, Ware JH, Berkey CS, Dockery DW, Spiro A, Speizer FE (1985) Effects of passive smoking on health of children. *Environ Health Perspect* 62: 285–295

80 Taylor B, Wadsworth J (1987) Maternal smoking during pregnancy and lower respiratory tract illness in early life. *Arch Dis Child* 62: 786–791

81 Fergusson DM, Horwood LJ, Shannon FT, Taylor B (1981) Parental smoking and lower respiratory illness in the first three years of life. *J Epidemiol Community Health* 35: 180–184

82 Fergusson DM, Horwood LJ, Shannon FT (1980) Parental smoking and respiratory illness in infancy. *Arch Dis Child* 55: 358–361

83 Wright AL, Holberg C, Martinez FD, Taussig LM (1991) Relationship of parental smoking to wheezing and nonwheezing lower respiratory tract illnesses in infancy. *J Pediat* 118: 207–214

84 Rona RJ, Chinn S (1993) Lung function, respiratory illness, and passive smoking in British primary school children. *Thorax* 48: 21–25

85 Cunningham J, Dockery DW, Speizer FE (1994) Maternal smoking during pregnancy as a predictor of lung function in children. *Am J Epidemiol* 139: 1139–1152

86 Tager IB, Weiss ST, Munoz A, Rosner B, Speizer FE (1983) Longitudinal study of the effects of maternal smoking on pulmonary function in children. *N Engl J Med* 309: 699–703

87 Woolcock AJ, Leeder SR, Peat JK, Blackburn CRB (1979) The influence of lower respiratory illness in infancy and childhood and subsequent cigarette smoking on lung function in Sydney schoolchildren. *Am Rev Respir Dis* 120: 5–14

88 Gold DR, Tager IB, Weiss ST, Tosteson TD, Speizer FE (1989) Acute lower respiratory illness in childhood as a predictor of lung function and chronic respiratory symptoms. *Am Rev Respir Dis* 140: 877–884

89 Shaheen SO, Barker DJP, Holgate ST (1995) Do lower respiratory tract infections in early childhood cause chronic obstructive pulmonary disease? *Am J Respir Crit Care Med* 151: 1649–1652

90 Paoletti P, Prediletto R, Carrozzi L, Viegi G, Di Pede F, Carmignani G et al (1989) Effects of childhood and adolescence-adulthood respiratory infections in a general population. *Eur Respir J* 2: 428–436

91 Shaheen SO, Barker DJ, Shiell AW, Crocker FJ, Wield GA, Holgate ST (1994) The relationship between pneumonia in early childhood and impaired lung function in late adult life. *Am J Respir Crit Care Med* 149: 616–619

92 Hanrahan JP, Tager IB, Segal MR, Tosteson TD, Castile RG, Van Vunakis H et al (1992) The effect of maternal smoking during pregnancy on early infant lung function. *Am Rev Respir Dis* 145: 1129–1135

93 Stick SM, Burton PR, Gurrin L, Sly PD, Lesouef PN (1996) Effects of maternal smoking during pregnancy and a family history of asthma on respiratory function in newborn infants. *Lancet* 348: (9034)1060–1064

94 Collins MH, Moessinger AC, Kleinerman J, Bassi J, Rosso P, Collins AM et al (1985) Fetal lung hypoplasia associated with maternal smoking: a morphometric analysis. *Pediatric Research* 19: 408–412

95 Dodge R (1982) The effects of indoor air pollution on Arizona children. *Arch Environ Health* 37: 151–155

96 Dijkstra L, Houthuijs D, Brunekreef B, Akkerman I, Boleij JSM (1990) Respiratory health effects of the indoor environment in a population of Dutch children. *Am Rev Respir Dis* 142: 1172–1178

97 Strachan DP (1988) Damp housing and childhood asthma: validation of reporting of symptoms. *Br Med J* 297: 1223–1226

98 Ware JH, Dockery DW, Spiro A, Speizer FE, Ferris BG (1984) Passive smoking, gas cooking, and respiratory health in children living in six cities. *Am Rev Respir Dis* 129: 366–374

99 Stoddard JJ, Miller T (1995) Impact of parental smoking on the prevalence of wheezing respiratory illness in children. *Am J Epidemiol* 141: 96–102

100 Dekker C, Dales R, Bartlett S, Brunekreef B, Zwanenburg H (1991) Childhood asthma and the indoor environment. *Chest* 100: 922–926

101 Goren AI, Hellmann S (1995) Respiratory conditions among schoolchildren and their relationship to environmental tobacco smoke and other combustion products. *Arch Dis Child* 50: 112–118

102 Chilmonczyk BA, Salmun LM, Megathlin KN, Neveux LM, Palomaki GE, Knight GJ et al (1993) Association between exposure to environmental tobacco smoke and exacerbations of asthma in children. *N Engl J Med* 328: 1665–1669

103 Murray AB, Morrison BJ (1986) The effect of cigarette smoking from the mother on bronchial hyperresponsiveness and severity of symptoms in children with asthma. *J Allergy Clin Immunol* 77: 575–581

104 Murray AB, Morrison BJ (1990) It is children with atopic dermatitis who develop asthma more frequently if the mother smokes. *J Allergy Clin Immunol* 86: 732–739

105 Jensen EJ, Pedersen B, Schmidt E, Dahl R (1992) Serum IgE in nonatopic smokers, nonsmokers, and recent exsmokers: Relation to lung function, airway symptoms, and atopic predisposition. *J Allergy Clin Immunol* 90: 224–229

106 Ericsson CH, Svartengren M, Mossberg B, Camner P (1993) Bronchial reactivity, lung function, and serum innumoglobulin e in smoking-discordant monozygotic twins. *Am Rev Respir Dis* 147: 296–300

107 Sherrill DL, Halonen M, Burrows B (1994) Relationships between total serum IgE, atopy, and smoking: A twenty-year follow-up analysis. *J Allerg Clin Immunol* 94: 954–962

108 Venables KM, Topping MD, Howe W, Luczynska CM, Hawkins R, Newman Taylor AJ (1985) Interaction of smoking and atopy in producing specific IgE antibody against a hapten protein conjugate. *Br Med J* 290: 201–204

109 Strachan DP, Harkins LS, Johnston IDA, Anderson HR (1997) Childhood antecedents of allergic sensitisation in young British adults. *J Allergy Clin Immunol* 99: 6–12

110 Vonmutius E, Martinez FD, Fritzsch C, Nicolai T, Reitmeir P, Thiemann H (1994) Skin test reactivity and number of siblings. *Br Med J* 308: 692–695

111 Soyseth V, Kongerud J, Boe J (1995) Postnatal maternal smoking increases the prevalence of asthma but not of bronchial hyperresponsiveness or atopy in their children. *Chest* 107: 389–394

112 Rona RJ, Gulliford MC, Chinn S (1993) Effects of prematurity and intrauterine growth on respiratory health and lung function in childhood. *Br Med J* 306: 817–820

113 Greenough A, Maconochie I, Yuksel B (1990) Recurrent respiratory symptoms in the first year of life following preterm delivery. *J Perinatal Med* 18: 489–494

114 Schwartz J, Gold D, Dockery DW, Weiss ST, Speizer FE (1990) Predictors of asthma and persistent wheeze in a national sample of children in the United States. *Am Rev Respir Dis* 142: 555–562

115 Chen Y (1994) Environmental tobacco smoke, low birth weight, and hospitalization for respiratory disease. *Am J Respir Crit Care Med* 150: 54–58

116 Kelly YJ, Brabin BJ, Milligan P, Heaf DP, Reid J, Pearson MG (1995) Maternal asthma, premature birth, and the risk of respiratory morbidity in schoolchildren in Merseyside. *Thorax* 50: 525–530

117 Seidman DS, Laor A, Gale R, Stevenson DK, Danon YL (1991) Is low birth weight a risk factor for asthma during adolescence. *Arch Dis Child* 66: 584–587

118 Mansell AL, Driscoll JM, James LS (1987) Pulmonary follow-up of moderately low birth weight infants with and without respiratory distress syndrome. *J Pediat* 110: 111–115

119 Lodrup Carlsen KC, Magnus P, Carlsen K (1994) Lung function by tidal breathing in awake healthy newborn infants. *Eur Respir J* 7: 1660–1668

120 Merth IT, Dewinter JP, Borsboom GJJM, Quanjer PH (1995) Pulmonary function during the first year of life in healthy infants born prematurely. *Eur Resp J* 8: 1141–1147

121 Doyle W, Crawford MA, Wynn AHA, Wynn SW (1989) Mternal nutrient intake and birthweight. *J Hum Nutr Diet* 2: 415–422

122 Wynn AHA, Crawford MA, Doyle W, Wynn SW (1991) Nutrition of women in anticipation of pregnancy. *Nutr Health* 7: 69–88

123 Kramer MS (1987) Determinants of low birth weight:methodological assessment and meta-analysis. *Bull WHO* 65: 663–737

124 Lowe CR (1959) Effect of mother's smoking habits on birth weight of their children. *Br Med J* 4: 673–676

125 Berkowitz GS, Papiernik E (1993) Epidemiology of preterm birth. *Epidemiol Rev* 15: 414–443

126 Tenovuo AH, Kero PA, Korvenranta HJ (1988) Risk factors associated with severely small for gestational age neonates. *Am J Perinatol* 5: 267–271

127 Martinez FD, Wright AL, Holberg CJ, Morgan WJ, Taussig LM (1992) Maternal age as a risk factor for wheezing lower respiratory illnesses in the first year of life. *Am J Epidemiol* 136: 1258–1268

128 Anderson HR, Bland JM, Peckham CS (1987) Risk factors for asthma up to 16 years of age. *Chest* 91: 127S–130S

129 Strachan DP, Taylor EM, Carpenter RG (1996) Family structure, neonatal infection, and hay fever in adolescence. *Arch Dis Child* 74: (5)422–426

130 Strachan DP (1995) Epidemiology of hay fever: Towards a community diagnosis. *Clin Experiment Allergy* 25: 296–303

131 Naeye RL (1981) Teenaged and pre-teenaged pregnancies: consequences of the fetal-maternal competition for nutrients. *Pediatrics* 67: 146–150

132 Strachan DP (1989) Hay fever, hygiene, and household size. *Br Med J* 299: 1259–1260

133 Bjorksten F, Suoniemi I (1976) Dependence of immediate hypersensitivity on the month of birth. *Clin Allergy* 6: 165–171

134 Bjorksten F, Suoniemi I, Koski V (1980) Neonatal birch-pollen contacts and subsequent allergy to birch-pollen. *Clin Allergy* 10: 585–591

135 Sears MR, Holdaway MD, Flannery EM, Herbison GP, Silva PA (1996) Parental and neonatal risk factors for atopy, airway-hyperresponsiveness, and asthma. *Arch Dis Child* 75: 392–398

136 Korsgaard J, Dahl R (1983) Sensitivity to house dust mite and grass pollen. Influence of the month of birth. *Clin Allergy* 13: 529–536

137 Arshad SH, Matthews S, Gant C, Hide DW (1992) Effect of allergen avoidance on development of allergic disorders in infancy. *Lancet* 339: 1493–1497

138 Hide DW, Matthews S, Tariq S, Arshad SH (1996) Allergen avoidance in infancy and allergy at 4 years of age. *Allergy* 51: 89–93

139 Venables KM, Dally MB, Burge PS, Pickering CAC, Newman Taylor AJ (1985) Occupational asthma in a steel coating plant. *BJIM* 42: 517–524

140 Sporik R, Holgate ST, Platts-Mills TAE, Cogswell JJ (1990) Exposure to house-dust mite allergen (Der p I) and the development of asthma in childhood. *N Engl J Med* 323: 502–507

141 Kabasawa Y, Lishi A, Minata H, Takaoka M (1976) Clinical significance of the housedust mite in asthmatic children in Japan. *Acta Allergologica* 31: 442–446

142 Warner JA, Little SA, Pollock I, Longbottom JL, Warner JO (1991) The influence of exposure to house dust mite on sensitization in asthma. *Paediatr Allergy Immunol* 1: 79–86

143 Peat JK, Tovey E, Toelle BG, Haby MM, Gray EJ, Mahmic A et al (1996) House dust mite allergens: A major risk factor for childhood asthma in Australia. *Am J Respir Crit Care Med* 153: (1)141–146

144 Custovic A, Taggart SCO, Francis HC, Chapman MD, Woodcock A (1996) Exposure to house dust mite allergens and the clinical activity of asthma. *J Allerg Clin Immunol* 98: (1)64–72

145 Chanyeung M, Manfreda J, Dimichward H, Lam J, Ferguson A, Warren P et al (1995) Mite and cat allergen levels in homes and severity of asthma. *Am J Respir Crit Care Med* 152:

(6)1805–1811

146 Carswell F, Birmingham K, Oliver J, Crewes A, Weeks J (1996) The respiratory effects of reduction of mite allergen in the bedrooms of asthmatic children: A double-blind controlled trial. *Clin Experiment Allergy* 26: (4)386–396

147 Sporik R, Ingram JM, Price W, Sussman JH, Honsinger RW, Plattsmills TAE (1995) Association of asthma with serum IgE and skin test reactivity to allergens among children living at high altitude: Tickling the dragon's breath. *Am J Respir Crit Care Med* 151: 1388–1392

148 Strachan DP, Carey IM (1995) Home environment and severe asthma in adolescence: A population based case-control study. *Br Med J* 311: 1053–1056

149 Baldacci S, Viegi G, Carozzi L, Modena P, Pedreschi Fd Paoletti P et al (1993) Respiratory effects due to the presence of pets in the home environment: an epidemiological evaluation. *Proc Ind Air* 1: 175–179

150 Lindfors A, Wickman M, Hedlin G, Pershagen G, Rietz H, Nordvall SL (1995) Indoor environmental risk factors in young asthmatics: A case-control study. *Arch Dis Child* 73: (5)408–412

151 Brunekreef B, Groot B, Hoek G (1992) Pets, allergy and respiratory symptoms in children. *Int J Epidemiol* 21: 338–342

152 Shaheen SO, Aaby P, Hall AJ, Barker DJP, Heyes CB, Shiell AW et al (1996) Measles and atopy in Guinea-Bissau. *Lancet* 347: (9018)1792–1796

153 Strachan DP, Sanders CH (1989) Damp housing and childhood asthma: respiratory effects of indor air temperature and relative humidity. *J Epidemiol Community Health* 43: 7–14

154 Brunekreef B, Dockery DW, Speizer FE, Ware JH, Spengler JD, Ferris BG (1989) Home dampness and respiratory morbidity in children. *Am Rev Respir Dis* 140: 1363–1367

155 Verhoeff AP, Vanstrien RT, Vanwijnen JH, Brunekreef B (1995) Damp housing and childhood respiratory symptoms: The role of sensitization to dust mites and molds. *Am J Epidemiol* 141: 103–110

156 Williamson IJ, Martin CJ, McGill G, Monie RDH, Fennerty AG (1997) Damp housing and asthma: a case-control study. *Thorax* 52: 229–234

157 Brunekreef B, Verhoeff AP, van Strien RT, van Wijnen JH (1993) The role of sensitization to dust mites and moulds in explaining the relationship between home dampness and childhood respiratory symptoms. *Proc Ind Air* 1: 153–158

158 Hide DW, Matthews S, Matthews L, Stevens M, Ridout S, Twiselton R et al (1994) Effect of allergen avoidance in infancy on allergic manifestations at age two years. *J Allerg Clin Immunol* 93: 842–846

159 Chandra RK, Puri S, Cheema PS (1985) Predictive value of cord blood IgE in the development of atopic disease and role of breast-feeding in its prevention. *Clin Allergy* 15: 517–522

160 Lucas A, Brooke OG, Morley R, Cole TJ, Bamford MF (1990) Early diet of preterm infants and development of allergic or atopic disease: randomised prospective study. *Br Med J* 300: 837–840

161 Saarinen UM, Kajosaari M (1995) Breastfeeding as prophylaxis against atopic disease: Prospective follow-up study until 17 years old. *Lancet* 346: 1065–1069

162 Arshad SH, Hide DW (1992) Effect of environmental factors on the development of allergic disorders in infancy. *J Allergy Clin Immunol* 90: 235–241

163 Lilja G, Dannaeus A, Foucard T, Graff-Lonnevig V, Johansson GO, Oman H (1989) Effects of maternal diet during late pregnancy and lactation on the development of atopic diseases in infants up to 18 months of age—*in vivo* results. *Clin Exp Allergy* 19: 473–479

164 Taylor B, Wadsworth J, Golding J, Butler N (1983) Breast feeding, eczema, asthma, and hayfever. *J Epidemiol Community Health* 37: 95–99

165 Van Asperen PP, Kemp AS, Mellis CM (1984) Skin test reactivity and clinical allergen sensitivity in infancy. *J Allergy Clin Immunol* 73: 381

166 Rowntree S, Cogswell JJ, Platts-Mills TAE, Mitchell EB (1985) Development of IgE and IgG antibodies to food and inhalant allergens in children at risk of allergic disease. *Arch Dis Child* 60: 727–735

167 Chandra RK, Puri S, Hamed A (1989) Influence of maternal diet during lactation and use of formula feeds on development of atopic eczema in high risk infants. *Br Med J* 299: 228–230

168 Burr ML, Miskelly FG, Butland BK, Merrett TG, Vaughan-Williams E (1989) Environmental factors and symptoms in infants at high risk of allergy. *J Epidemiol Community Health* 43: 125–132

169 Burr ML, Limb ES, Maguire MJ, Amarah L, Eldridge BA, Layzell JC et al (1993) Infant feeding, wheezing and allergy: a prospective study. *Arch Dis Child* 68: 724–728

170 Wright AL, Holberg CJ, Taussig LM, Martinez FD (1995) Relationship of infant feeding to recurrent wheezing at age 6 years. *Arch Pediatr Adolesc Med* 149: 758–763

171 Wright AL, Holberg CJ, Martinez FD, Morgan WJ, Taussig LM (1989) Breast feeding and lower respiratory tract illness in the first year of life. *Br Med J* 299: 946–949

172 Beaudry M, Dufour R, Marcoux S (1995) Relation between infant feeding and infections during the first six months of life. *J Pediat* 126: 191–197

173 Committee on the medical effects of air pollutants (1995) Asthma and outdoor air pollution. London: HMSO

174 Ishizaki T, Koizumi K, Ikemori R, Ishiyama Y, Kushibiki E (1987) Studies of prevalence of Japanese cedar pollinosis among the residents in a densely cultivated area. *Ann Allergy* 58: 265–270

175 Wjst M, Reitmeir P, Dold S, Wulff A, Nicolai T, Vonloeffelholzcolberg EF et al (1993) Road traffic and adverse effects on respiratory health in children. *Br Med J* 307: 596–600

176 Oosterlee A, Drijver M, Lebret E, Brunekreef B (1996) Chronic respiratory symptoms in children and adults living along streets with high traffic density. *Occup Environ Medicine* 53: (4)241–247

177 Weiland SK, Mundt KA, Ruckmann A, Keil U (1994) Self reported wheezing and allergic rhinitis in children and traffic density on street of residence. *Ann Epidemiol* 4: 79–83

178 Edwards J, Walters S, Griffiths RK (1994) Hospital admissions for asthma in preschool children: relationship to major roads in Birmingham, United Kingdom. *Arch Environ Health* 49: 223–227

179 Schwartz J (1995) Short term fluctuations in air pollution and hospital admissions of the elderly for respiratory disease. *Thorax* 50: 531–538

180 Higgins BG, Francis HC, Yates CJ, Warburton CJ, Fletcher AM, Reid JA et al (1995) Effects of air pollution on symptoms and peak expiratory flow measurements in subjects with obstructive airways disease. *Thorax* 50: 149–155

181 Weinmann GG, Bowes SM, Gerbase MW, Kimball AW, Frank R (1995) Response to acute ozone exposure in healthy men: Results of a screening procedure. *Am J Respir Crit Care Med* 151: 33–40

182 Buchdahl R, Parker A, Stebbings T, Babiker A (1996) Association between air pollution and acute childhood wheezy episodes: Prospective observational study. *Br Med J* 312: (7032)661–665

183 Molfino NA, Wright FC, Katz I, Tarlo S, Silverman F, Mcclean PA et al (1991) Effect of low concentrations of ozone on inhaled allergen responses in asthmatic subjects. *Lancet* 338: 199–203

184 Hoek G, Fischer P, Brunekreef B, Lebret E, Hofschreuder P, Mennen MG (1993) Acute effects of ambient ozone on pulmonary function of children in the Netherlands. *Am Rev Respir Dis* 147: 111–117

185 Schwartz J, Dockery DW, Neas LM, Wypij D, Ware JH, Spengler JD et al (1994) Acute effects of summer air pollution on respiratory symptom reporting in children. *Am J Respir Crit Care Med* 150: 1234–1242

186 Neas LM, Dockery DW, Koutrakis P, Tollerud DJ, Speizer FE (1995) The association of ambient air pollution with twice daily peak expiratory flow rate measurements in children. *Am J Epidemiol* 141: 111–122

187 Austin JB, Russell G, Adam MG, Mackintosh D, Kelsey S, Peck DF (1994) Prevalence of asthma and wheeze in the highlands of Scotland. *Arch Dis Child* 71: 211–216

188 Devereux G, Ayatollahi T, Ward R, Bromly C, Bourke SJ, Stenton SC et al (1996) Asthma, airways responsiveness and air pollution in two contrasting districts of northern England. *Thorax* 51: (2)169–174

189 Strachan DP, Anderson HR, Limb ES, O'Neill A, Wells N (1994) A national survey of asthma prevalence, severity, and treatment in Great Britain. *Arch Dis Child* 70: 174–178

190 Speizer FE, Ferris BG, Bishop YMM, Spengler JD (1980) Respiratory disease rates and pulmonary function in children associated with NO_2 exposure. *Am Rev Respir Dis* 121: 3–10

191 Melia RJW, Florey Cd Altman DG, Swan AV (1977) Association between gas cooking and respiratory disease in children. *Br Med J* 2: 149–152

192 Melia RJW, Florey cd Chinn S (1979) The relation between respiratory illness in primary schoolchildren and the use of gas for cooking; I. Results from a national survey. *Int J Epidemiol* 8: 333–338

193 Melia RJW, Florey cd Chinn S (1980) The relation between indoor air pollution from nitrogen dioxide and respiratory illness in primary schoolchildren. *Clin Resp Physiol* 16: 7P–8P

194 Vonmutius E, Illi S, Nicolai T, Martinez FD (1996) Relation of indoor heating with asthma, allergic sensitisation, and bronchial responsiveness: Survey of children in South Bavaria. *Br Med J* 312: (7044)1448–1450

195 Seaton A, Godden DJ, Brown K (1994) Increase in asthma—a more toxic environment or a more susceptible population. *Thorax* 49: 171–174

196 Gregory J, Foster K, Tyler H, Wiseman M (1990) The dietary and nutritional survey of British Adults. London: HMSO

197 Burney PGJ, Britton JR, Chinn S, Tattersfield AE, Platt HS, Papacosta AO et al (1986) Response to inhaled histamine and 24 h sodium excretion. *Br Med J* 292: 1483–1486

198 Schwartz J, Weiss ST (1990) Dietary factors and their relation to respiratory symptoms. *Am J Epidemiol* 132: 67–76

199 Pistelli R, Forastiere F, Corbo GM, Dell'Orco V, Brancato G, Agibiti N et al (1993) Respiratory symptoms and bronchial responsiveness are related to dietary salt intake and urinary potassium excretion in male children. *Eur Respir J* 6: 517–522

200 Javaid A, Cushley MJ, Bone MF (1988) Effect of dietary salt on bronchial reactivity to histamine. *Br Med J* 297: 454

201 Burney PGJ, Neild JE, Twort CHC, Chinn S, Jones TD, Mitchell WD et al (1989) Effect of changing dietary sodium on the airway response to histamine. *Thorax* 44: 36–41

202 Carey OJ, Locke C, Cookson JB (1993) Effect of alterations of dietary sodium on the severity of asthma in men. *Thorax* 48: 714–718

203 Sparrow D, O'Connor GT, Rosner B, Weiss ST (1991) Methacholine airway responsiveness and 24-hour urine excretion of sodium and potassium. *Am Rev Respir Dis* 144: 722–725

204 Britton J, Pavord I, Richards K, Knox A, Wisniewski A, Weiss S et al (1994) Dietary sodium intake and the risk of airway hyperreactivity in a random adult population. *Thorax* 49: 875–880

205 Britton J, Pavord I, Richards K, Wisniewski A, Knox A, Lewis S et al (1994) Dietary magnesium, lung function, wheezing, and airway hyperreactivity in a random adult population sample. *Lancet* 344: 357–362

206 Strachan DP, Cox BD, Erzinclioglu SW, Walters DE, Whichelow MJ (1991) Ventilatory function and winter fresh fruit consumption in a random sample of British adults. *Thorax* 46: 624–629

207 Schwartz J, Weiss ST (1994) The relationship of dietary fish intake to level of pulmonary function in the first national health and nutrition survey (NHANES I). *Eur Respir J* 7: 1821–1824

208 Editorial (1989) Fish oil revisited. *Lancet* 2(8666): 810–812

209 Britton J (1995) Dietary fish oil and airways obstruction. *Thorax* 50:S11–S15

210 Peat JK, Hodge L, Salome CM, Woolcock AJ (1995) Dietary fish intake and asthma in children. *Am J Respir Crit Care Med* 151: A469

211 Demissie K, Ernst P, Donald KG, Joseph L (1996) Usual dietary salt intake and asthma in children: A case-control study. *Thorax* 51: (1)59–63

212 Powell CVE, Nash AA, Powers HJ, Primhak RA (1994) Antioxidant status in asthma. *Pediatrics* 18: 34–38

213 Godfrey M, Barker DJP, Osmond C (1994) Disproportionate fetal growth and raised IgE concentration in adult life. *Clin Exp Allergy* 24: 641–648

214 Gurwitz D, Mindorff C, Levison H (1981) Increased incidence of bronchial reactivity in children with a history of bronchiolitis. *J Pediat* 98: 551–555

215 Pullan CR, Hey EN (1982) Wheezing, asthma, and pulmonary dysfunction 10 years after infection with respiratory syncytial virus in infancy. *Br Med J* 284: 1665–1669

216 Stokes GM, Milner AD, Hodges IGC, Groggins RC (1981) Lung function abnormalities after acute bronchiolitis. *J Pediat* 98: 871–874

217 Voter KZ, Henry MM, Stewart PW, Henderson FW (1988) Lower respiratory illness in early childhood and lung function and bronchial reactivity in adolescent males. *Am Rev Respir Dis* 137: 302–307

218 Wittig HJ, Glaser J (1959) The relationship between bronchiolitis and childhood asthma. A follow-up study of 100 cases of bronchiolitis in infancy. *J Allergy* 30: 19–23

219 Martinez FD, Stern DA, Wright AL, Taussig LM, Halonen M, Bean J et al (1995) Association of non-wheezing lower respiratory tract illnesses in early life with persistently diminished serum IgE levels. *Thorax* 50: 1067–1072

220 Martinez FD (1994) Role of viral infections in the inception of asthma and allergies during childhood: Could they be protective? *Thorax* 49: 1189–1191

221 Matricardi PM, Rosmini F, Ferrigno L, Nisini R, Rapicetta M, Chionne P et al (1997) Cross sec-

tional retrospective study of prevalence of atopy among Italian military students with antibodies against hepatitis A virus. *Br Med J* 314: 999–1003

222 Shirakawa T, Enomoto T, Shimazu S, Hopkin J (1997) The inverse association between tuber- culin responses and atopic disorder. *Science* 275: 77–79

223 Moqbel R, Pritchard DI (1990) Parasites and allergy: evidence for a "cause and effect" relation- ship. *Clin Exp Allergy* 20: 611–618

CHAPTER 3
Is Chronic Use of β2-Agonists Detrimental in the Treatment of Asthma?

D. Robin Taylor[1] and Malcolm R. Sears[2]

[1] Department of Medicine, Dunedin School of Medicine, University of Otago, Dunedin, New Zealand
[2] Firestone Regional Chest and Allergy Unit, St.Joseph's Hospital, McMaster University, Hamilton, Ontario, Canada L8N 4A6

1. Introduction

A plethora of recent reviews testify to the controversy that has been generated in recent years by laboratory, clinical and epidemiological data challenging the wisdom of regular use of the short-acting β2-agonists which traditionally have formed the mainstay of treatment for bronchial asthma [1–5]. Although all national and international guidelines for the management of asthma now recommend anti-inflammatory therapy for most patients with chronic symptoms [6–9], short-acting β2-agonists are still the most widely prescribed and most frequently used form of asthma treatment, and so the issue remains an important one. The prompt symptom relief afforded by these agents, together with the apparent lessening of side-effects such as tremor and tachycardia as more selective agents became available, led to almost universal acceptance of β2-agonist therapy in any required dosage to control clinical manifestations of asthma. Surprisingly, this occurred in the absence of any substantial controlled clinical trials demonstrating their long-term efficacy or safety. A 1-week crossover trial of four times daily *versus* as-needed inhalation of salbutamol in 18 patients whose evening peak flow rates improved, but whose symptoms of cough and wheezing did not change, seems to have provided the basis for recommending regular use of β_2-agonists as maintenance treatment in asthma [10].

In this chapter we will review the evidence that this confidence in the efficacy and safety of regular use of short-acting β_2-agonists was misplaced, and that chronic use has detrimental effects which can lead to increased morbidity and even mortality from asthma. Studies over the last decade have shown that chronic β_2-agonist inhalation may result in increased airway inflammation, increased airway responsiveness to allergen, exercise and non-specific bronchoconstrictor agents, tolerance to non-bronchodilator effects, impaired lung function, and thus ultimately to poorer control of asthma. Furthermore there is substantial epidemiological evidence for a link between patterns of increased β_2-agonist use and asthma morbidity and mortality, including temporal relationships during epidemics of mortality [11], and a substantial parallel decrease in morbidity and mortality when a potent β_2-agonist was withdrawn from use [12]. These data converge to form the case against chronic use of short-acting β_2-agonists in the management of asthma. While very important in acute asthma for relief of symptoms, chronic use confers no important long-term benefit and is potentially harmful.

2. Evidence that Chronic Use of β_2-Agonists is Detrimental in Asthma

2.1. Increased Airway Inflammation

Asthma is a disease of the airways in which both acute and chronic exposure to trigger factors such as inhaled allergens gives rise to airway inflammation, which is responsible for airway narrowing and reactive bronchospasm. While the latter is effectively relieved using as-needed single doses of inhaled β_2-agonist, recent evidence suggests that airway inflammation may be increased as a direct consequence of regular exposure to β_2-agonists.

In controlled studies in guinea pigs, Wang et al. demonstrated that enhanced bronchial hyper-responsiveness (BHR) [13] and airway smooth muscle contractility and remodelling [14] occurred following chronic exposure to inhaled fenoterol. The magnitude of these changes was similar to those which resulted from chronic antigen exposure (ovalbumin). In other *in vitro* experiments, interleukin-4-mediated production of IgE by human mononuclear cells has been shown to be potentiated in a dose-dependent manner by the presence of the β_2-agonists salbutamol and fenoterol [15].

These experimental data are consistent with the results of a placebo-controlled study in humans in which, following regular inhalation of salbutamol by 11 asthmatic patients for 16 weeks, bronchial biopsies and lavage fluid contained significantly greater numbers of eosinophils and increased quantities of eosinophilic cationic protein respectively [16]. Similarly, Gauvreau et al. showed that, compared to placebo, regular treatment with 800 µg inhaled salbutamol daily significantly ($p < 0.02$) increased blood eosinophils and the influx of metachromatic cells into induced sputum 24 h after allergen challenge in patients with mild asthma [17].

Hence both animal and human data suggest that chronic exposure to inhaled β_2-agonists may increase airway inflammation. Thus, paradoxically, despite their capacity to alleviate reactive bronchospasm, one of the major pathophysiological consequences of asthma, β_2-agonists may simultaneously be potentiating the underlying disease process.

2.2. Increased Airway Responsiveness to Exercise, Allergen and Non-Specific Bronchoconstrictors

If chronic use of inhaled β_2-agonists enhances airway inflammation, then patients so treated would be expected to demonstrate increased bronchial responsiveness to a variety of exogenous stimuli as a measurable consequence of that effect. There is now a substantial body of evidence to support this relationship.

2.2.1. Exercise Provocation: In a study of 10 asthmatic patients with predominantly exercised-induced symptoms, Inman and O'Byrne showed that following 7 days of treatment with regular salbutamol, a standardised exercise challenge resulted in a mean post-exercise fall in FEV_1 averaging 390 ml. greater than after 7 days treatment with placebo [18]. In addition, the protective effect afforded by a single dose of inhaled salbutamol against exercise-induced asthma was attenuated after regular treatment. One of the most frequent indications for the use of short-acting β_2-agonists is to protect against exercise-induced bronchospasm. It is therefore illogical and, we would argue, counterproductive to prescribe regular inhaled β_2-agonist to control exercise-induced asthma, as regular use potentiates the clinical problem it is designed to treat. Furthermore, if the therapeutic effect of a single dose to treat exercise-induced symptoms is attenuated by regular use, the most appropriate use of β_2-agonist for EIA is "as-needed" and not on a scheduled regimen.

2.2.2. Allergen Provocation: Several studies suggest that the airway response to inhaled allergen is enhanced by regular β_2-agonist therapy. Lai et al. demonstrated that regular treatment with inhaled rimiterol permitted five of eight patients with mild asthma to develop a late asthmatic response to an allergen challenge where none had previously occurred, the explanation being that rimiterol treatment allowed a higher dose of allergen to be inhaled before a early response warning occurred [19]. However β_2-agonists may also enhance the

response to a constant dose of allergen. The early asthmatic response to a constant allergen stimulus was increased following 2 weeks of regular salbutamol [20]. There was a near two-fold shift in allergen PC_{20} after regular treatment, together with a significant reduction in the protective effect of a single-dose of salbutamol. In another placebo-controlled investigation, the same authors have demonstrated that the late asthmatic response to a constant dose of allergen was significantly increased in atopic dual-responding asthmatic subjects who received regular salbutamol for 1 week [21].

2.2.3. Increased Responsiveness to Non-Specific Bronchoconstrictors:
Assessing airway inflammation directly in asthmatic patients is difficult, and most studies are carried out in small numbers of selected patients. However, the measurement of non-specific bronchial hyper-responsiveness (BHR) correlates significantly with other more direct measures of airway inflammation [22]. Thus if regular β_2-agonist treatment has an adverse effect on the pathology of asthma, this ought to be reflected in adverse changes in non-specific BHR during chronic use. This is indeed the overall result from a substantial number of studies using different β_2-agonists in different populations of asthmatics.

The mean doubling dose shift in PC_{20} for methacholine or histamine during regular β_2-agonist treatment compared with values obtained during treatment with placebo or at baseline in 18 studies are shown in Figure 1. In 12 BHR increased, in two there was no detectable change, and in four there was a decrease in BHR. If only those with a statistically significant result are analysed, all but one study show an increase in BHR on regular treatment. The one exception, a study of effects of terbutaline vs budesonide in newly diagnosed asthma, had a substantial number of dropouts in the terbutaline treated arm. As most dropped out because of worsening asthma, the loss of these subjects may have biased the BHR towards not showing a deleterious effect. Hence the weight of evidence points to a deterimental effect of β_2-agonists as a class on BHR.

In some studies [23, 25] increased BHR was maximal immediately after the withdrawal of inhaled β_2-agonist treatment, although this so-called "rebound" phenomenon is not a consistent finding [40]. Nevertheless, it raises the additional possibility that in circumstances where regularly treated patients abruptly discontinue their β_2-agonist therapy, they become even more susceptible to trigger factors, and hence to instability of their asthma.

It has been argued that the magnitude of these observed changes in PC_{20} is not clinically significant [41, 42]. In eight studies [23–30] a doubling dose or concentration shift of greater than 0.5 was observed, a change considered to be clinically important. However, the magnitude of the change is not the sole criterion by which these observations ought to be judged. The direction of the change in BHR seen in the majority of studies is also important, especially as it contrasts sharply with the consistent increase in PC_{20} (decreased BHR) which follows regular use of inhaled corticosteroids such as budesonide [31,

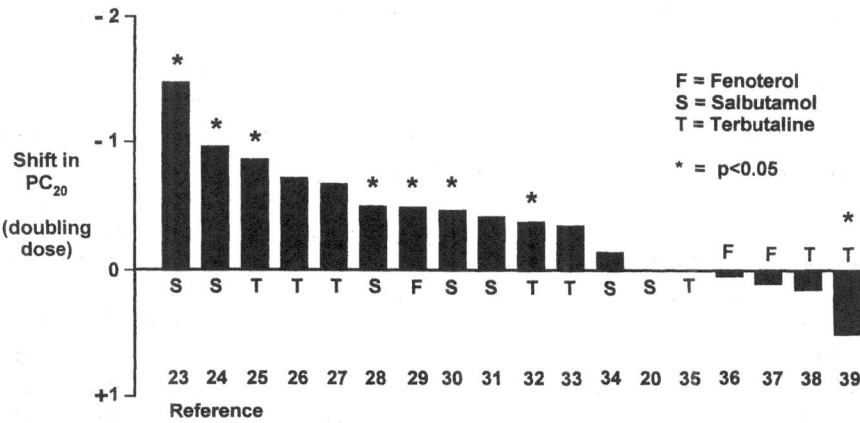

Figure 1. Mean doubling dose shift in PC$_{20}$ for methacholine or histamine during regular β-agonist treatment compared with values at baseline or during placebo treatment, in 18 studies. Key: F = fenoterol, S = salbutamol, T = terbutaline, * $p < 0.05$.

43]. The contrast between worsening BHR during β₂-agonist treatment and improved BHR during inhaled corticosteroid treatment, which is known to reduce airway inflammation, suggests that in many patients receiving regular inhaled β₂-agonists airway inflammation is increased. Certainly it is not reduced. These contrasting observations argue strongly against the regular use of β₂-agonists in the long-term treatment of airway inflammation.

2.3. Tolerance to the Non-Bronchodilator Effects of β₂-Agonists

In addition to acting on airway smooth muscle, β₂-agonists exhibit non-bronchodilator effects on the airways, notably suppression of mast cell mediator release. These combined actions are thought to be responsible for the benefits of inhaled β₂-agonist treatment. Indeed, it may be that the latter effect is the more important in offering protection against stimuli which cause bronchoconstriction by indirect means e.g. cold air, exercise, allergen.

It is generally agreed that tolerance to the bronchodilator actions of β₂-agonists does not occur or is minimal and insignificant [44]. However, tolerance to the non-bronchodilator effects occurs after relatively short periods of regular β₂-agonist treatment. O'Connor et al. demonstrated that following 2 weeks of regular treatment with inhaled terbutaline, the protective effect of a single dose against methacholine- and AMP-induced bronchoconstriction was reduced by 19% and 55% respectively [45]. Similarly, it has been demonstrated that as well as enhancing the airway response to exercise [18] or inhaled allergen [20, 21] when given regularly, the bronchoprotective benefits of single-dose pre-treatment with inhaled salbutamol are diminished by regular treatment, albeit modestly [46]. Thus theoretically the chronic use of β_2-agonist may be doubly hazardous: susceptibility to trigger factors may be increased, and the effectiveness of single "rescue" doses of the drug to treat resultant bronchoconstriction may be decreased.

The clinical relevance of tolerance to non-bronchodilator effects has not been clarified and it may or may not explain why poorer control of asthma results from regular β_2-agonist inhalation [29]. In each of the investigations reporting the development of tolerance to non-bronchodilator effects, standard doses of inhaled β_2-agonist have been administered. However, a dose-response relationship for such effects has been demonstrated, in that while there was a trend for a decreasing geometric mean allergen PC_{20} at 200 and 400 µg salbutamol daily, this became significant at 800 µg daily [47]. Thus in individual patients inhaling large quantities of β_2-agonist, these effects are likely to be more apparent.

2.4. Changes in Lung Function

If short-acting β_2-agonists had only a short-acting effect on bronchial smooth muscle, then lung function as measured either by pre-bronchodilator morning peak expiratory flow rates or FEV_1 ought to be no different from baseline or placebo in controlled studies of regular β_2-agonist treatment. However, this is not the case. A comprehensive review of this topic has recently been published [1]. In the majority of studies in which a significant result was reported, a *fall* in either FEV_1 or morning PEFR was observed (Tab. 1). For FEV_1, the mean decrease ranged from −0.15 l [48] to as much as −0.48 l [49]. In more recently published placebo-controlled studies of inhaled salbutamol, non-significant but none the less negative changes in pre-bronchodilator lung function have been observed [28, 55].

The results of some of these studies deserve closer examination. In the first lengthy double blind, placebo-controlled, cross-over study of regular vs. as-needed β_2-agonist (29, 48), inhaled fenoterol 1600 µg daily for 24 weeks resulted in a mean change in FEV_1 of −0.15 litres in 64 patients with mild to moderate asthma ($p < 0.05$). In the placebo-controlled parallel-group study of Drazen et al. [28], in which 255 patients with mild asthma received either inhaled salbutamol 720 µg daily or placebo for 16 weeks, the changes in morning PEFR and FEV_1 were consistently negative in the actively treated group. This was associated with an increase in BHR to methacholine (0.5 doubling doses). In the study by D'Alonzo et al. [55], the fall in mean morning peak flow rate in 108 patients with mild asthma during regular treatment with inhaled salbutamol was −13 l/min compared to the placebo group. The statistical significance of this last result was not reported.

Table 1. Effects of regular inhaled or oral β-agonist on lung function in asthmatics[*]

Drug	Duration (weeks)	Variable	Baseline value	Regular treatment	p	Reference
Fenoterol	24	FEV_1	2.46	2.29	<0.05	29, 48
Salbutamol	12	PEFR	352	289	NS	49
Salbutamol	4	FEV_1	2.30	2.08	NS	50
Salbutamol	4	FEV_1	3.68	3.33	<0.05	51
Fenoterol	4	FEV_1	2.76	2.43	<0.05	52
		PEFR	377	317	<0.02	
Salbutamol	2–5	PEFR	63%	57%	NS	53
Salbutamol	95	FEV_1	79%	76%	<0.0001	31
Salbutamol (oral)	4–20	PEFR	61%	53%	NS	53
Fenoterol (oral)	12	FEV_1	2.53	2.05	<0.05	54
Ephedrine (oral)	12	FEV_1	2.25	2.08	<0.05	54
Salbutamol	12	PEFR (A.M.)	NR	−13 L/min	NR	55

[*]FEV_1 (L), PEFR (L/min), or as percent predicted FEV_1 or PEFR, FEV_1 = Forced expiratory volume in 1 s; PEFR = peak-expiratory flow rate.
NS = Not significant; NR = not reported.

The pattern of results emerging from these more recent studies is consistent. Although it is possible to interpret the results of some studies as indicating no statistically significant difference between regular inhaled β_2-agonist and placebo, there is overall consistency in the direction of the reported changes. Differences in their magnitude and thus the statistical significance of the outcomes may be explained by the fact that some subjects being studied had milder asthma, as judged by baseline characteristics and use of inhaled corticosteroids, and that the dose of inhaled β_2-agonist being given was less than in some other investigations.

In summary, negative rather than no changes in pre-bronchodilator lung function during regular β_2-agonist therapy are the most frequent outcome in controlled studies. This overall picture is consistent with the view that their chronic use is detrimental.

2.5. Control of Asthma

The first reports to highlight the possibility that regular β_2-agonist treatment might give rise to deterioration in asthma control were published in the late 1960s. At that time aerosols containing relatively high doses of isoprenaline or adrenaline became available. No prospective or controlled investigations were carried out. However, in three case-based studies, worsening asthma was attributed to the use of inhaled adrenergic drug therapy [56–58]. Improvement was achieved in many cases by withdrawing the inhaled drug treatment.

In the more recent literature, whereas lung function is usually carefully documented, control of asthma as a study end-point has been largely neglected. The New Zealand study of regular inhaled fenoterol treatment in which asthma control was the primary end-point provided the first prospective experimental evidence concerning the effects of chronic β_2-agonist therapy on asthma control (29, 48). Forty of the 64 patients who completed the study had better asthma control during the as-needed treatment period ($p = 0.003$). Exacerbations were more frequent during the period of regular β_2-agonist treatment. The median time to first exacerbation was only 33 days during regular treatment compared with 66 days during placebo treatment ($p = 0.008$).

That poorer overall control of asthma ought to coincide with negative changes in mean pre-bronchodilator lung function may appear self-evident. In the New Zealand study, the deterioration in asthma control which occurred with regular fenoterol use was associated with a mean fall in pre-bronchodilator FEV_1 of -0.15 l ($p < 0.05$). Hence although the mean change in pre-bronchodilator lung function observed in many studies during regular β_2-agonist use may appear small, it reflects significant deterioration in overall asthma control. In many of the studies which we have reviewed [1], serious exacerbations of asthma requiring intervention with additional treatment, notably oral corticosteroid, are reported. However, the numbers of these events have usually been insufficiently large for statistical comparisons to be made. This highlights the importance of designing long-term studies in which control of asthma and occurrence of exacerbations rather than simply lung function measurements are primary study end points.

3. Epidemiological Evidence for a Link Between β_2-Agonist Use and Asthma Morbidity and Mortality

3.1. Mortality Epidemics Associated with the Introduction of Potent Agonists

Two major epidemics of asthma mortality have occurred in New Zealand during the last 30 years. The first began in the mid 1960s in England and Wales, Australia and New Zealand, and was associated in time with the introduction of a high-dose formulation of the non-selective β_2-agonist isoprenaline [59, 60]. More recently, a second New Zealand epidemic began in 1976 and concluded in 1990, in this instance coinciding closely with the introduction of the inhaled β_2-agonist fenoterol in a relatively high-dose formulation. From a rate of approximately 1.5 per 100 000 per annum, asthma mortality in the 5–34 age group rose dramatically to over 4.0 per 100 000 per annum over a 3-year period from 1976. This rise occurred in parallel with a steep rise in the prescription of inhaled fenoterol when compared to other β_2-agonist drugs [61] (Fig. 2).

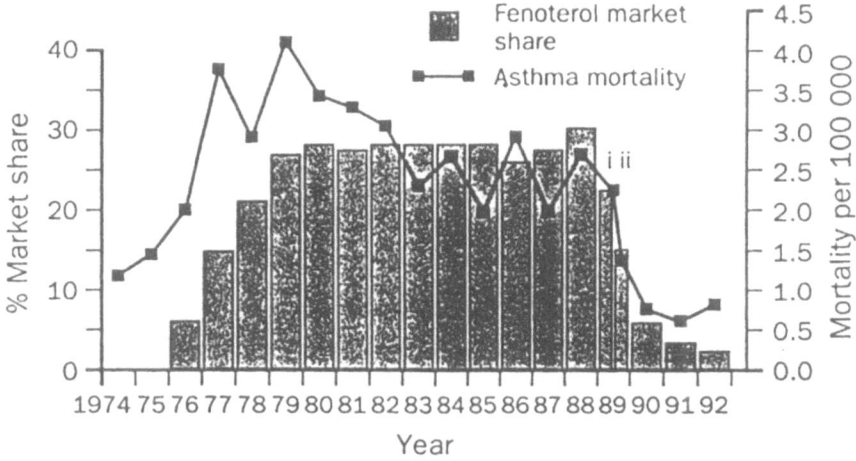

Figure 2. Inhaled fenoterol market share and annual asthma mortality in persons aged 5–34 years. (The data for 1989 are divided into two 6-month periods because the first Department of Health warnings about the safety of fenoterol were issued in mid-1989) (from [61]).

It has been argued that the introduction of other β₂-agonist drugs such as salbutamol and terbutaline and the continuing increase in their use has not been associated with similar epidemics. There are clinically important differences in intrinsic pharmacological efficacy between the different β₂-agonist drugs [62], which may be of importance in explaining apparent differences in the frequency and magnitude of adverse effects associated with the different agents, and hence differences in epidemiological data. While the strong temporal relationship between the introduction of isoprenaline and fenoterol and increases in asthma mortality is not seen for the other agents, asthma mortality and β₂-agonist use have both risen over time. However a causal relationship between these observations cannot be proven using epidemiological data alone [63].

3.2. Case Control Studies of Asthma Mortality

In 1989, the first of three New Zealand case control studies investigating the risk of death from asthma in relation to the prescription of β₂-agonist medication was published [64]. The odds ratio for death from asthma in patients prescribed inhaled fenoterol was 1.55 ($p = 0.03$), increasing in patients also receiving continuous oral corticosteroids to 6.45 ($p < 0.01$). Two subsequent case-control studies were published to address criticisms of the design of the first study: similar results were obtained [65, 66]. The consistent finding that adjustment for markers of severity increased rather than decreased the odds ratios for risk of death associated with prescription of fenoterol was used to refute the suggestion that the link with fenoterol was due to confounding by severity.

In order to confirm or negate the New Zealand findings, further epidemiological studies were conducted by Spitzer et al. using computerized prescribing data from the province of Saskatchewan, Canada [67]. In a nested case control study in which data from 12 301 patients for the period 1978–1987 were obtained, 129 cases of death or near-death from asthma and 655 selected controls were compared. Adjusted odds ratios for the relationship between the index event and the prescription of fenoterol and salbutamol were calculated. For fenoterol a highly significant result was obtained (O.R. 6.1, 95% CI 3.1–12.2). When adjusted for dose equivalence, there was no difference in the odds ratio for a major event between high users of fenoterol (>12 canisters during the 12 months prior to the index event; O.R. 22.7 (95% CI; 8.1–63.3)) and high users of salbutamol (>24 canisters; O.R. 24.0 (95% CI; 9.0–64.1)). Further analysis revealed a dose response relationship between the number of aerosol canisters of β_2-agonist prescribed and the risk of death or near death from asthma, and that the pattern of use i.e. whether decreasing or increasing, appears to be a very important predictor for the subsequent index event [68].

A major consideration in the interpretation of these data is whether the apparent relationship between drug prescribing and asthma morbidity and mortality is due to "confounding by severity" i.e. the possibility that patients with more severe asthma were prescribed more frequent and more potent β_2-agonist. These concerns have been addressed by a number of authors but opinion remains divided. The second and third New Zealand case control studies, in which controlling for asthma severity was more rigorously applied, continued to show a significantly increased risk of asthma death associated with prescription of fenoterol (O.R. 2.66 (95% CI; 1.74–4.06)) [65, 66]. Similarly, re-analysis of the Saskatchewan data using additional clinical information relating to asthma severity, did not significantly reduce the odds ratio for asthma death or near death for either fenoterol or salbutamol (2.5 and 2.0 respectively) [69]. If adjustment for severity does not reduce the relationship between prescribed β_2-agonist therapy and important asthma-related events, but rather increases the odds ratios (as in the New Zealand studies), confounding by severity seems unlikely.

On the other hand, Garrett et al. [70] reported that among 655 patients admitted to hospital with acute asthma during the period 1986–1987, the risk of subsequent admission to the ICU or death from asthma during the subsequent 2 years after controlling for several indices of severity was no different for those patients taking inhaled fenoterol compared to those taking salbutamol. However, while this analysis is helpful in distinguishing the relative risks associated with different β_2-agonist drugs, this study fails to address whether or not β_2-agonist use *per se* is a risk factor for increased asthma morbidity and mortality.

3.3. Reduction in Morbidity and Mortality Associated with Withdrawal of Fenoterol

In the early and mid 1980s a concerted campaign was mounted in New Zealand to control the dramatic rise in asthma mortality and morbidity. This included a wide variety of public health measures and therapeutic recommendations [71]. However, although the measures undertaken appear to have been somewhat successful, their impact on asthma mortality, which fell only modestly during the mid-1980s to an average annual rate of 2.3 per 100 000, was disappointing. First hospital admission rates remained unchanged throughout this period (Fig. 3).

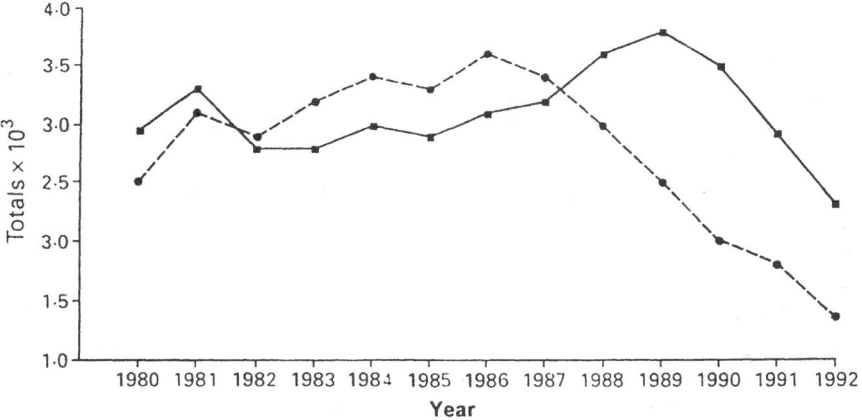

Figure 3. First admissions (■—■) and readmissions (●—●) per calendar year for asthma in 5–54 year old New Zealanders 1980–92 (from [71]).

In 1990, following the publication of the New Zealand case control studies [64–66], fenoterol was withdrawn from the prescribed medicines list by the Department of Health in New Zealand. Thereafter asthma mortality rates fell dramatically. Within 1–2 years mortality rates declined to be comparable to most other Western countries (approximately 0.8 per 100 000 for each of the 3 years 1990–1992) (Fig. 4). In addition, first hospital admissions for asthma were also reduced for the first time since 1981 (Fig. 3).

The importance of these epidemiological data has been debated [11, 71]. The striking and repeated temporal relationship between the introduction of the high-potency β$_2$-agonist preparations and significant changes in asthma mortality and morbidity on two occasions provides strong circumstantial evidence that the relationship is a causal one [11]. Even stronger support for this view is obtained from observing the changes which occurred following the

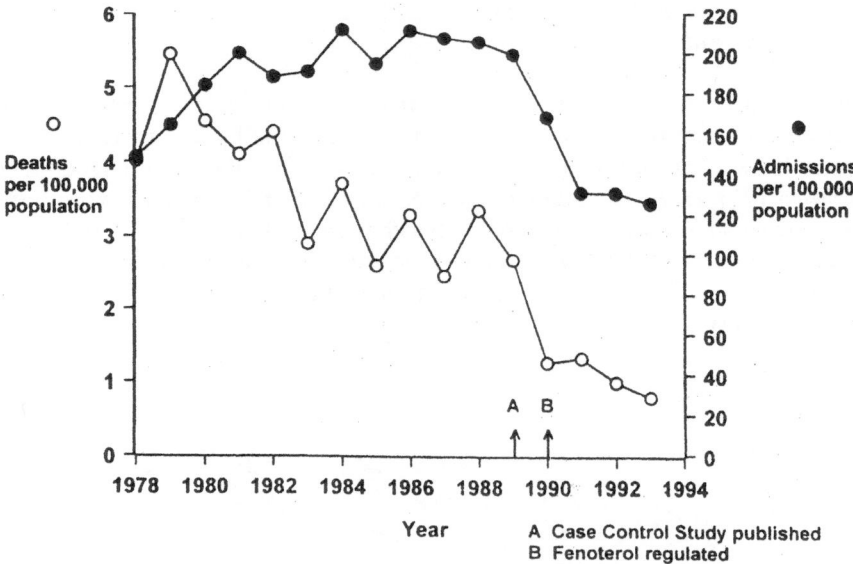

Figure 4. Abrupt decrease in asthma-related hospital admissions and mortality in New Zealanders aged 15 to 44 years following withdrawal of fenoterol in 1990 (from [12]).

withdrawal of fenoterol, when an even greater rate of change in asthma deaths and hospital admissions occurred—this time downwards—than occurred upwards immediately after its introduction [12]. This cannot otherwise be explained unless another major factor predisposing to increased asthma severity was simultaneously brought under control and there is no evidence for this. The disparity between the improvements in the rates for asthma death and rates for first hospital admission during the period 1984–1989 argues that despite an intensive response to the "asthma problem" in New Zealand, medical measures alone were insufficient to reduce morbidity and mortality to baseline. Withdrawal of the potent β_2-agonist clearly defined the end of the epidemic.

4. Conclusion

In his address to the Royal Society of Medicine in 1965 [72], Sir Austin Bradford Hill, Emeritus Professor of Medical Statistics at the University of London proposed a number of criteria to answer the question "*Upon what basis should we proceed to pass from an observed association to a verdict of causation?*" He cited nine: *strength, plausibility, consistency, specificity, temporality, biological gradient, coherence, experiment,* and *analogy*. Interestingly, statistical analyses were relegated by Bradford Hill to a subordinate role: "*Tests of significance contribute nothing to the proof of our hypothesis*".

In this chapter we have presented evidence which supports the hypothesis that chronic β_2-agonist use is detrimental to patients with bronchial asthma. The *strength* and *consistency* of the evidence are found in the repeatability of studies, both clinical and epidemiological, which have demonstrated an adverse outcome when inhaled β_2-agonists are used regularly. The *plausibility* of the hypothesis has been substantiated by studies demonstrating increased airway inflammation both *in vitro* and *in vivo* following chronic drug exposure, as well as increased responsiveness to trigger factors such as exercise and allergen. *Temporality* is demonstrated in that not one but two epidemics of asthma mortality have accompanied the introduction of potent agents, and that morbidity and mortality associated with the second epidemic was dramatically reduced when fenoterol was withdrawn.

The case presented is also *coherent:* there is a logical relationship between various categories of evidence. Increases in airway inflammation reasonably and logically ought to give rise to enhanced bronchial responsiveness, impairment of lung function, poorer control of asthma and adverse trends in asthma morbidity and mortality. Likewise, where the hypothesis that chronic β_2-agonist use is detrimental has been prospectively tested in an appropriate clinical setting over a sufficient period of time, the results have yielded *experimental* support. That these effects are not universally observed is a function of *biological gradient*: there is a dose-response relationship between cause and effect, and the effects on morbidity and mortality are greatest among those using high doses of the most potent β_2-agonists.

Few commentators now advocate the regular use of short-acting β_2-agonists to treat asthma. Nevertheless the detrimental effects associated with these drugs should not be forgotten, particularly when dealing with the difficult asthmatic whose "as-needed" use remains high. Their inappropriate use and overuse remains a risk factor for unstable and potentially life-threatening bronchial asthma.

References

1 Taylor DR, Sears MR, Cockcroft DW (1996) The β_2-agonist controversy. *Med Clin N Am* 80(4): 719–747
2 Giuntini CG, Paggiaro PL (1995) Present state of the controversy about regular inhaled β_2-agonists in asthma. *Eur Respir J* 8(5): 673–8
3 McFadden ER (1995) The β_2-agonist controversy revisited. *Ann Allergy Asthma Immunol* 75(2) 173–6
4 Lipworth BJ (1992) The β_2-agonist controversy: fact or fiction? *Clin Exp Allergy* 22: 659–664
5 Nelson HS, Szefler SJ, Martin RJ (1991) Regular inhaled β_2-adrenergic agonists in the treatment of bronchial asthma: beneficial or detrimental? *Am Rev Respir Dis* 144: 249–250
6 British guidelines on asthma management Review, position statement (1997) *Thorax* 52: Suppl 1
7 US Department of Health, Human Services National asthma education program: executive summary Guidelines for the diagnosis, management of asthma (1991) NIH Publication No 91–3042A
8 US Department of Health, Human Services NIH (1992) International consensus report on diagnosis and management of asthma. NIH Publication No. 92–3091

9 Global initiative for asthma (1995) NHLBI/WHO Workshop report, NIH Publication No. 95–3659

10 Shepherd GL, Hetzel MR, Clark TJH (1981) Regular *versus* symptomatic aerosol bronchodilator treatment of asthma. *Br J Dis Chest* 75: 215–7

11 Sears MR, Taylor DR (1994) The β_2-agonist controversy: observations, explanations and relationship to asthma epidemiology. *Drug Safety* 11: 259–283

12 Sears MR (1996) Epidemiological trends in asthma. *Cancer Res* 3: 261–8

13 Wang ZL, Bramley AM, McNamara A, Pare PD, Bai TR (1994) Chronic fenoterol exposure increases *in vivo* and *in vitro* airway response in guinea pigs. *Am J Respir Crit Care Med* 149(4): 960–965

14 Wang ZL, Walker BA, Weir TD, Yarema MC, Roberts CR, Okazawa M, Pare PD, Bai TR (1995) Effect of chronic antigen and β_2-agonist exposure on airway remodelling in guinea pigs. *Am J Respir Crit Care Med* 152(6): 2097–2104

15 Coqueret O, Dugas B, Mencia-Huerta JM, Braquet P (1995) Regulation of IgE production from human mononuclear cells by β_2-adrenoceptor agonists. *Clin Exp Allergy* 15: 304–311

16 Manolitsas ND, Wang J, Devalia JL, Trigg CJ, McAulay AE, Davies RJ (1995) Regular albuterol, nedocromil sodium, and bronchial inflammation in asthma. *Am J Respir Crit Care Med* 151: 1925–1930

17 Gauvreau GM, Watson RM, Jordana M, Cockcroft DW, O'Byrne PM (1995) The effect of regular inhaled salbutamol on allergen-induced airway responses and inflammatory cells in blood and induced sputum. *Am J Respir Crit Care Med* 151:A39

18 Inman MD, O'Byrne PM (1996) The effect of regular inhaled albuterol on exercise-induced bronchoscontriction. *Am J Respir Crit Care Med* 153: 65–69

19 Lai CKW, Twentyman OP, Holgate ST (1989) The effect of an increase in inhaled allergen dose after rimiterol hydrobromide on the occurrence and magnitude of the late asthmatic response and the associated change in non-specific bronchial responsiveness. *Am Rev Respir Dis* 140: 917–923

20 Cockcroft DW, McParland CP, Britto SA, Swystun VA, Rutherford BC (1993) Regular inhaled salbutamol and airway responsiveness to allergen. *Lancet* 342: 833–837

21 Cockcroft DW, O'Byrne PM, Swystun VA (1995) Regular use of inhaled albuterol and the allergen-induced late asthmatic response. *J Allerg Clin Immunol* 96: 44–49

22 Jatakanon A, Lim S, Chung KF, Barnes PJ (1997) Correlation between exhaled nitric oxide, sputum eosinophils and methacholine responsiveness. *Am J Respir Crit Care Med* 155: A819

23 Wahedna I, Wong CS, Wisniewski AFZ, Pavord ID, Tatterfield AE (1993) Asthma control during and after cessation of regular β_2-agonist treatment. *Am.Rev.Respir.Crit Care Med* 148: 707–712

24 Valente S, De Rosa M, Corbo GM et al (1993) Effect of treatment with β-agonist on the bronchial responsiveness and lung function in mild asthma. *Eur Respir J* 6(Suppl 17): 420s

25 Vathenen AS, Knox AJ, Higgins BG, Britton JR, Tattersfield AE (1988) Rebound increase in bronchial responsiveness after treatment with inhaled terbutaline. *Lancet* 1: 554–558

26 Kerrebijn KF, van Essen-Zandvliet EEM, Neigens HJ (1987) Effect of long-term treatment with inhaled corticosteroids and β-agonists on the bronchial responsiveness in children with asthma. *J Allerg Clin Immunol* 79: 653–9

27 O'Connor BJ, Aikman SL, Barnes PJ (1992) Tolerance to the nonbronchodilator effects of inhaled β_2-agonists in asthma. *N Engl J Med* 327: 1204–8

28 Drazen JM, Israel E, Boushey HA, Chinchilli VM, Fahy JV, Fish JE, Lazarus SC, Lemanske RF, Martin RJ, Peters SP et al (1996) Comparison of regularly scheduled with as-needed use of albuterol in mild asthma. *N Engl J Med* 335: 841–847

29 Sears MR, Taylor DR, Print CG (1990) Regular inhaled β-agonist treatment in bronchial asthma. *Lancet* 336: 1391–1396

30 van Schayck CP, Graafsma SJ, Visch MB, Dompeling E, van Weel C, van Herwaarden CLA (1990) Increased bronchial hyperresponsiveness after inhaling salbutamol during 1 year is not caused by subsensitization to salbutamol. *J Allerg Clin Immunol* 86: 793–800

31 Van Essen Zandvliet EE, Hughes MD, Waalkens HJ, Duiverman EJ, Pocock SJ, Kerrebijn KF (1992) Effects of 22 months of treatment with inhaled corticosteroids and/or β_2-agonists on lung function, airway responsiveness, and symptoms in children with asthma. *Am Rev Respir Dis* 146: 547–554

32 Kraan J, Koeter GH, v d Mark ThW, Sluiter HJ, de Vries K (1985) Changes in bronchial hyper-

reactivity induced by 4 weeks of treatment with antiasthmatic drugs in patients with allergic asthma: a comparison between budesonide and terbutaline. *J Allerg Clin Immunol* 76: 628–36

33 Waalkens HJ, Gerritsen J, Koeter GH, Krouwels FH, van Adlderen WMC, Knol K (1991) Budesonide and terbutaline or terbutaline alone in children with mild asthma: effects on bronchial hyperresponsiveness and diurnal variation in peak flow. *Thorax* 46: 499–503

34 Peel ET, Gibson GJ (1980) Effects of long-term inhaled salbutamol therapy on the provocation of asthma by histamine. *Am Rev Respir Dis* 121: 973–8

35 Wong CS, Wahedna I, Pavord ID, Tattersfield AE (1992) Effect of regular budesonide and terbutaline on bronchial reactivity to allergen challenge. *Am Rev Respir Dis* 145:A54

36 Raes M, Mulder P, Kerrebijn KF (1989) Long-term effect of ipratropium bromide and fenoterol on the bronchial hyperresponsiveness to histamine in children with asthma. *J Allerg Clin Immunol* 84: 874–9

37 Town I, O'Donnell TV, Purdie G (1991) Bronchial responsiveness during regular fenoterol therapy: a 4 months prospective study. *N Z Med J* 104: 3–5

38 Kerstjens HAM, Brand PLP, Hughes MD et al (1992) A comparison of bronchodilator therapy with or without inhaled corticosteroid therapy for obstructive airways disease. *N Engl J Med* 327: 1413–9

39 Haahtela T, Jarvinen M, Kava T, Kiviranta K, Koskinen S, Lehtonen K, Nikander K, Persson T, Reinikainen K, Selroos O et al (1991) Comparison of a β₂-agonist, terbutaline with an inhaled corticosteroid, budesonide, in newly detected asthma. *N Engl J Med* 325: 388–92

40 DeJong JW, Van der Mark TW, Koeter GH, Postma DS (1996) Rebound airway obstruction and responisveness after cessation of terbutaline: effects of budesonide. *Am J Respir Crit Care Med* 153: 70–75

41 VanSchayck CP, Van Heerwaarden CLA (1993) Do bronchodilators adversely affect the prognosis of bronchial hyper-responsiveness? *Thorax* 48: 470–473

42 McFadden ER (1995) Perspectives in β₂-agonist therapy: Vox clamantis in deserto vel lux in tenebris? *J Allerg Clin Immunol* 95: 641–51

43 Juniper EF, Kline PA, Vansieleghem MA (1990) Effect of long-term treatment with an inhaled corticosteroid (budesonide) on airway hyper-responsiveness and clinical asthma in non-steroid dependent asthmatics. *Am Rev Respir Dis* 142: 832–836

44 Grove A, Lipworth BJ (1995) Tolerance with β₂-adrenoceptor agonists: time for re-appraisal. *Br J Clin Pharmacol* 39: 109–118

45 O'Connor BJ, Aikman SL, Barnes PJ (1992) Tolerance to the non-bronchodilator effects of inhaled β₂-agonists in asthma. *N Engl J Med* 327: 1204–1208

46 Cockcroft DW, Swystun VA (1996) Functional antagonism: tolerance produced by inhaled β₂-agonists. *Thorax* 51: 1051–1056

47 Bhagat R, Swystun VA, Cockcroft DW (1996) Salbutamol-induced increased airway responsiveness to allergen and reduced protection vs. methacholine: dose-response. *J Allerg Clin Immunol* 97: 47–52

48 Taylor DR, Sears MR, Herbison GP, Flannery EM, Print CG, Lake DC, Yates DM, Lucas MK, Li Q (1993) Regular inhaled β-agonist in asthma: effects on exacerbations and lung function. *Thorax* 48: 134–138

49 Beswick KBJ, Pover GM, Sampson S (1986) Long-term regularly inhaled salbutamol. *Curr Med Res* 10: 228–34

50 Patakas D, Maniki E, Tsara V, Daskalopoulou E (1988) Intermittent and continuous salbutamol rotacaps inhalation in asthmatic patients. *Respiration* 54: 174–8

51 Harvey JE, Tattersfield AE (1982) Airway response to salbutamol: effect of regular salbutamol inhalations in normal, atopic and asthmatic subjects. *Thorax* 37: 280–7

52 Trembath PW, Greenacre JK, Anderson M, Dimmock S, Mansfield L, Wadsworth J, Green M (1979) Comparison of four weeks' treatment with fenoterol and terbutaline aerosols in adult asthmatics. *J Allerg Clin Immunol* 63: 395–400

53 Gibson GJ, Greenacre JK, Konig P, Conolly ME, Pride NB (1978) Use of exercise challenge to investigate possible tolerance to β-adrenoceptor stimulation in asthma. *Br J Dis Chest* 72: 199–206

54 Van Arsdel PP, Schaffrin RM, Rosenblatt J (1978) Evaluation of oral fenoterol in chronic asthmatic patients. *Chest* 73: 997–998

55 D'Alonzo GE, Nathan RA, Henochowicz S (1994) Salmeterol xinafoate as maintenance therapy compared with albuterol in patients with asthma. *JAMA* 271: 1412–1416

56 Keighley JF (1966) Iatrogenic asthma associated with adrenergic aerosols. *Ann Intern Med* 65: 985–995
57 Van Metre TE (1969) Adverse effects of inhalation of excessive amounts of nebulised isoproterenol in status asthmaticus. *J Allergy* 43: 101–113
58 Reisman RE (1970) Asthma induced by adrenergic aerosols. *J Allergy* 46: 162–177
59 Stolley PD, Schinnar R (1978) Association between asthma mortality and isoproterenol aerosols: a review. *Prev Med* 7: 319–338
60 Stolley PD Asthma mortality Why the United States was spared an epidemic of deaths due to asthma (1972) *Am Rev Respir Dis* 105: 883–90
61 Pearce N, Beasley R, Crane J, Burgess C, Jackson R (1995) End of the New Zealand asthma mortality epidemic. *Lancet* 345: 41–43
62 Dickey BF, Clark RC, Barber R (1996) Partial β_2-agonists and their impartial assessment. *Chest* 110: 1131–1132
63 Taylor DR, Sears MR (1994) Regular β-adrenergic agonists. Evidence, not reassurance, is what is needed. *Chest* 106: 552–9
64 Crane J, Pearce NE, Flatt A, Burgess C, Jackson R, Kwong T, Ball M, Beasley R (1989) Prescribed fenoterol and death from asthma in New Zealand, 1981–1983: a case-control study. *Lancet* 1: 917–922
65 Pearce NE, Grainger J, Atkinson M, Crane J, Burgess C, Culling C, Windom H, Beasley R (1990) Case-control study of prescribed fenoterol and death from asthma in New Zealand, 1977–1981. *Thorax* 45: 170–175
66 Grainger J, Woodman K, Pearce NE, Crane J, Burgess C, Keane A, Beasley R (1991) Prescribed fenoterol and death from asthma in New Zealand 1981–1987: a further case control study. *Thorax* 46: 105–111
67 Spitzer WO, Suissa S, Ernst P, Horwitz RI, Habbick B, Cockcroft DW, Boivin JF, McNutt M, Buist AS, Rebuck AS (1992) The use of β-agonists and the risk of death and near death from asthma. *N Engl J Med* 336: 501–506
68 Suissa S, Blais L, Ernst P (1994) Patterns of increasing β-agonist use and the risk of fatal and near-fatal asthma. *Eur Respir J* 7: 1602–1609
69 Ernst PE, Habbick B, Suissa S, Hemmelgarn B, Cockcroft D, Buist AS, Horwitz RI, McNutt M, Spitzer WO (1993) Is the association between inhaled β-agonist use and life-threatening asthma because of confounding by severity? *Am Rev Respir Dis* 148: 75–79
70 Garrett JE, Lanes SF, Kolbe J, Rea HH (1996) Risk of severe life-threatening asthma and β-agonist type: an example of confounding by severity. *Thorax* 51: 1093–1099
71 Garrett J, Kolbe J, Richards G, Whitlock T, Rea H (1995) Major reduction in asthma morbidity and continued reduction in asthma mortality in New Zealand: what lessons have we learned? *Thorax* 50: 303–311
72 Bradford-Hill A (1965) The environment and disease: association or causation? President's address. *Proc R Soc Med* 58: 295–300

CHAPTER 4
Assessment of Airway Inflammation in Asthma Using Non-Invasive Methods

K. Parameswaran and F.E. Hargreave

Asthma Research Group, St. Joseph's Hospital and McMaster University, Hamilton, Ontario, Canada L8N 3Z5

1. Introduction

1.1. Invasive versus Non-Invasive Clinical Measurements in Medicine

Clinical measurement has become an essential complement to traditional physical diagnosis. An ideal clinical measurement should be quantitative, have a high level of reliability and accuracy, be safe, acceptable to the patient, easy to perform and non-invasive. The latter demands that the technique should not break the skin or the lining epithelium and should be devoid of effects on the tissues of the body by the dissipation of energy or the introduction of infection [1]. It is therefore logical that for a given measurement, a non-invasive test will be preferred if it provides the same information with the same accuracy and precision.

In the following sections, we will discuss the role of various non-invasive or relatively non-invasive methods to assess airway inflammation in asthma and concentrate on the only direct method of induced sputum examination.

1.2. Why Is Assessment of Airway Inflammation Important in Asthma?

Inflammation is a localized protective response elicited by injury or destruction of tissues which serves to destroy, dilute or wall off both the injurious agent and the injured tissue [2]. The role of inflammation in asthma was recognized long ago. In his textbook *The Principles and Practice of Medicine*, in 1892, Sir William Osler described "bronchial asthma... in many cases is a special form of inflammation of the smaller bronchioles... characterized by hyperaemia and turgescence of the mucosa of the smaller bronchial tubes and a peculiar exudate of mucin..." [3]. The classical clinical signs of heat, redness, swelling and pain first described by Celsus [4] have been observed in the airway. These are caused by the release of various mediators which cause an increase in vascular flow and permeability, exudation of serum, mucus secretion, stimulation of sensory nerve endings and inflammatory cell infiltration. Because these, with the exception of cell infiltration, can occur with the release of vasodilatory (and bronchoconstrictor) mediators, an inflammatory cell infiltration is usually considered necessary before it can said that inflammation is present.

According to current knowledge airway inflammation is the primary cause of airway diseases including asthma, the cause of exacerbations, and the cause of persistent or progressive airway hyperresponsiveness and chronic airflow limitation. Airway inflammation has many different causes, these result in different types of inflammation and these different types respond differently to treatment. Hence, theoretically, measurements should be necessary in order to be certain of the presence and type of airway inflammation as well as its severity. Measurements should be required to guide antiinflammatory treatment. The importance of airway inflammation have led to its inclusion in consensus guidelines and definitions of asthma [5, 6]. The treatment guidelines recommend that therapy for asthma should control the inflammatory process in addition to relieving symptoms. It is reasonable to state that inflammation cannot be effectively controlled if it cannot be accurately assessed. The measurement of different components of inflammation is therefore critical to improve the understanding of asthma and its treatment.

1.3. What Are the Different Methods to Assess Airway Inflammation?

The presence and severity of airway inflammation has been gauged by different indirect and direct methods, some of which are invasive and others non-invasive [7].

The indirect indices include worsening of symptoms, FEV_1, variability in peak expiratory flow (PEF) and airway responsiveness and increased bronchodilator requirement, blood eosinophil and basophil counts and sputum production. When symptoms are absent or require the least bronchodilator treatment, and the FEV_1 and airway responsiveness are normal or the best possible, inflammation is considered to be controlled. Alternatively, when the symptoms or need for bronchodilator treatment are increased, airflow limitation is present or worse and airway responsiveness is abnormal or heightened from best measurements, inflammation is considered to be present or increased. These objective measurements are non-invasive and cause little distress to the patients but they may be misinterpreted.

Another recent development has been the introduction of measurement of exhaled nitric oxide (ENO) to assess airway inflammation non-invasively [8]. Although this provides information on the presence or absence of inflammation, it does not provide information on the cellular or molecular components. Other indirect relatively non-invasive methods that have been employed in research include lung imaging using ventilation and perfusion scanning [9] and computerized tomographic scanning [10].

The direct methods of assessing inflammation using fibreoptic bronchoscopy are invasive. They include bronchoscopic biopsy, bronchial washings and brushings and bronchoalveolar lavage (BAL). The only direct non-invasive method is examination of sputum. Therefore, sputum examination is the logical assessment tool if it "performs" well in different clinical situations. In the following sections, we will present evidence for the performance and utility of improved methods of sputum examination and compare them with those of the other direct but invasive methods.

2. What Determines a Good Measurement Tool?

A good measurement tool should be accurate, precise, responsive to changes, and acceptable to the subject [11]. The cost and risk involved should also be taken into account in the assessment of the test. A measurement may be evaluated depending on what it is used for, as a tool to identify the normal from the abnormal or as a diagnostic test to make a diagnosis of a diseased state (evaluative), or to differentiate between different types of abnormalities (discriminative). There are several criteria for making these assessments:

2.1. Performance of a Measurement

2.1.1 Validity (Accuracy): This is the degree to which the data measures what is intended. For example, the results of measurement of sputum cell counts and fluid phase indices correspond to the airway inflammation being measured. For clinical observations that can be measured by physical means, it is relatively easy to establish validity. However, there is no gold standard for the measurement of airway inflammation. In such a situation, there are three strategies for establishing the validity of measurements:
1) Content validity is the extent to which a particular method of measurement includes all the dimensions of the construct one intends to measure and nothing more (e.g. different aspects of inflammation such as inflammatory cells, mediators, microvascular leakage, etc.
2) Construct validity is the extent to which the measurement is consistent with other measurements of the same phenomenon such as clinical severity indicated by airflow limitation and airway hyperresponsiveness, or other direct measurements like BAL and bronchial biopsies.
3) Criterion validity is a measure of the extent to which the measurement predicts a directly observable phenomenon. For example, changes in sputum measurements with different severities of asthma, correlation of sputum cell counts with specific corresponding markers of cell activation and differences in sputum measurements in different airway diseases.

2.1.2 Reliability (Precision): This is the extent to which repeated measurements of a stable phenomenon, e.g., airway inflammatory indices, measured by different people and instruments, and at different times and places, are similar.

2.1.3 Responsiveness: An instrument is responsive to the extent that its results change as conditions change. For example, when glucocorticoid treatment improves asthma, sputum inflammatory indices are reduced.

2.1.4 Sensitivity and Specificity: These refer to the relationship between a diagnostic test (e.g. sputum meaurement) and the actual presence or absence of the disease (e.g. asthma). Sensitivity is the the proportion of people with the disease who have a positive test for the disease. Specificity is the proportion of people without the disease who have a negative test.

2.2. Utility (Cost and Risk)

An important aspect of any measurement that could alter patient management is utility of the test. This takes into consideration the cost of the test and the risks involved, as well as assumptions about the patient's preferences for quality of life, length of life and the pleasant and unpleasant aspects of the test from the patient's point of view.

3. Performance of Various Non-Invasive Methods Other than Sputum

3.1. Clinical

The severity of symptoms is an important indicator of the severity of an asthma exacerbation. However, for some patients the onset of symptoms is a very sensitive indicator and can develop several days before significant changes in PEF or spirometry [12], symptoms are non-specific and an imprecise measure of the severity of the airflow limitation, airway responsiveness and airway inflammation [13].

3.2. Spirometry

Spirometry has traditionally been used to monitor the degree of airflow limitation and guide the treatment changes in asthma. A decrease in FEV_1 (indicating worse airflow limitation) has been observed to correlate with an increase in sputum and blood eosinophilia [12]. However, it is not true for all ranges of severity of the disease, particularly the more severe forms of the disease. Pizzichini and co-workers have demonstrated this in two groups of patients [14, 15] in whom sputum eosinophilic counts were observed before symptoms and FEV_1 worsened and persisted long after clinical parameters improved. In a group of prednisone dependent asthmatics who had normal sputum eosinophilia and best FEV_1, slow reduction of the dose of prednisone caused an increase in sputum eosinophils before worsening of symptom, PEF or FEV_1 [14]. In another study, in which the kinetics of inflammatory indices in sputum were observed after treatment with prednisone for a severe exacerbation of asthma, symptoms and FEV_1 improved before the improvement in sputum eosinophils [15]. These observations suggest that eosinophilic inflammation begins before worsening of symptoms or deterioration in airflow limitation and tends to lag behind clinical improvement. They indicate that spirometric measurements of airflow limitation do not necessarily reflect the true nature of airway inflammation.

3.3. Airway Responsiveness

Chronic [16, 17] and acute [18, 19] inflammatory processes in the airways
have been associated with airway hyperresponsiveness. However, some studies have suggested that exacerbations of asthma, as measured by increased
symptoms and variable airflow limitation, is not always associated with
changes in the severity of airway hyperresponsiveness [20]. Moreover, airway
hyperresponsiveness can occur without sputum eosinophilia and sputum
eosinophilia can occur without airway hyperresponsiveness. These observations suggest that more objective and direct evidence of inflammation is
required.

3.4. Exhaled Nitric Oxide

Measurement of levels of ENO has recently been recognized as a non-invasive
method to assess airway inflammation [21]. An increase in ENO in patients
with asthma has been reported and NO levels have been shown to correlate
with early and late asthmatic responses in spirometry after allergen challenge
[22]. The cellular source of NO in the lower respiratory tract is not yet certain
and therefore ENO does not give any information about the type of inflammation e.g., eosinophilic or neutrophilic. Exhaled NO, despite provoking considerable interest as a non-invasive means of measuring airway inflammation, has
not been validated by comparing it with more direct measurements like BAL
or bronchial biopsies. Modest correlations have been observed between ENO
and sputum eosinophil counts ($r = 0.42$, $p = 0.01$) in a small study on unselected sputum [23]. The measurement moreover is not specific for disease and
can be increased not only in asthma but also in bronchiectasis [24], and respiratory tract infections [25]. Until the methodology is validated, its clinical use
in patient management will remain uncertain.

3.5. Imaging: Computerized Tomography (CT), Position Emission
Tomography (PET)

High-resolution CT abnormalities have been compared in patients with allergic and non-allergic asthma of similar duration in an attempt to correlate structural abnormalities with symptoms (Aas score) and FEV_1 [10]. The extent of
airway remodelling was assessed indirectly by comparing permanent CT-scan
abnormalities (cylindric and varicose bronchiectasis, emphysema, bronchial
linear shadows) between allergic and non-allergic asthmatics who had asthma
for a similar duration. The data demonstrated that the extent of airway remodelling could be quantified by CT scans and there was a significant increase in
the extent of persistent abnormalities with increasing severity and duration of
asthma. However high-resolution CT does not provide any information on the

presence or type of current airway inflammation. It provides anatomical information but not cytological.

Positron emission tomography has also been employed to image the airway inflammation in asthma. Taylor et al. [26] demonstrated that [18]FDG uptake in the airway after segmental allergen challenge could be visualized using PET scan. However it provides no information about the cellular localization of the signal and the technique is expensive and not widely available.

4. Induced Sputum

Sputum is defined as secretions from the lower respiratory tract and contains both cellular and non-cellular elements. The specific anatomical origin of cells collected in sputum is not known, but they are believed to originate from the larger as well as smaller airways. When it is expectorated, it is often mixed with saliva.

In this section, we will present evidence to show that induced sputum examination is the most validated minimally invasive method to assess airway inflammation. It provides direct information on the presence and type of inflammation which is not provided by the other indirect non-invasive methods.

4.1. Evaluation of the Methodology

The examination of sputum was previously thought to be difficult and unreliable. Recent developments have shown that it can be processed to give repeatable, valid and responsive results for an increasing number of measurements.

Two methods have been used to induce sputum with an aerosol of hypertonic saline in stable or mildly exacerbated asthmatics, smokers with non-obstructive bronchitis and healthy people [27]. In one, the subject is pretreated with inhaled salbutamol 200 µg to prevent airway constriction and the hypertonic saline is then inhaled from an ultrasonic nebulizer. The concentration of saline and the duration of inhalation is either 3% for up to 20–21 min [28] or 3% followed by 4%, followed by 5% each for 7 min [29]. In the other method, the hypertonic saline (4.5%) is given without pretreatment and inhaled for doubling times from 30 s to 8 min [30]

The success of sputum induction is dependent on a number of possible factors related to the subject characterisitics (cigarette smoking, whether the subject is healthy or has disease and the degree of airway inflammation), components of the induction procedure (nebulizer output and particle size, concentration of saline, duration of inhalation, β_2-agonist pretreatment and the encouragement given to cough up sputum) and the success of processing sputum (selection of sputum from saliva and the effectiveness of dithiothreitol treatment) [31]. The procedure is successful in about 80% of stable asthmatics or healthy subjects who are unable to produce sputum spontaneously and in whom sputum is selected from saliva and processed for cell and fluid phase measurements by the method described by Pizzichini et al. [32]. The success can be 100% when the induction is performed in asthmatics with uncontrolled asthma, in previously healthy subjects with a current respiratory infection or in smokers or ex-smokers.

Sputum induction with an ultrasonic nebulizer is more successful than a jet nebulizer which has a lower output [31]. Moreover, between ultrasonic nebulizers the output required for maximum success may be relatively low. For example, the Fisoneb ultrasonic nebulizer (also called the Medix or Universal Ultrasonic nebuliser, Clement Clarke International Ltd.) with an output of 0.87 ml/min and mass median aerodynamic diameter (mmad) of 5.58 μm has comparable success but less side-effects than the DeVilbiss Ultraneb 99 with an output of 2.17 ml/min and mmad of 4.14 μm. However the effect of the output on repeated inductions and the cellular and fluid phase measurements is not well understood and is currently being studied. Hypertonic saline is more successful than isotonic saline and pretreatment with salbutamol does not influence the success [31].

The induction of sputum in asthmatics who can produce sputum spontaneously does not influence the cell content but might reduce the levels of some of the fluid phase measurements perhaps because of the dilution with inhaled saline [33]. Induced sputum gives a higher recovery of viable cells and cytospins of better quality. Cell viability does not affect the repeatability of cell counts by the same observer [32]. However, samples with cell viability <50% and squamous cell contamination >20% have lower interobserver agreement than those with cell viability >50% and squamous contamination <20%. The fluid phase measurements obtained from spontaneous and induced sputum can only be used interchangeably when both samples have a cell viability of >50%.

Details of the methods that we follow to induce and process sputum have been described elsewhere. Laboratory details are given in a video and booklet [34] available from the Canadian Thoracic Society.

4.2. Evaluation of the Test

4.2.1. Content Validity: Airway inflammation in asthma has different components, namely cellular infiltration, mediator release, microvascular leakage, cytokine and chemokine interplay, mucosal oedema and mucus hypersecretion. These different aspects of inflammation have been successfully measured in induced sputum. The normal values for total and differential cell counts (Tab. 1) and some of the fluid-phase measurements (Tab. 2) have been established by studying relatively few healthy subjects [35]. They need further validation from studies in a larger number of randomly selected, well characterized subjects. The various measurements that can be made in the fluid phase

Table 1. Normal values for total and differential cell counts (proportions and absolute number) based on the examination of 10 samples of induced sputum from healthy subjects

Proportions %		95% Confidence interval		
	Mean	Lower limit	Upper limit	Median
Neutrophils	24.3	14.9	33.7	24.1
Eosinophils	0.6	0.2	1.0	0.5
Macrophages	65.2	49.8	80.6	62.9
Lymphocytes	1.4	0.3	2.5	1.3
Bronchial epithelial cell	0.6	0.06	1.2	0.3
Metachromatic cells	0	0	0.1	0
Total cell count $\times 10^6$	3.8	0.02	0.06	0.03
Neutrophils $\times 10^6$	0.87	0.30	1.45	0.6
Eosinophils $\times 10^6$	0.02	0.5	0.04	0.02
Macrophages $\times 10^6$	2.25	1.28	3.22	1.66
Lymphocytes $\times 10^6$	0.08	0.0	0.27	0.03

Efthimiadis A, Pizzichini E, Pizzichini MMM, Hargreave FE (197)Sputum examination for indices of airway inflammation: laboratory procedures. Astra Draco AB, Lund, Sweden.

Table 2. Normal values for fluid-phase indices based on the examination of 10 samples of induced sputum from healthy subjects

		95% Confidence interval			
	Mean	Lower limit	Upper limit	Median	Kit/antibody source
ECP, µg/L	405.0	165.0	655.0	288.0	Pharmacia
MBP, µg/L	445.0	37.0	852.0	304.0	Dr. GJ. Gleich
EDN, µg/L	570.0	57.0	1082.0	448.0	Dr. GJ. Gleich
Tryptase, IU/L	15.4	10.8	19.8	12.8	Pharmacia
Fibrinogen, µg/L	728.0	180.0	1275.0	440.0	Dako
Albumin, µg/L	380.0	173.0	588.0	288.0	Dako
MPO, µg/L	4360.0	2890.0	5380.0	5880.0	Pharmacia
Elastase, ng/mL	248.0	62.0	395.0	286.0	Dr. GJ. Gleich
IL-5, pg/mL	ULD	ULD	UDL	UDL	R&D

ULD: Under limit of detection. See Appendix 2 for kits.
Efthimiadis A, Pizzichini E, Pizzichini MMM, Hargreave FE (1997) Sputum examination for indices of airway inflammation: laboratory procedures. Astra Draco AB, Lund, Sweden.

of sputum include 1) cell products [35], e.g. eosinophil cationic protein (ECP), major basic protein (MBP), esoinophil derived neurotoxin (EDN), myeloperoxidase (MPO), elastase and human neutrophil lipokalin [36], 2) cytokines

[15, 35, 37], e.g. IL-5 and IL-8, 3) chemokines [38], e.g. RANTES, MIP-1α and eotaxin, 4) tachykinins [39], e.g. substance P, 5) adhesion molecules [40], e.g. ICAM-1, 6) fibrinogen, albumin and α-2 macroglobulin as measures of microvascular leakage [41], 7) mediators, e.g. leukotrienes [42], and 8) mucus secretion [43], e.g. mucin-like glycoprotein.

The validity has been further examined by observing the strong correlations between the different markers of inflammation (Tab. 3)

Table 3. Correlation (rs)* matrix for sputum eosinophils and fluid phase markers

	ECP	EDN	MBP	Albumin	Fibrinogen	IL-5
Eosinophils	0.89	0.75	0.81	9.8	0.54	0.97
ECP		0.9	0.81	0.7	0.64	
EDN			0.89	0.7	0.62	
MBP				0.66	0.67	
Albumin					0.61	

p values for all correlations <0.001.
only in asthmatic subjects
For the correlations between ECP and albumin with eosinophils, the Spearman correlation coefficient was obtained by linear regression and the best fitted curve was estimated based on a cubic relationship.
Pizzichini E et al. (1996) Indices of airway inflammation in induced sputum: reproducibility and validity of cell and fluid phase measurements. *Am J Respir Crit Care Med* 154: 308–317.

4.2.2. Criterion Validity: The sputum cell counts have been examined in asthma of differing severity and in different airway diseases. Few eosinophils are present in healthy subjects [35]. The eosinophil count increases in uncontrolled asthma [44]. An increase in eosinophils have also been observed in severe exacerbations of asthma [15] and in prednisone-dependent asthmatics [14]. However, increase in sputum eosinophils has also been observed in eosinophilic bronchitis without the physiological abnormalities of asthma [45]. Asthma exacerbations can also occur without an increase in eosinophil counts. For example, neutrophils counts have also been reported to increase in some asthma exacerbations [46, 47].

The criterion validity has been further established by examining the cell and fluid-phase measurements in healthy and abnormal airways, for example, healthy and asthmatic subjects, and smokers with non-obstructive bronchitis [35]. Asthmatics had an increase of the proportion of eosinophils, metachromatic cells and neutrophils and of the eosinophilic proteins, tryptase, fibrinogen and IL-5. In smokers with non-obstructive bronchitis, the proportion of neutrophils and the concentration of fibrinogen and albumin are increased in comparison with healthy subjects (Fig. 1). The total cell counts are also increased in other conditions e.g. respiratory infections, particularly bacterial infections. The proportion of neutrophils is higher in smokers' obstructive

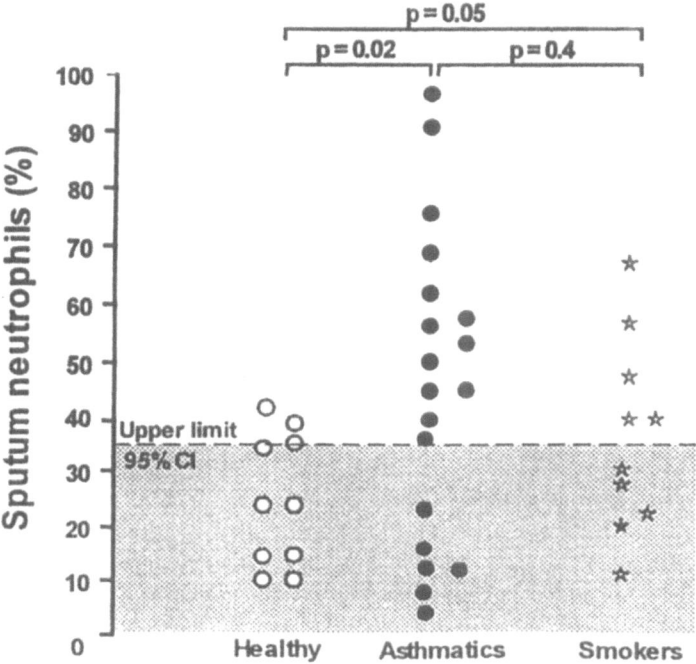

Figure 1. Indices of airway inflammation in induced sputum: reproducibility and validity of cell and fluid phase measurements. Pizzichini E et al (1996) *Am J Respir Crit Care Med* 154: 308–317.

bronchitis than in nonobstructive bronchitis and asthma, and is highest in infections.

Criterion validity is also supported by observing the high correlations between the inflammatory cells and their activation products in the sputum supernatant. Pizzichini et al. [35] reported correlation coefficients of 0.89 and 0.81 between eosinophils and ECP and EDN respectively. They also observed a correlation between sputum metachromatic cells and tryptase (rs = 0.71, p = 0.001). Similarly, a high correlation has been observed between neutrophil cell counts and the levels of free neutrophil elastase activity in sputum in asthmatics with an exacerbation (rs = 0.8, p = 0.003) [47].

4.2.3. Construct Validity: Construct validity has been established by observing the correlations between sputum indices and clinical indices of asthma severity such as symptoms, measures of airflow limitation (FEV_1, FEV_1/VC) and airway responsiveness (PC_{20} methacholine) [35] (Tab. 4). In symptomatic patients, eosinophils, ECP, MBP, EDN and albumin were higher than in asymptomatic patients.

Table 4. Correlation (rs)* matrix for sputum and clinical measurements

	Symptomscores	FEV$_1$% pred	FEV$_1$/VC%	PC$_{20}$mg/ml
Eosinophils	−0.68	−0.68	−0.50	−0.66
ECP	−0.57	−NS	−0.62	NS
EDN	−0.67	−0.62	−0.73	−0.56
MBP	−0.63	−0.52	−0.53	−0.50
Albumin	−0.60	NS	−0.57	NS
Fibrinogen	NS	NS	NS	NS

* p values for all correlations <0.01.
Symptoms were recorded only in asthmatics
NS: Non signifcant with an rs < 0.50 and p > 0.01.
Pizzichini E et al. (1996) Indices of airway inflammation in induced sputum: reproducibility and validity of cell and fluid phase measurements. *Am J Respir Crit Care Med* 154: 308–317.

Construct validity has been further tested by comparing the cellular and fluid phase measurements in sputum with more direct measurements obtained by bronchoscopy and lavage. Fahy and co-workers [28] demonstrated that the proportions of nonsquamous cells in sputum plus saliva more closely resembled those in bronchial washings than BAL but the agreement between the methods was not reported. Maestrelli et al. [48] observed that the agreement of the number of eosinophils in induced sputum and bronchial biopsy was better than the agreement of the same measurement between BAL and biopsy. We have demonstrated that sputum contains more cells especially neutrophils and CD4$^+$ T-cells compared to BAL in mild stable asthma [49]. Parameswaran et al. [50] observed that the sputum measurements of cell counts were reflected in the histopathological examination of the resected lung specimen in a patient presumed to have prednisone dependent asthma but who had bronchiectasis and chronic airflow limitation. Clinical deterioration was not associated with sputum eosinophilia, but rather with neutrophilia. The resected lung specimen did not show any airway eosinophilic infiltration or structural changes consistent with typical asthmatic inflammation.

4.2.4. Repeatability: The repeatability of cell counts has been examined in different ways and expressed either as intra class correlation coefficient (ICC) or as coefficient of variation. Repeatability has been examined on two different days (within subject variability), between two observers on the same sample (interobserver variability) and by the same observer on one sample which was separated into two portions (within sample variability). There are only three reports using ICC. Pizzichini et al. [35] (on sputum selected from saliva, within subject), In't Veen et al. [51] (unselected sputum sample, within subject) and Iredale et al. [30] (unselected sputum sample, interobserver and within sample) observed high ICC with the exception of total count and proportion of lymphocytes. Good repeatability has also been demonstrated in flow cytometry for lymphocyte markers [52].

There are only two reports of within subject variability of the fluid phase measurements reported as ICC. Pizzichini et al. [35] observed high ICC for ECP (0.85), MBP (0.80), EDN (0.86), albumin (0.94), fibrinogen (0.86), tryptase (0.60) and IL-5 (0.69). In't Veen et al. [51] observed high ICC in the fluid phase of unselected sputum sample for ECP (0.82), albumin (0.71) and fibrinogen (0.88).

This good repeatability identifies the reliability of these measurements (Tab. 5).

4.2.5. Responsiveness: The responsiveness of the methods of sputum examination have been investigated by following the results after inflammation has been induced or treated. Eosinophil counts and ECP concentrations are increased by exposure to allergens or diisocyanates in sensitized subjects and by reduction of steroid treatment [12,] [53, 54] and decreased by treatment with corticosteroids [15,] [55]. Similar observations have been made in prednisone dependent asthmatics [56]. When the prednisone is reduced, the eosinophilic inflammation returns. Regular treatment with inhaled steroid has also been shown to prevent the rise in eosinophils and metachromatic cells, 7 and 24 h after allergen exposure [57]. These observations indicate that the methods of sputum examination are responsive to change.

4.2.6. Sensitivity and Specificity: Traditionally, blood eosinophil counts have been used to monitor disease activity in asthma. Pizzichini et al. [58] compared the diagnostic utility of peripheral blood eosinophil counts and ECP levels with similar measurements in sputum by constructing receiver operating characteristic curves and comparing the area under the curves (AUC). Comparisons of the AUCs showed that percentage of eosinophils in sputum were significantly more sensitive and specific than blood eosinophils or ECP in the differentiation of patients with asthma from control subjects. Sputum eosinophilia of 2% had 100% specificity and 63% sensitivity. These results indicate that sputum eosinophils have better discriminative properties than the same indices in peripheral blood. Sensitivity and specificity of measurements in bronchial biopsies or BAL have not been investigated.

4.2.7. Risks: Inhalation of hypertonic saline aerosol can cause airway constriction [59]. This is inhibited by pretreatment with salbutamol [15]. However the degree of protection will depend on a number of factors including subject characteristics, the amount of saline inhaled and the amount of a recent β_2-agonist used. When asthma is uncontrolled, airway responsiveness is severely increased, the dose of saline is greater, or a short acting β_2-agonist has been used three or more times in the past 24 h or a long acting β_2-agonist is in use, and the protection by inhaled salbutamol against bronchoconstriction is likely to be less.

Table 5. Repeatability of sputum fluid phase indices expressed as median and interquartile range

Subjects (n)	ECP µg/L		MBP µg/L		EDN µg/L		Albumin µg/L		Fibrinogen ng/L		Tryptase U/L	
	Day 1	Day 2	Day 1	Day 2	Day 1	Day 2	Day 1	Day 2	Day 1	Day 2	Day 1	Day 2
Healthy	288	376	304	76	448	328	288	384	440	732	13	12
(10)(338)	(332)	(602)	(876)	(376)	(622)	(318)	(298)	(756)	(1220)	(11.2)	(8.2)	
Asthmatics	1040	800	1176	2488	1512	4976	704	592	1080	1440	21	15
(19)(3008)	(6240)	(1984)	(2552)	(4016)	(6584)	(1176)	(1664)	(3440)	(2832)	(17.6)	(15.2)	
Smokers	352	596	160	480	272	456	452	464	708	940	12	13
(10)(725)	(398)	(512)	(708)	(464)	(448)	(238)	(370)	(1676)	(1074)	(3.0)	(6.4)	
R0.85		0.80	0.86	0.94		0.86		0.60				

R = Intraclass correlation coefficient

Pizzichini E et al. (1996) Indices of airway inflammation in induced sputum: reproducibility and validity of cell and fluid phase measurements. *Am J Respir Crit Care Med* 154: 308–317

The present methods of sputum induction with hypertonic saline in increasing concentrations is safe in subjects with mild stable or mildly exacerbated asthma [27,] [60]. Induction with an aerosol of isotonic saline given cautiously for shorter time periods can also be safe in patients with a severe exacerbation of asthma [15] or with severe airflow limitation [61]. However, the technique is still generally a research method and must be used cautiously. It should only be used by staff trained to perform the procedure safely.

4.2.8. Cost Utility, Patient Acceptance: It is logical to assume that patients would prefer a noninvasive test like sputum induction to an invasive procedure like bronchoscopy. However there are no scientific studies which have examined patient acceptance of sputum induction compared to other methods. Likewise, economic analysis of cost utility, cost effectiveness or cost minimization of sputum examination compared with other methods of assessing airway inflammation have not been conducted.

5. Sputum Compared with Bronchoscopic Procedures

Direct measurements of airway inflammation by bronchoscopy are considered to be the "gold standards" for assessing airway inflammation. However, their performance has not been investigated to the same extent as sputum examination and they are impractical in practice. Two studies have examined the safety of bronchoscopy and biopsy in bronchial asthma. Djukanovic and co-workers [62] concluded that fiberoptic bronchoscopy with BAL and endobronchial biopsy can be conducted safely in asthmatics under careful monitoring of oximetry except in patients with severe airway hyperresponsiveness. The safety of the procedure was also examined by Van Vyve and colleagues [63], who demonstrated significant deterioration in FEV_1 (75.6% of predicted to 55.3% of predicted) and VC (86.2% of predicted to 64.0% of predicted) in a group of asthmatics with a range of severity of airflow obstruction. However they concluded that the procedure was safe because there was no correlation between the physiological deterioration and clinical severity and because similar deteriorations were observed in normal controls (FEV_1 decreased from a mean 97.1% of predicted to 80.3% of predicted).

There have been only four published studies comparing sputum with these direct measurements. Fahy et al. [28] compared cells and soluble markers in the whole expectorate of induced sputum with BAL and bronchial washings of 10 asthmatics and 10 healthy subjects. The proportion of nonsquamous cells in sputum plus saliva more closely resembled those in washings than in BAL. Maestrelli et al. [48] observed that the agreement of the number of eosinophils in induced sputum and bronchial biopsies was better than the agreement of the same measurement between BAL and biopsies. Keatings and co-workers [64], in a study of 16 asthmatics, showed that the sputum is richer in neutrophils and eosinophils and poor in lymphocytes. Modest correlations were observed between eosinophils and neutrophils in sputum and washings, but not in BAL. Grootendorst and co-workers [65] compared the cellular compositions of hypertonic saline-induced sputum, BAL, bronchial washings and biopsies in 18 clinically stable mild atopic asthmatics, 10 of whom were on regular inhaled steroids. Sputum cell differentials were not significantly different between the patients with and without inhaled steroids. Sputum had higher neutrophil counts (median 28.7%) than washings (2.3%) and BAL (1.4%). The percentage eosinophils in sputum was significantly correlated with the percentage in washings (rs = 0.52, p = 0.03) and BAL (rs = 0.55, p = 0.02). The correlation between the number of eosinophils in sputum and the number of $EG2^+$ eosinophils (/mm^2 lamina propria in bronchial biopsies) however was not significant (rs = 0.44, p = 0.07). The percentage of $CD4^+$ lymphocytes correlated between sputum and BAL (rs = 0.55, p = 0.03).

We have compared the cell (differentially and metachromatically), lymphocyte subsets and fluid phase ECP, fibrinogen and tryptase in induced sputum and BAL [49]. Our results confirmed the previous observations that sputum contained higher proportions of neutrophils and lower proportions of macrophages and higher concentrations of ECP; others have shown higher levels of albumin and mucin-like glycoprotein [28]. In contrast to previous observations, we did not observe correlations between sputum and BAL eosinophil count (ICC 0.4). Furthermore, we observed that both the absolute number and the proportion of eosinophils and the fluid-phase ECP in sputum, but not in BAL, were highly correlated.

These differences in observations between induced sputum measurements and BAL may be accounted for by two factors: firstly, the two methods of investigation provide information about the inflammatory processess in two different airway compartments. BAL particularly samples the peripheral airway and sputum is believed to mostly sample the larger airways. Secondly, BAL results will be influenced by the dilution effect of the fluid used for lavage, and the variable amount of fluid used in different studies makes comparisons difficult. The excellent correlations between the absolute number or proportion of eosinophils and fluid-phase ECP in induced sputum in the absence of similar correlations in BAL may be due to this dilution phenomenon. Sputum measurements, in the expectorate separated from saliva, has a known dilution factor, which overcomes this problem.

Finally, both BAL and bronchial biopsies do not have the same discriminative properties as induced sputum. The repeatability of both measurements have been reported to be poor [66, 67] The high intra-subject variability of BAL measurements makes it a less precise measurement tool than sputum. The results have not been reported as intraclass correlation coefficient, making it difficult to compare them with the repeatability of other instruments such as sputum.

The differences and lack of correlation between sputum measurements and BAL and biopsies do not decrease the construct validity of sputum measurements. This may simply be a reflection of the differences in the discriminative properties of the measurement tools and the type of airway sampling. Moreover, some of the differences may be accounted for by the different techniques involved in processing induced sputum. For example, Pizzichini et al. [49] use sputum selected from saliva, Fahy et al. [28] use whole expectorate, and Keatings et al. [64] and Maestrelli et al. [48] use whole sputum with attempts to minimize salivary contamination.

6. Clinical Usefulness of Sputum Examination

Sputum examination for inflammatory indices is still primarily a research tool. Its place in clinical practice still needs to be evaluated. However, there are theoretical reasons why it should be required as little or as much as any other objective measurement.

As Lord Kelvin has said "When you can measure what you are speaking about and express it in numbers you know something about it; but when you cannot measure it, when you cannot express it in numbers, your knowledge is of a meagre and unsatisfactory kind: it may be the beginning of knowledge, but you have scarcely, in your thoughts, advanced to the stage of *science*, whatever the matter may be [68]". Of course, measurements of airway inflammation must be made accurately, otherwise they will not be reliable and will not be useful in practice. At present, fresh sputum needs to be examined within about 2 h. This can be accomplished by obtaining specimens at the hospital where the processing of sputum and examination is carried out. The measurements require a registered technologist, haematologically trained; in Canada, this is a prerequisite for reporting on clinical specimens in research or practice. The processing and examination of sputum for cell counts, with automation of rocking and staining, takes about 30–45 min of technician time. At present these measurements are simple and robust and, as such, they resemble the FEV_1 in measuring the presence and severity of airflow limitation and have already been introduced in our own practice.

The clinical uses of sputum examination can be considered in relation to diagnosis, causes of inflammation, prediction of response to glucocorticoid or antibiotic treatment, and helping to establish optimum treatment (including the minimum regular treatment required).

6.1. Diagnosis of Eosinophilic Bronchitis

Eosinophilic bronchitis can be defined as the presence of sputum eosinophilia without evidence of peripheral respiratory disease [69]. It occurs in asthma defined as variable airflow limitation [44]. It can occur when variable airflow limitation and airway hyperresponsiveness are only mildly abnormal and also in patients without asthma [45]. The latter has only recently been recognized because it requires measurement of airway inflammation to be diagnosed.

Eosinophilic bronchitis without asthma usually presents with a chronic cough with or without sputum [69]. It can also be associated with chest tightness, wheezing and a feeling of dyspnea when these are not associated with variable airflow limitation. It can occur in cigarette smokers [61] and in atopic or nonatopic subjects. It can be caused by airway reactions to inhaled allergens [53, 57] or occupational chemical sensitizers [54,] [70]. If left untreated, it can become associated with asthma (as indicated by the development of airway hyperresponsiveness) [45,] [71] or with progressive airflow limitation without reversibility to a β_2-agonist or hyperresponsiveness.

Eosinophilic bronchitis, whether it is associated with asthma or not, usually responds to treatment with inhaled glucocorticoids [45, 57]. However, it may require treatment with prednisone [69, 71] and it may be prednisone-dependent [56]. When asthma is not present, inhaled bronchodilators are not required.

6.2. Recognition of the Type of Airway Inflammation and its Cause

The type of airway inflammation may be categorized as eosinophilic, neutrophilic or lymphocytic depending on whether the proportion of eosinophils, neutrophils or lymphocytes respectively are increased. An increase in eosinophils can be caused by reactions to inhaled allergens [53] or chemical sensitizers [54, 70]. It is a common feature of asthma and is exacerbated in steroid-dependent patients when the steroid is reduced below the dose required to suppress it [14, 56].

Serial measurements of sputum cell counts can be useful to confirm occupational allergy or chemical sensitization causing eosinophilic bronchitis without asthma [70] or occupational asthma [72]. If these are present, periods at work are associated with sputum eosinophilia and periods away from work by a reversal of this.

Exacerbations of asthma are usually considered to be eosinophilic. However, they can be neutrophilic [46, 47] and result from viral [73] or bacterial infections [50] or, perhaps, other stimuli. Clinical judgements of the type of inflammation often do not agree with sputum cell counts [74]. Without sputum examination, this will not be recognized and inappropriate treatment may be prescribed.

6.3. Prediction of Response to Treatment with Glucocorticoids

Sputum eosinophilia responds to glucocorticoid treatment in patients with chronic cough without asthma [45], in patients with asthma [15, 55] and in smokers with chronic airflow limitation [61]. Those patients without eosinophilia do not seem to respond. The latter has been prospectively investigated in chronic cough [75] and in a pilot study of smokers with moderate to severe chronic airflow limitation [61]. Amongst asthmatics, there is supportive evidence [15] but no prospective investigation.

These observations are clearly important in interpreting research trials to investigate drugs in the treatment of airway diseases. If subjects are selected without sputum eosinophilia, drugs with anti-eosinophilic effects but no bronchodilator or bronchoprotective effects will be ineffective. This is one of the reasons that patients on regular treatment with inhaled steroid who have uncontrolled symptoms are more likely to benefit from added inhaled long-acting β-agonists than from the addition of inhaled steroid.

6.4. To Monitor the Effects of Antiinflammatory Drugs in Difficult-to-Control Asthma

Patients who seem to require regular treatment with prednisone (e.g. prednisone-dependent asthma) may benefit from serial objective measurements of sputum cell counts as well as from spirometry. Patients who are truly prednisone-dependent [14, 56], have sputum eosinophilia when on suboptimal treatment. When they are given an adequate high dose, sputum eosinophilia usually disappears [56]. When the dose of prednisone is reduced, sputum eosinophilia recurs before a clinical and physiological exacerbation and before the development of blood eosinophilia. Serial measurements may therefore be useful to establish the minimum regular dose of prednisone that is required. Some patients who are thought to be prednisone-dependent are not [50]. In these sputum eosinophilia is not a feature and exacerbations are neutrophilic. Because of the latter, exacerbations may be treated without additional prednisone.

The value of monitoring sputum cell counts in treating airway disease in general needs to be investigated.

7. Summary

Sputum examination has become an established tool to assess airway inflammation. It is the most evaluated of all measurement tools available for this purpose. It is valid, repeatable, responsive and safe. Sputum induction takes about 30–45 min and sputum examination about 2 h. The procedure can be performed at any time of day, at random, in more severe forms of airway disease, and performed repeatedly. There are some recent data suggesting that repeated sputum examination within 24 h affects the cell differential counts, but these have yet to be confirmed. Sputum examination may be handled by any haematology laboratory. However it is important to adequately train the laboratory personnel and to establish regular quality control so that the reliability of results is ensured. The method is non-invasive and has comparable, if not better, discriminative properties to the invasive direct methods of assessing airway inflammation, and is therefore a logical alternative to these. The role of measuring airway inflammation in general, and sputum examination in particular, in routine clinical practice now needs proper investigation.

Acknowledgments

This chapter is dedicated to the memory of the late Professor Jerry Dolovich who was actively involved in our research program. Drs. Emilio and Marcia Pizzichini conducted most of the recent original research reported in this chapter. The research has received funding from the Medical Research Council of Canada, Ontario Thoracic Society, Father Sean O'Sullivan Research Centre, Astra Pharma Inc., Boehringer-Ingelheim (Canada) Inc., and GlaxoWellcome. We gratefully acknowledge the help and expertise of all members of the Asthma Research Group and of our clinical and blood and sputum research laboratories. We are grateful to Lori Burch for her secretarial assistance.

References

1　Taylor DEM, Whamond J (1977) *Non-invasive clinical measurement*. University Park Press, London, ix–xv
2　*Dorland's Illustrated Medical Dictionary* (1988) WB Saunders Company, Philadelphia, p 835
3　Osler W (1892) *The principles and practice of medicine*. Appleton and Co, New York, p 497
4　Weissman G (1988) Inflammation: Historical perspectives. *In*: JI Gallin et al. (eds): *Inflammation—Basic principles and clinical correlates*. Raven Press, New York, 5
5　Ernst P, FitzGerald JM, Spier S (1996) Canadian asthma consensus conference: summary of recommendations. *Can Respir J* 3: 89–100
6　Sheffer AL, Bousquet J, Busse WW et al (1992) International consensus report on the diagnosis and management of asthma. Publication 92-3091, US Department of Health and Human Services, National Institute of Health, Bethesda, Maryland,. *Eur Respir J* 5: 601–41
7　O'Byrne PM, Hargreave FE (1994) Non-invasive monitoring of airway inflammation. *Am J Respir Crit Care Med* 150: S100–2
8　Kharitonov SA, Yates D, Robbins RA, Logan-Sinclair R, Shinebourne EA, Barnes PJ (1994) Increased nitric oxide in exhaled air of asthmatic patients. *Lancet* 343: 133–5
9　Iikura Y, Yamada T, Akasawa A, Ebisawa M, Katasunuma T (1993) Monitoring of inflammation in relation to pathophysiology. *Allergy* 48: 138–42
10　Paganin F, Seneterre E, Chanez P et al (1996) Computed tomography of the lungs in asthma: influence of disease severity and etiology. *Am J Respir Crit Care Med* 153: 110–4
11　Fletcher FH, Fletcher SW, Wagner EH (1996) *In*: *Clinical Epidemiology-the essentials*. Williams and Wilkins 19–42
12　Gibson PG, Wong BJO, Hepperle MJE, Kline PA, Girgis-Gabardo A, Guyatt G et al (1992) A research method to induce and examine a mild exacerbation of asthma by withdrawal of inhaled corticosteroid. *Clin Exp Allergy* 22: 525–32
13　Kendrick AH, Higgs CMB, Whitfield MJ, Laszlo G (1993) Accuracy of perception of severity of asthma: patients treated in general practice. *BMJ* 307: 422–4
14　Pavord ID, Pizzichini MMM, Clelland L, Efthimiadis A, Hargreave FE (1996) Sputum inflammatory cell characteristics of prednisone dependent asthma. *Am J Respir Crit Care Med* 153: A293
15　Pizzichini MMM, Pizzichini E, Clelland L, Efthimiadis A, Mahony J, Dolovich J, Hargreave FE (1997) Sputum in severe exacerbations of asthma: kinetics of inflammatory indices after prednisone treatment. *Am J Respir Crit Care Med* 155: 1501–8
16　Kirby JG, Hargreave FE, Gleich GJ, O'Byrne PM (1987) Bronchoalveolar cell profiles of asthmatic and non-asthmatic subjects. *Am Rev Respir Dis* 136: 379–83
17　Wardlaw AJ, Dunnette S, Gleich GJ, Collins JV, Kay AB (1988) Eosinophils and mast cells in bronchoalveolar lavage in subjects with mild asthma. *Am Rev Respir Dis* 137: 62–9
18　Cartier A, Thompson NC, Frith PA, Roberts R, Hargreave FE (1982) Allergen-induced increase

in bronchial responsiveness to histamine: relationsihp to the late asthmatic response and change in airway calibre. *J Allerg Clin Immunol* 70: 170–7

19 Twentyman OP, Holgate ST (1988) The temporal development of increased bronchial responsiveness following allergen challenge and its relationship to the late asthmatic reaction. *Am Rev Respir Dis* 137: 135

20 Josephs LK, Gregg I, Mullee MA, Holgate ST (1989) Nonspecific bronchial reactivity and its relationship to the clinical expression of asthma. *Am Rev Respir Dis* 140: 350–7

21 Barnes PJ, Kharitonov SA (1996) Exhaled nitric oxide: a new lung function test. *Thorax* 51: 233–7

22 Kharitonov SA, O'Connor BJ, Evans DJ, Barnes PJ (1995) Allergen induced late asthmatic reactions are associated with elevation of exhaled nitric oxide. *Am J Respir Crit Care Med* 151: 1894–9

23 Jatakanon A, Lim S, Kharitonov SA, Chung KF, Barnes PJ (1998) Correlation between exhaled nitric oxide, sputum eosinophils and metacholine responsiveness in patients with mild asthma. *Thorax 53: 91–95*

24 Kharitonov SA, Wells AU, O'Connor BJ, Hansell DM, Cole PJ, Barnes PJ (1995) Elevated levels of exhaled nitric oxide in bronchiectasis. *Am J Respir Crit Care Med* 151: 1889–93

25 Kharitonov SA, Yates D, Barnes PJ (1995) Increased nitric oxide in exhaled air or normal human subjects with upper respiratory tract infections. *Eur Respir J* 8: 295–297

26 Taylor IK, Hill AA, Hayes B et al (1996) Imaging allergen-invoked airway inflammation in atopic asthma with [18F]-flurodeoxyglucose and positron emission tomography. *Lancet* 347: 937–940

27 Kips JC, Fahy JV, Hargreave FE, Ind PW, in't Veen JCCM (1998) Position paper on methods for sputum induction and analysis of induced sputum as a method for assessing airway inflammation in asthma. *Eur Respir J* 11(Suppl. 26): 9S–12S

28 Fahy JV, Wong H, Liu J, Boushey HA (1995) Comparison of samples collected by sputum induction and bronchoscopy from asthmatic and healthy subjects. *Am J Respir Crit Care Med* 152: 53–8

29 Pin I, Gibson PG, Kolendowicz et al (1992) Use of induced sputum cell counts to investigate airway inflammation in asthma. *Thorax* 47: 25–9

30 Iredale MJ, Wanklyn SAR, Philips IP, Krauz T, Ind PW (1994) Non-invasive assessment of bronchial inflammation in asthma: no correlation between eosinophilia of induced sputum and bronchial responsiveness to inhaled hypertonic saline. *Clin Exp Allergy* 24: 940–5

31 Popov TA, Pizzichini E, Kolendowicz R et al (1995) Some technical factors influencing the induction of sputum for cell analysis. *Eur Respir J* 8: 559–65

32 Pizzichini E, Pizzichini MMM, Efthimiadis A, Hargreave FE, Dolovich J (1996) Measurement of inflammatory indices in induced sputum: effects of selection of sputum to minimize salivary contamination. *Eur Respir J* 9: 1174–80

33 Pizzichini MMM, Popov T, Efthimiadis A et al (1996) Spontaneous and induced sputum to measure indices of airway inflammation. *Am J Respir Crit Care Med* 154: 866–9

34 Efthimiadis A, Pizzichini E, Pizzichini MMM, Hargreave FE (1997) Sputum examination for indices of airway inflammation: laboratory procedures. Astra Draco AB, Lund, Sweden

35 Pizzichini E, Pizzichini MMM, Efthimiadis A et al (1996) Indices of inflammation in induced sputum: reproducibility and validity of cell and fluid phase measurements. *Am J Respir Crit Care Med* 154: 308–17

36 Keatings VM, Barnes PJ (1997) Granulocyte activation markers in induced sputum: comparison between chronic obstructive pulmonary disease, asthma and normal subjects. *Am J Respir Crit Care Med* 155: 449–53

37 Keatings VM, Collins PD, Scott DM, Barnes PJ (1996) differences in interleukin-8 and tumor necrosis factor-α in induced sputum from patients with chronic obstructive pulmonary disease or asthma. *Am J Respir Crit Care Med* 153: 530–4

38 Kurashima K, Mukaida N, Fujimura M et al (1996) Increase of chemokine levels in sputum precedes exacerbation of acute asthma attacks. *J Leukocyte Biol* 59: 313–6

39 Tomaki M, Ichinose M, Miura M et al (1995) Elevated substance P content in induced sputum from patients with asthma and patients with chronic bronchitis. *Am J Respir Crit Care Med* 151: 613–7

40 Louis R, Shute J, Biagi S et al (1997) Cell infiltration, ICAM-1 expression and eosinophil chemotactic activity in asthmatic sputum. *Am J Respir Crit Care Med* 155: 466–72

41 Schoonbrood DFM, Lutter R, Habets FJM et al (1994) Analysis of plasma-protein leakage and

local secretion in sputum from patients with asthma and chronic obstructive pulmonary disease. *Am J Respir Crit Care Med* 150: 1519-27

42 Evans DJ, Barnes PJ, Spaethe SM et al (1996) Effect of a leukotriene B4 receptor antagonist LY293111 on allergen induced responses in asthma. *Thorax* 51: 1178-84

43 Fahy JV, Steiger DJ, Liu J, Basbaum CB, Finkbeiner WE, Boushey H (1993) Markers of mucus secretion and DNA levels in induced sputum from asthmatic and from healthy subjects. *Am Rev Respir Dis* 147: 1132-7

44 Gibson PG, Girgis-Gabardo A, Hargreave FE et al (1989) Cellular characteristics of sputum from patients with asthma and chronic bronchitis. *Thorax* 44: 693-9

45 Gibson PG, Hargreave FE, Girgis-Gabardo A, Morris MM, Denburg JA, Dolovich J (1995) Chronic cough with eosinophilic bronchitis and examination for variable airflow obstruction and response to corticosteroid. *Clin Exp Allergy* 25: 127-32

46 Turner MO, Hussack P, Sears MR, Dolovich J, Hargreave FE (1995) Exacerbations of asthma without sputum eosinophilia. *Thorax* 50: 1057-61

47 Fahy JV, Kim KW, Liu J, Boushey HA (1995) Prominent neutrophilic inflammation in sputum from subjects with asthma exacerbation. *J Allerg Clin Immunol* 95: 843-52

48 Maestrelli P, Saetta M, Di Stefanno A et al (1995) Comparison of leukocyte counts in sputum, bronchial biopsies and bronchoalveolar lavage. *Am J Respir Crit Care Med* 152: 1926-31

49 Pizzichini E, Pizzichini MMM, Kidney JC, Efthimiadis A, Popov T, Cox G, Dolovich J, O'Byrne PM, Hargreave FE (1998) Induced sputum, bronchoalveolar lavage and blood from mild asthmatics: inflammatory cells, lymphocyte subsets and soluble markers compared. *Eur Respir J* 11: 828-834

50 Parameswaran K, Pizzichini MMM, Li D, Pizzichini E, Jeffery PK, Hargreave FE (1998) Serial sputum cell counts in the management of chronic airflow limitation. *Eur Respir J* 11: 1405-1408

51 In't Veen JCCM, de Gouw HWFM, Smits HH et al (1996) Repeatability of cellular and soluble markers of inflammation in induced sputum from patients with asthma. *Eur Respir J* 9: 2441-7

52 Kidney JC, Wong AG, Efthimiadis A et al (1996) Elevated B-cells in sputum of asthmatics: close correlation with eosinophils. *Am J Respir Crit Care Med* 153: 540-4

53 Pin I, Freitag AP, O'Byrne PM et al (1992) Changes in the cellular profile of induced sputum after allergen-induced asthmatic responses. *Am Rev Respir Dis* 145: 1265-9

54 Maestrelli P, Calcagni PG, Saetta M et al (1994) Sputum eosinophilia after responses induced by isocyanates in sensitized subjects. *Clin Exp Allergy* 24: 29-34

55 Claman DM, Boushey DA, Liu J, Wong H, Fahy JV (1994) Analysis of induced sputum to examine the effects of prednisone on airway inflammation in asthmatic subjects. *J Allerg Clin Immunol* 94: 861-9

56 Pizzichini MMM, Pizzichini E, Clelland E, Efthimiadis A, Pavord I, Dolovich J, Hargreave FE (1999) Prednisone dependent asthma: inflammatory indices in induced sputum. *Eur Respir J* 13: 15-21

57 Gauvreau GM, Doctor J, Watson RM, Jordana M, O'Byrne PM (1996) Effects of inhaled budesonide on allergen induced airway responses and inflammation. *Am J Respir Crit Care Med* 154: 1267-71

58 Pizzichini E, Pizzichini MMM, Efthimiadis A, Dolovich J, Hargreave FE (1997) Measuring airway inflammation in asthma: eosinophils and eosinophilic cationic protein in induced sputum compared with peripheral blood. *J Allerg Clin Immunol* 99: 539-44

59 Anderson SD, Smith CM, Rodwell LT, du Toit JI, Riedler J, Robertson CF (1995) The use of non-isotonic aerosols for evaluating bronchial hyperresponsiveness. *In*: CL Spector (ed): *Provocation testing in clinical practice*. Marcel Dekker, New York, 249-78

60 Wong HH, Fahy JV (1997) Safety of one method of sputum induction. Am Rev Respir *Crit Care Med* 156: 299-303

61 Pizzichini E, Pizzichini MMM, Gibson P, Parameswaran K, Gleich GJ, Berman L, Dolovich J, Hargreave FE (1998) Sputum eosinophilia predicts benefit from prednisone in smokers with chronic obstructive bronchitis. *Am J Respir Crit Care Med* 158: 1511-1517

62 Djukanovic R, Wilson JW, Lai CKW, Holgate ST, Howarth PH (1991) The safety aspects of fiberoptic bronchoscopy, bronchoalveolar lavage, and endobronchial biopsy in asthma. *Am Rev Respir Dis* 143: 772-7

63 Van Vyve T, Chanez P, Bousquet J, Lacoste J, Michel F, Godard P (1992) Safety of bronchoalveolar lavage and bronchial biopsies in patients with asthma of variable severity. *Am Rev Respir Dis* 146: 116-21

64 Keatings VM, Evans DJ, O'Connor BJ (1997) Cellular profiles in asthmatic airways: a comparison of induced sputum, bronchial washings and bronchoalveolar lavage fluid. *Thorax* 52: 372–4
65 Grootendorst DC, Sont JK, Willems LNA et al (1997) Comparison of inflammatory cell counts in asthma: induced sputum vs bronchoalveolar lavage and bronchial biopsies. *Clin Exp Allergy* 27: 769–79
66 Ward C, Gardiner PV, Booth H, Walters EH (1995) Intrasubject variability in airway inflammation sampled by bronchoalveolar lavage in stable asthmatics. *Eur Respir J* 8: 1866–71
67 Richmond I, Booth H, Ward C, Walters EH (1996) Intrasubject variability in airway inflammation in biopsies in mild to moderate stable asthma. *Am J Respir Crit Care Med* 153: 899–903
68 Thomson Sir Wm (Lord Kelvin). (1891) Electrical units of measurement. *In: Popular lectures and addresses*. MacMillan and Co, London, 80–143
69 Gibson PG, Dolovich J, Denburg J, Ramsdale EH, Hargreave FE (1989) Chronic cough: eosinophilic bronchitis without asthma. *Lancet* 1346–8
70 Lemiere C, Efthimiadis A, Hargreave FE (1997) Occupational eosinophilic bronchitis without asthma: an unknown occupational airway disease. *J Allergy Clin Immunol* 100: 852–853
71 Wong AG, Pavord ID, Sears MR, Hargreave FE (1996) A case for serial examination of sputum inflammatory cells. *Eur Respir J* 9: 2174–5
72 Lemiere C, Pizzichini MMM, Balkissoon R, Efthimiadis A, Clelland L, O'Shaughnessy D, Dolovich J, Hargreave FE (1999) Diagnosing occupational asthma: use of induced sputum. *Eur Respir J* 13: 482–488
73 Pizzichini E, Pizzichini MMM, Johnston S, Hussack P, Efthimiadis A, Mahony J, Dolovich J, Hargreave FE (1998) Asthma and natural colds: inflammatory indices in induced sputum. A feasibility study. *Am J Respir Crit Care Med* 158: 1178–1184
74 Parameswaran K, Pizzichini E, Pizzichini MMM, Hussack P, Efthimiadis A, Hargreave FE (1999) Clinical judgement of airway inflammation *versus* sputum cell counts in patients with asthma. *Eur Respir J*; *in press*
75 Pizzichini MMM, Pizzichini E, Parameswaran K, Clelland L, Efthimiadis A, Dolovich J, Hargreave FE (1999) Non-asthmatic chronic cough: no effect of treatment with an inhaled corticosteroid in patients without sputum eosinophilia. *Can Respir J* 6: 323–330

CHAPTER 5
Treatment of Asthma in Children: the Case for Inhaled Corticosteroids as First Line Agents

Søren Pedersen

University of Odense, DK-5000 Odense, Denmark

1. Introduction

Decisions about the use of a drug in any group of patients should be based upon the knowledge about beneficial and adverse effects. Appropriate data is obtained through controlled clinical trials in patients of a similar age and disease severity as the group in which the drug is being considered for use. Abundant, high quality clinical efficacy and safety data have been obtained on the use of inhaled corticosteroids in children >3 years of age with mild, moderate and severe asthma. Our knowledge about the use of inhaled corticosteroids and other drugs in children ≤3 years is more limited. Therefore, recommendations about pharmacological asthma management in the ≤3 age group are based upon less evidence than the recommendations for older children.

Several issues must be considered when positioning a drug in asthma management. Some of the more important are:
- The aims and outcome measures of asthma treatment
- The dose of drug which is required to achieve these aims

- Comparison of the clinical efficacy of a particular drug with the efficacy of other treatments or no treatment at all
- Influence of timing on the clinical effect
- Cost-effectiveness
- The risk of clinically important side-effects at doses required to control the disease to the same extent as other treatments

In the following, these issues will be briefly discussed and summarized in order to provide the reader with some important information for therapeutic decision making.

2. Aims and Outcome Measures of Treatment

The choice of treatment to a great extent depends on which goals (outcomes) the physician wants to achieve. Over the years the aims of asthma management have changed markedly from effective prn. treatment of symptoms and exacerbations towards more use of continuous prophylactic treatment. This change seems to have become widespread judging by the various international guidelines. With the new therapeutic strategy definition of the aims of treatment and assessment of optimal asthma control has become much more complex and difficult.

The goals of asthma treatment of children are twofold (Tab. 1). *The immediate aim* is to produce the maximum achievable effect on all outcome parameters. *The long-term aim* is to prevent complications of the disease or its pharmacological treatment. If the immediate aim is not achieved the risk of also missing the long-term aim is increased. On this basis the *undertreatment of asthma* can be clearly defined (Fig. 1) as:

I. The maximum effect on an outcome is not achieved by the treatment

II. An insufficient number of outcomes is affected by the treatment

Table 1. The goals of asthma treatment of children are dual. The *immediate aims* are to produce a maximum achievable effect on all outcome parameters. The *long-term aim* is to prevent complications by the disease or its pharmacological treatment

---

Important for choice of first-line therapy:

Achieve optimal control

    Maximal effect

    Effect on as many outcome parameters as possible

Prevent complications

    Interference with normal social interactions and development

    Consequences of airway remodelling

    Clinical side-effects of the treatment

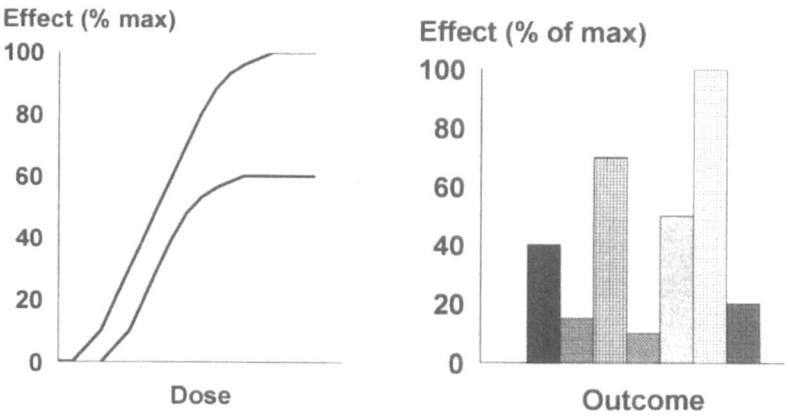

Figure 1. Undertreatment of asthma is seen 1) When the maximum effect on an outcome is not achieved by the treatment, or 2) when an insufficient number of outcomes is affected by the treatment. Inhaled corticosteroids beneficially affect more outcome parameters to a greater extent than any other asthma drug in the majority of children with asthma.

In day to day management most physicians would agree that an optimally controlled child with asthma lives a normal life without *any* restrictions in physical activity and without *any* asthma symptoms or exacerbations. Lung functions are "normal" and increase over time as in healthy non-asthmatic children. Furthermore, the child has good knowledge about the disease, is confident about self-management and experiences no side-effects from the treatment. This level of control probably requires that bronchial reactivity is within the normal range and that inflammatory changes in the airways are minimal.

Though these objectives seem pretty straightforward, and are achievable in the majority of children clinical experience and review of the literature suggest that they are not fulfilled in many children and that undertreatment is common [14]. The main reason for this seems to be variations in the perception and definition of the terms *symptom free, normal lung functions and inaccurate assessment of the daily physical activity and degree of restriction of lifestyle of the child.* Several studies have shown that asthma severity and the impact of disease on daily life are often greatly underestimated because of the difficulty in correctly assessing symptoms and the extent to which the child has adapted his or her lifestyle to avoid symptoms [1, 3, 4]. As a consequence many children are undertreated, optimal asthma control is not achieved and effective treatment is either not prescribed or prescribed after the asthmatic condition has progressed for a number of years.

Historically, the most extensively studied outcome parameters for anti-asthma drugs has been improvement in 1) symptoms and 2) lung function. However, during recent years, other outcome parameters have been recognized to be of similar or even greater importance than improvement in symptoms and peak expiratory flow rate. These include 3) reduction in frequency and severity of acute exacerbations, 4) reduction in mortality and morbidity, 5) control of airway hyperresponsiveness, 6) normalization of the chronic inflammatory changes in the airways, 7) improvement in quality of life, 8) normalisation of physical activity 9) prevention of airway remodelling and 10) normal growth of lung function. Furthermore, the question of whether early intervention with treatment can 11) change the natural course or even 12) cure the underlying disease are important issues to consider when the response to treatment is evaluated.

Our understanding of the effect of various drugs on these different aspects of control of disease is at a very early stage. The *dose* of drug sufficient to normalize lung function may be quite different from the dose required to control other outcomes. Furthermore, a certain *drug* may produce excellent control of one outcome such as symptoms without having any significant effects upon another such as exacerbations [5]. Finally, the *time-course* of the effect on the various parameters differs. Improvements in lung function and symptoms often precede and reach a plateau before the maximum reduction in responsiveness [6].

Because of this complexity and difficulty with correct monitoring in daily clinical practice it is important to choose a prophylactic therapy, which has been shown in controlled clinical trials to affect as many outcomes as much as possible and to a greater extent than other available therapies. If this is not done the risk of undertreatment will be substantial.

3. Effects of Inhaled Corticosteroids on Various Clinical Outcome Measures

In the clinical situation it is almost impossible for the prescribing physician to accurately to assess if all the goals have been achieved. At present the best outcome or clinically most important combination of outcome parameters is not known. Therefore, it is *important to choose a first-line treatment which has been shown to influence as many outcome parameters as possible*. Such strategy is likely to reduce the risk of undertreatment. In this respect inhaled steroids normally have a significant and greater effect upon more outcome parameters than any other anti-asthma drug in patients with asthma regardless of disease severity. Inhaled corticosteroids have been documented in controlled trials in both children and adults to have a significant and often marked effects upon outcome parameters 1–10. Continuous use improves day- and night-time symptoms and lung function, reduces morbidity, mortality, the frequency of acute exacerbations and the number of hospital admissions, improves bronchial hyperreactivity, quality of life and capacity for physical activity, reduces chronic inflammatory changes in the airways, airway remodelling and restrictions in daily activities, and ensures normal growth of lung function [1, 2, 5–46]. Furthermore, some studies have suggested that inhaled steroids may also have an effect upon the natural course of the disease [2, 47, 48].

Controlled trials of all other asthma drugs in the chronic treatment of children have mainly shown a significant and reproducible effects on parameters 1 and 2 and, infrequently, a limited effect on parameters 7 and 8.

Undoubtedly, many of the outcomes are to some extent related to the degree of airway inflammation, which has been shown to exist in *all* disease severities. However, at present we do not have the tools to measure all aspects of airway inflammation in the day to day management of the disease in children. Furthermore, it is not clear to what extent the inflammatory process must be suppressed or which aspects of inflammation need to be controlled to influence the various parameters. While most drugs possess some anti-inflammatory actions no other drug has been shown in controlled studies to affect the chronic inflammation of the airways to the same extent as inhaled corticosteroids. Inhaled corticosteroids produce anti-inflammatory effects which are superior to those of all other anti-asthma drugs. The only component of the disease which may not respond to inhaled corticosteroids is the increased airway responsiveness caused by structural changes in the airways. In contrast to other drugs, steroids not only shift the dose response curve to spasmogens to the right, but also limit the maximum narrowing in response to spasmogens [49].

4. The Inhaled Steroid Dose Required to Achieve Treatment Aims

The dose of inhaled steroid required to achieve the aims of treatment seems to depend upon:
• The outcome measure studied
• The duration of administration of the inhaled steroid
• The severity of the disease
• The drug/inhaler combination used for the administration
• The age of the patient
• The duration of asthma when treatment is initiated

As a consequence, each child may have her/his own individual dose-response curve. However, some general, superior conclusions about inhaled corticosteroid dose-response relationships can be made:

Marked and rapid clinical improvements and changes in symptoms and lung function are seen at very low daily doses (around 100 µg) of inhaled steroids in most children with moderate and severe asthma [34, 35, 50, 51]. These improvements in lung function and symptoms precede and reach a plateau before a reduction in airway responsiveness is seen [52]. Additional improvement in these parameters with increasing doses is rather small, often taking an additional four-fold increase in dose to produce further significant effect. Therefore, low doses are clinically so effective that even very large, well conducted studies normally fail to show any statistically significant or clinically relevant additional effect on symptoms and lung function when the dose is increased beyond 100 µg per day [51].

The dose-response curve for other outcome parameters is less thoroughly studied. It may be less steep in children with moderate and severe asthma [50] although this is probably not the case in children with mild asthma, who seem to reach the top of the dose-response curve with low daily doses of inhaled steroids [1, 53, 54]. Thus, in children with moderate and severe asthma, 4 weeks treatment with a daily dose of 400 µg budesonide from a spacer (equivalent to 200 µg from Turbuhaler or 200 µg fluticasone propionate) produces about 85% of the maximum achievable protection against exercise induced asthma [50, 54]. No dose response studies on the anti-inflammatory effects have been performed in children. Budesonide at a daily dose of 400 µg has been shown to normalize NO levels in exhaled air [55]. In a biopsy study in adults fluticasone propionate 500 µg/day had a marked antiinflammatory effect and also seemed to influence airway remodelling [46], indicating that quite marked anti-inflammatory effects are also seen at low doses. However, further studies are needed.

This means that the vast majority of school children will achieve optimal symptom control and maximum effect on peak expiratory flow rates, and a marked and clinically significant effect on other outcome parameters at daily doses of <400 µg/day of inhaled steroids [1, 26, 31, 32, 34, 35, 50, 52, 54, 56–58]. Thus a recent dose reduction trial on 216 children with moderate asthma found that the minimal effective daily dose of inhaled corticosteroid required to maintain optimal lung function and clinical control, and prevent exercise induced asthma was 188 µg budesonide from Turbuhaler and 180 µg fluticasone propionate from Diskhaler [54]. The marked efficacy of low doses of inhaled steroids has also been confirmed in clinical trials and dose-response studies in adults [51, 59, 61].

5. Clinical Efficacy and Comparisons with Other Anti-Asthma Drugs

The beneficial effects of inhaled steroids in children are more pronounced than for any other anti-asthma drug as shown in a number of studies [1, 2, 5, 24, 25, 33, 38, 39, 44, 45, 62–64]. In two recent studies, including one from general practice, children with mild and moderate asthma achieved markedly better symptom control, significantly higher morning and evening peak expiratory flow rates and clinical lung function, and reported fewer adverse events during treatment with 50 µg fluticasone propionate twice daily as compared with children treated with DSCG 20 mg four times daily [1, 45] (Fig. 2). Similar results were also reported with budesonide 400 µg/day from a spacer [25, 64]. In three other studies, 200 and 400 µg beclomethasone propionate per day was significantly more effective than continuous theophylline treatment administered in optimal doses in combination with inhaled bronchodilators [38, 39, 62]. Furthermore, inhaled budesonide 400 µg/day was better than nedocromil

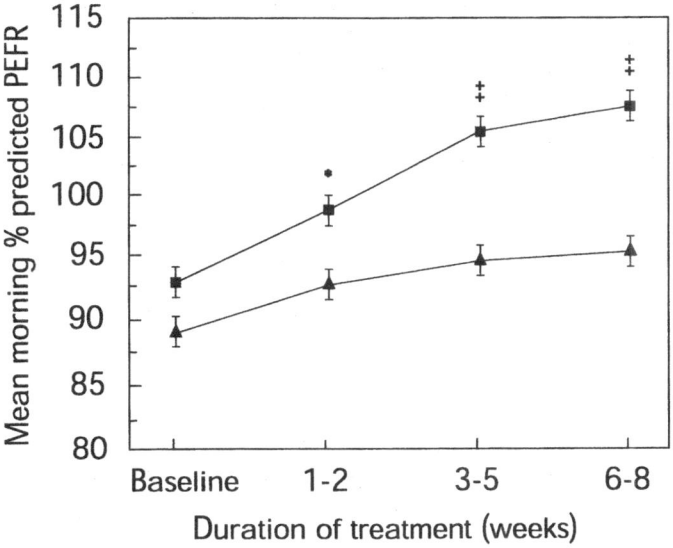

Figure 2. Mean morning (SE) peak expiratory flow rate (PEFR) expressed as percent of that predicted in children with mild asthma treated with ■ = fluticasone propionate, 50 μg b.i.d (n = 110), ▲ = cromolyn sodium, 20 mg qid (n = 115); *$p < 0.05$; ++$p < 0.0001$ [1].

[33], sodium cromoglycate [44], salmeterol 50 μg b.i.d [55, 65] or combinations of all other asthma drugs [2]. Finally, beclomethasone 400 μg/day was recently shown in two long-term studies to be clinically more effective than salmeterol 50 μg b.i.d on a variety of outcome parameters, including symptoms, lung functions, exacerbations and bronchial hyperreactivity [5, 63]. In all these studies, a fixed dose of inhaled corticosteroid was used (dose titration was not performed); in light of the dose-response relationships described earlier, it is likely that similar results could have been achieved at lower doses of inhaled corticosteroid in many of the studies. This assumption is indirectly supported by the similarity between the findings of studies using daily doses of 100 μg and studies using doses of 400 μg/day.

So far, no controlled clinical studies have found other drugs to be more effective than inhaled steroids in children or adults with asthma.

6. Timing—Early Treatment Produces Better Results

A recent long-term study provided interesting information about the beneficial clinical effects associated with long-term continuous use of inhaled steroids [2]. The improvement in lung function was significantly greater in children who started budesonide treatment early (within 2 years) after the onset of

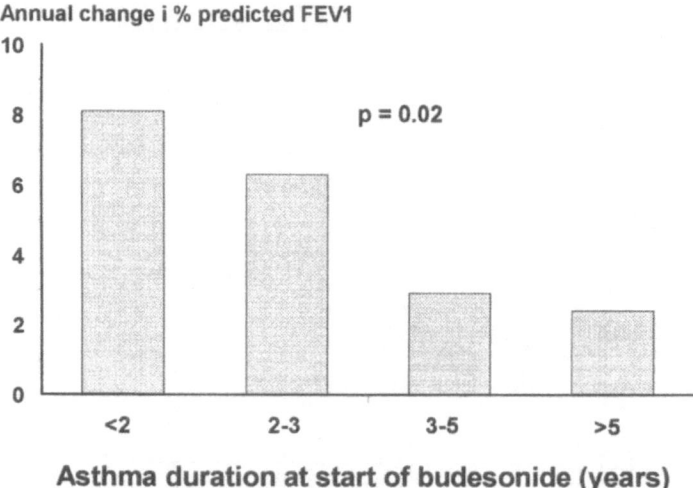

Annual change i % predicted FEV1

p = 0.02

Asthma duration at start of budesonide (years)

Figure 3. Annual increase (i%) predicted FEV₁ in relation to the duration of asthma at the time when treatment with inhaled budesonide was initiated [2].

asthma than in children who did not start the treatment until some years after onset of asthma symptoms (Fig. 3). In addition, children who started early had better lung function at a lower accumulated dose of budesonide during the first 4.5 years of treatment than children in whom inhaled steroids were not initiated until after more than 5 years of symptoms. The development of the lung functions in the group of children who did not receive inhaled corticosteroids, was slower inthe group of the corticosteroid-treated children. The average annual "loss" of lung function was around 1% in FEV_1, compared with the expected growth over time. These findings strongly suggest that early treatment with inhaled steroids may prevent airway remodelling and the development of irreversible structural changes in the airways. Recently, similar findings have been reported in other studies of children and adults where early introduction of inhaled corticosteroids produced a better clinical effect compared with late introduction [47, 48, 6670]. The findings of these studies speak strongly for introducing inhaled steroid treatment early rather than late in the treatment schedule. Similar findings have not been reported with other drugs in controlled prospective studies.

7. Cost-Effectiveness Considerations

When the effects of therapy on disease are assessed, it is important to consider not only effectiveness in modifying the physiological parameters of disease, but also the influence on health-care costs. If two treatments are equally effective and safe, other factors, including the costs of the two alternatives, are important to consider when choosing therapy.

A number of studies have evaluated the cost effectiveness of intervention with inhaled corticosteroids in children. In a detailed analysis of costs involved in adding an inhaled corticosteroid to inhaled β_2-agonists, there was an expected increase in drug costs, but this was compensated for by savings in the use of medical services. Furthermore, for similar costs patients experienced significant advantages in terms of symptom control and increased activity [71]. These findings concur with the results of another prospective study which compared inhaled budesonide and placebo in preschool children with wheeze [43]. This study found that total health-care costs were higher in the placebo group due to greater indirect and other direct expenses incurred in that group. For each US$ spent on budesonide total costs were reduced by 2.6 US$.

Inhaled budesonide has also been compared with other non-steroidal anti-asthma treatments in a long-term (up to 7 years) study of 278 children. In that study, inhaled budesonide treatment was associated with a greater than 50% reduction in annual direct health care costs per child and provided improved asthma control compared with other non-steroidal anti-asthma treatments [72]. Each US$ spent on budesonide was associated with a reduction in health-care costs of 2.9 US$.

These results agree with the findings of a recent study comparing inhaled fluticasone treatment with sodium cromoglycate in children with mild and moderate asthma: The inhaled steroid was found to be makedly more cost-effective than sodium cromoglycate [73]. It was calculated that the cost of one symptom-free day was 1 US$ in the fluticasone group and 2.5 US$ in the sodium cromoglycate group.

These four studies and several studies in adults clearly show that treatment with inhaled corticosteroids is very cost-effective, not only in children with severe asthma but also in children with moderate and mild disease severity. Inhaled corticosteroids are normally more cost-effective than other anti-asthma treatment. This conclusion seems to be true not only for industrialized countries but also for developing countries.

8. Risk of Side-Effects

The occurrence of systemic effects has been extensively studied over the past 20 years without a clear definition of the various terms. Often no distinction is made between a a measurable systemic effect and a clinically relevant systemic side-effect. Whether a systemic effect is measurable or not depends entirely upon the sensitivity of the method used for the measurement: when more sensitive methods are utilized, more systemic effects become measurable. Thus, for a given drug or inhaler, there will always be a dose below which no systemic effects can be detected no matter which method is used. As the dose increases, there will be a dose range within which systemic effects are measurable in one or more systems. However, more often than not, these measurable effects merely reflect small changes within the normal range of the normal biological feedback system or are chance findings without clinical relevance. For example, studies have found sodium cromoglycate treatment to be associated with significant effects upon the excretion of growth hormone in the urine [74] and markers of bone metabolism [75]. Treatment with inhaled β_2-agonists has also been found to adversely affect the secretion of growth hormone [76, 77]. Although statistically significant, these findings are probably not clinically relevant. The same is the case for some of the findings with inhaled steroids. Finally, there will be a dose level beyond which the drug may be associated with clinically important systemic side-effects in one or more systems.

Our knowledge about the dose level at which measurable systemic effects are seen is quite good. It varies with different steroid/inhaler combinations [51, 78] and conclusions from one drug/inhaler combination cannot be extrapolated to other drug/inhaler combinations. It can usually be assumed that doses which are not associated with any measurable systemic effects in sensitive laboratory test systems are also clinically safe.

A recent study suggested that significant differences may exist between findings in patients and healthy volunteers [79], the systemic effects being markedly higher in healthy volunteers than patients. Therefore, the results of studies of systemic activity of inhaled corticosteroids should preferably be performed in patients with moderate-to-severe asthma. For inhaled steroids, the vast majority of safety data has been obtained in school children with mild asthma who have not required the doses of inhaled corticosteroid under investigation to be optimally controlled. Furthermore, many studies have been conducted under artificial laboratory conditions which are very different from the actual conditions occurring during day-to-day treatment. Conclusions from such studies should be applied with great caution to the day-to-day treatment of patients with more severe disease who may require the doses used in these studies. Clinically relevant safety data should be obtained in clinical trials which tailor the dose of inhaled steroid to the severity of the disease. Often, the findings in such "dose-tailored" studies are different from the conclusions of studies carried out in the laboratory or from studies in which patients are overtreated due to a fixed (often high-dose) dosing regimen which does not allow for dose adjustments as indicated by the individual's clinical picture.

It is clear from efficacy studies in pediatric patients that 100–200 µg inhaled steroid per day is more effective than any other treatment in the majority of patients. Therefore, it is only relevant to assess the risk of clinically important systemic effects of such doses of inhaled steroids when comparing the clinical efficacy/side-effect ratio with other drugs. When reviewing the literature about the safety of low doses of inhaled steroids, it becomes clear that at present, no controlled studies have reported any clinically relevant systemic side-effects with such doses of inhaled corticosteroid [51, 80, 81].

8.1. Growth

Growth is a complex and variable process. Many studies have demonstrated poor correlations between short-term height velocity and annual height velocity [8286] and between steroid-induced changes in short-term lower leg growth rate and statural growth during the subsequent year. One month lower leg length velocity explains virtually nothing of the variation in annual statural height velocity [85, 86]. In addition, the correlation between two consecutive annual height velocity values for normal prepubescent children is also very poor. A low gain in 1 year is not necessarily followed by a low gain the next year and *vice versa* [85]. The correlation between 1- 2- 3- and 4-year values are only partially correlated with one another [85] and height velocity computed over a period of 3 or 4 years in childhood only explains 34% and 38%, respectively, of the variation in final height, respectively. *Therefore, the only clinically important outcome measure of human growth is the final height in relation to expected final height, allowing for gender and midparental height differences.* Few studies have assessed final height in children treated for long periods with inhaled corticosteroids. Two prospective studies found that long-term treatment with inhaled corticosteroids did not adversely affect final height [87, 88]. In agreement with this a meta-analysis of 21 studies concluded that inhaled corticosteroids did not adversely affect final height [89].

Over the years, a large number of intermediate-term studies studies have evaluated the effect of inhaled corticosteroids on statural growth. The vast majority have not found any adverse effect. However, over the last few years several studies have found growth retardation in children with mild asthma treated continuously for 1 year with a fixed daily dose of beclomethasone ≥400 µg [5, 38, 63, 81, 90]. This dose is markedly higher than the dose required to control mild asthma. Furthermore, a dry powder inhaler or a pMDI was used for the administration of beclomethasone. These devices deposit a large amount of drug in the oropharynx. Oral deposition of beclomethasone results in extensive absorption into the systemic circulation through the gastrointestinal tract with a subsequent increase in systemic effect. The reason for the discrepancy between the findings in these intermediate-term studies and the conclusion of the metaanalysis are not clear. It is known that the growth retarding effect of exogenous steroids is most pronounced during the first year of treatment. In addition, steroids also seem to retard bone maturation. If this occurs to the same extent as the retardation of growth, then final height is not expected to be adversely affected since bone age will correspond to height age. Such children will grow for a longer period than their peers and eventually attain normal final height.

Other prospective, high quality, controlled studies of ≥2 year's duration with budesonide pMDI and Turbuhaler and of 1 year's duration with fluticasone propionate found no adverse effect on growth [2, 45, 91, 92]. The two studies with fluticasone propionate were performed in children with mild asthma. Both confirmed that fluticasone doses which are markedly more effective than sodium cromoglycate do not adversely affect growth during 1 year's treatment [45, 92].

These findings emphasize two important issues:

I. Important differences exist between the various inhaled corticosteroids and inhalers [51], and

II. Growth retardation may be seen when a sufficiently high dose is administered for long periods without any adjustment in the light of disease severity.

8.2. Osteoporosis

The effect of exogenous steroids on bone can be evaluated by measurement of biochemical markers of bone metabolism (bone formation and degradation), bone mineral density (BMD) or frequency of fractures.

8.2.1. *Biochemical Markers:* Several studies have assessed markers of bone resorption and formation. They all found that only high daily doses of inhaled steroids (equivalent to 800 μg budesonide) have a detectable effect on these markers in children. Daily doses of 400 μg or less had no effect in any of the studies [75, 93, 100]. Measurements of markers of bone formation and degradation have always been done in short-term studies on patients with quite mild disease.

8.2.2. *Bone Mineral Density:* A recent long-term, prospective study found that total body bone mineral density (BMD) of children treated with 3–6 years of continuous inhaled budesonide at an average daily dose of around 500 μg was not different from the BMD of 112 children with asthma, who had never received inhaled or oral steroids [101]. These findings corroborated those reported in previously published cross-sectional studies of much smaller groups of children treated for shorter periods of time with inhaled steroids [94, 102, 104] and two longitudinal studies assessing the development of bone mineral density over a period of 6 months in 14 children [105] and 1 year in 21 children [106]. Although the latter studies may have been underpowered, the results are reassuring—there are no indications that standard paediatric doses adversely affect bone mineral density in children.

8.2.3. *Fracture:* At present there are no indications that long-term treatment with inhaled corticosteroids is associated with an increased risk of fracture in children.

8.3. Cataracts

Three to 6 years' treatment of 178 children with inhaled budesonide at an average daily dose of about 500 μg was not associated with an increased occurrence of posterior subcapsular cataract, bruises, tendency to bruise, hoarseness or other noticeable voice changes [107]. This finding corroborates those reported in previously published studies of smaller groups of less well-characterized children and of adolescent patients treated for shorter periods of time with inhaled glucocorticosteroids [108, 112]. These data strongly suggest that *long-term treatment with inhaled corticosteroids in the doses required to control mild and moderate asthma is unlikely to cause cataract formation.*

9. Summary

Inhaled steroids have been used for the treatment of asthma in children for more than 20 years. During this time, a substantial number of studies have evaluated the safety and efficacy of this therapy. Generally, the results have been reassuring. Inhaled corticosteroids have a marked effect on both immediate and long-term aims of asthma therapy. In patients with mild and moderate asthma, low daily doses of around 100–200 μg/day of inhaled steroid produce a clinical effect which, in most trials, is better than the effect of any other treatment to which it has been compared. No clinically important side-effects have been associated with treatment in this dose range. Inhaled corticosteroids beneficially affect more outcome parameters than any other asthma drug and use of inhaled corticosteroids as first-line prophylactic therapy reduces the risk of undertreatment. Furthermore, early intervention with inhaled steroids facilitates, and may be a precondition for, long-term optimal asthma control. Finally treatment with inhaled corticosteroids is very cost-effective, more so than the other treatments to which they have been compared.

10. Conclusions

The marked efficacy and many beneficial effects of low doses of inhaled steroids, combined with the lack of clinically important systemic side-effects, give this treatment a favorable benefit/risk ratio compared with other treatments. This supports placing this treatment as a first-line therapy in children with asthma requiring continuous prophylactic treatment.
- Since the occurrence of measurable systemic effects and risk of clinical side-effects increases with dose, the lowest dose which controls the disease should always be used. Furthermore, inhaler-steroid combinations with a high clinical efficacy/systemic effect ratio should be used.
- If a child is not sufficiently controlled on a low dose of inhaled steroid it might be better to add another drug to the low dose inhaled steroid treatment

rather than to increase the steroid dose. Further studies are needed to assess that and at which dose this should be done for the individual steroid-inhaler combinations.

Further studies are needed in children ≤3 years.

References

1　Price JF, Weller PH (1995) Comparison of fluticasone propionate and sodium cromoglycate for the treatment of childhood asthma. *Respir Med* 89: 363–368
2　Agertoft L, Pedersen S (1994) Effects of long term treatment with an inhaled corticosteroid on growth and pulmonary function in asthmatic children. *Respir Med* 88: 373–381
3　Speight AN, Lee DA, Hey EN (1983) Underdiagnosis and undertreatment of asthma in childhood. *BMJ* 286: 1253–1256
4　Anderson HR, Bailey PA, Cooper JS et al (1983) Morbidity and school absence caused by asthma and wheezing illness. *Arch Dis Child* 58: 777–784
5　Verberne AAPH, Frost C, Roorda RJ, van der Laag H, Kerrebijn KF (1997) One year treatment with salmeterol, compared with beclomethasone in children with asthma. *Am J Respir Crit Care Med* 156: 688–695
6　van Essen Zandvliet EE, Hughes MD, Waalkens HJ, Duiverman EJ, Pocock SJ, Kerrebijn KF (1992) Effects of 22 months of treatment with inhaled corticosteroids and/or beta-2-agonists on lung function, airway responsiveness, and symptoms in children with asthma. The Dutch Chronic Nonspecific Lung Disease Study Group. *Am Rev Respir Dis* 146: 547–554
7　Laitinen LA, Laitinen A, Haahtela T (1992) A comparative study of the effects of an inhaled corticosteroid, budesonide, and of a beta-2-agonist, terbutaline, on airway inflammation in newly diagnosed asthma. *J Allerg Clin Immunol* 90: 32–42
8　Djukanovic R, Wilson JW, Britten YM, Wilson SJ, Walls AF, Roche WF, Howarth PH, Holgate ST (1992) Effect of an inhaled corticosteroid on airway inflammation and symptoms of asthma. *Am Rev Respir Dis* 145: 699–674
9　Jeffery PK, Godfrey RW, Edelroth E, Nelson F, Rogers A, Johansson S (1992) Effect of treatment on airway inflammation and thickening of basement membrane reticular collagen in asthma. *Am Rev Respir Dis* 145: 890–899
10　Burke C, Power CK, Norris A, Condez A, Schmekel B, Poulter LW (1992) Lung function and immunopathological changes after inhaled corticosteroid therapy in asthma. *Eur Respir J* 5: 73–79
11　Barnes PJ (1990) Effect of corticosteroids on airway hyperresponsiveness. *Am Rev Respir Dis* 141: 70–76
12　Ernst P, Habbick B, Suissa S, Hemmelgarn B, Cockcroft D, Buist AS, Horwitz RI, McNutt M, Spitzer WO (1993) Is the association between inhaled betaagonist use and lifethreatening asthma because of confounding by severity? *Am Rev Respir Dis* 148: 75–79
13　Boner AL, Piacentini GL, Bonizzato C, Dattoli V, Sette L (1991) Effect of inhaled beclomethasone dipropionate on bronchial hyperreactivity in asthmatic children during maximal allergen exposure. *Pediat Pulmonol* 10: 2–5
14　Cockroft DW, Murdoch KY (1987) Comparative effects of inhaled salbutamol, sodium cromoglycate and BDP on allergeninduced early asthmatic responses, late asthmatic responses and increased bronchial responsiveness to histamine. *J Allerg Clin Immunol* 79: 734–740
15　Burge PS (1982) The effects of corticosteroids on the immediate asthmatic reaction. *Eur J Respir Dis* 63 (suppl 122): 163–166
16　Dahl R, Johansson S (1982) Importance of duration of treatment with inhaled budesonide on the immediate and late bronchial reaction. *Eur J Respir Dis* 62 (suppl 122): 5167–5175
17　De Baets FM, Goetyn M, Kerrebijn KF (1990) The effect of two months of treatment with inhaled budesonide on bronchial responsiveness to histamine and housedust mite antigen in asthmatic children. *Am Rev Respir Dis* 142: 581–586
18　De Baets FM, Goetyn M, Kerrebijn KF (1990) The effect of two months of treatment with inhaled budesonide on bronchial responsiveness to histamine and housedust mite antigen in asth-

matic children. *Am Rev Respir Dis* 142: 581–586
19 Molema J, van Herwaarden CLA, Folgering HTM (1989) Effect of longterm treatment with inhaled cromoglycate and budesonide on bronchial hyperresponsiveness in patients with allergic asthma. *Eur Respir J* 2: 308–316
20 Kraan J, Koeter GH, Van der Mark TW, Sluiter HJ, De Vries K (1985) Changes in bronchial hyperreactivity induced by 4 weeks of treatment with antiasthmatic drugs in patients with allergic asthma: a comparison between budesonide and terbutaline. *J Allerg Clin Immunol* 76: 628–636
21 Kerrebijn KF, van EssenZandvliet EEM, Neijens HL (1987) Effect of longterm treatment with inhaled corticosteroids and betaagonists on bronchial responsiveness in asthmatic children. *J Allerg Clin Immunol* 79: 653–659
22 Dutoit JI, Salome CM, Woolcock AJ (1987) Inhaled corticosteroids reduce the severity of bronchial hyperresponsiveness in asthma, but oral theophylline does not. *Am Rev Respir Dis* 136: 1174–1178
23 Bel EH, Timmers MC, Hermans JO, Dijkman JH, Sterk PJ (1990) The longer term effects of nedocromil sodium and beclomethasone dipropionate on bronchial responsiveness to methacholine in nonatopic asthmatic subjects. *Am Rev Respir Dis* 141: 21–28
24 Van EssenZandvliet EE, Hughes MD, Waalkens HJ, Duiverman EJ, Pocock SJ, Kerrebijn KF (1992) Effects of 22 months of treatment with inhaled corticosteroids and/or beta-2-agonists on lung function, airway responsiveness and symptoms in children with asthma. *Am Rev Respir Dis* 146: 547–554
25 Østergaard P, Pedersen S (1987) The effect of inhaled disodium cromoglycate and budesonide on bronchial responsiveness to histamine and exercise in asthmatic children: a clinical comparison. *In*: S Godfrey (ed): *Glucocorticosteroids in childhood asthma*. 55–65
26 Benoist MR, Brouard JJ, Rufin P, Waernessyckle S, de Blic J, Paupe J, Scheinmann P (1992) Dissociation of symptom scores and bronchial hyperreactivity: study in asthmatic children on longterm treatment with inhaled beclomethasone dipropionate. *Pediat Pulmonol* 13: 71–77
27 Bennati D, Piacentini GL, Peroni DG, Sette L, Testi R, Boner AL (1989) Changes in bronchial reactivity in asthmatic children after treatment with beclomethasone alone or in association with salbutamol. *J Asthma* 26: 359–364
28 Kraemer R, Sennhauser F, Reinhardt M (1987) Effects of regular inhalation of beclomethasone dipropionate and sodium cromoglycate on bronchial hyperreactivity in asthmatic children. *Acta Paediat Scand* 76: 119–123
29 Resnick A, Greenberger PA (1987) A corticosteroid program for prevention of hospitalization for status asthmaticus in children. *NER Allergy Proc* 8: 104–107
30 Eseverri JL, Botey J, Marin AM (1995) Budesonide: treatment of bronchial asthma during childhood. *Allerg Immunol* 27: 129–135
31 Ribeiro LB (1993) Budesonide: safety and efficacy aspects of its longterm use in children. *Pediatr Allergy Immunol* 4: 73–78
32 Boner AL, Comis A, Schiassi M, Venge P, Piacentini GL (1995) Bronchial reactivity in asthmatic children at high and low altitude: effect of budesonide. *Am J Respir Crit Care Med* 151: 1194–1200
33 Gonzalez PerezYarza E, Garmendia Iglesias A, Mintegui Aramburu J, Callen Blecua M, Albisu Andrade Y, Rubio Calvo E (1994) Prolonged treatment of mild asthma with inhaled antiinflammatory therapy: *An Esp Pediatr* 41: 102–106
34 Larsen JS, De Boisblanc BP, Schaberg A, Herie N, Baker K, Szymeczek J, Kellerman D (1994) Magnitude of improvement in FEV1 with fluticasone propionate. *Am J Respir Crit Care Med* 149:A214
35 MacKenzie CA, Weinberg EG, Tabachnik E, Taylor M, Havnen J, Crescenzi K (1993) A placebo controlled trial of fluticasone propionate in asthmatic children. *Eur J Pediatr* 152: 856–860
36 Perera BJ (1995) Efficacy and cost effectiveness of inhaled steroid in asthma in a developing country. *Arch Dis Child* 72: 312–316
37 Svedmyr J, Nyberg E, sbrink-Nilsson E, Hedlin G (1995) Intermittent treatment with inhaled steroids for deterioration of asthma due to upper respiratory tract infections. *Acta Paediatr Int J Paediatr* 84: 884–888
38 Tinkelman DG, Reed CE, Nelson HS, Offord KP (1993) Aerosol beclomethasone dipropionate compared with theophylline as primary treatment of chronic, mild to moderately severe asthma in children [see comments]. *Pediatrics* 92: 64–77

39 Meltzer EO, Orgel HA, Ellis EF, Eigen HN, Hemstreet MPB (1992) Longterm comparison of three combinations of albuterol, theophylline, and beclomethasone in children with chronic asthma. *J Allerg Clin Immunol* 90: 211

40 White MP, MacDonald TH, Garg RA (1988) Ketotifen in the young asthmatic a double blind placebo controlled trial. *J Int Med Res* 16: 107–113

41 Hargreave FE, Dolovich J, Newhouse MT (1990) The assessment and treatment of asthma: a conference report. *J Allerg Clin Immunol* 85: 1098–1111

42 Pedersen S, Agertoft L (1993) Effect of longterm budesonide treatment on growth, weight and lung function in children with asthma. *Am Rev Respir Dis* 147:A265

43 Connett GJ, Lenney W, McConchie SM (1993) The cost effectiveness of budesonide in severe asthmatics aged one to 3 years. *Br J Med* 6: 127–134

44 Edmunds AT, Goldberg RS, Duper B, Devichand P, Follows RM (1994) A comparison of budesonide 800 micrograms and 400 micrograms via Turbohaler with disodium cromoglycate via Spinhaler for asthma prophylaxis in children. *Br J Clin Res* 5: 11–23

45 Price J, Russell G, Hindmarsh P, Weller P, Heaf D (1996) One year growth velocity in asthmatic children receiving fluticasone propionate 50 µg bid or sodiumcromoglycate 20 mg qid. *Am J Respir Crit Care Med* 153 (4): 409

46 Olivieri D, Chetta A, Del Donno M, Bertorelli G, Casalini A, Pesci A, Testi R, Foresi A (1997) Effect of shortterm treatment with lowdose inhaled fluticasone propionate on airway inflammation and remodeling in mild asthma: a placebocontrolled study. *Am J Respir Crit Care Med* 155: 1864–1871

47 Haahtela T, Järvinen M, Kava T, Kiviranta K, Koskinen S, Lehtonen K, Nikander K, Persson T, Selroos O, Sovijärvi A, SteniusAarniala B, Svahn T, Tammivaara R, Laitinen LA (1994) Effects of reducing or discontinuing inhaled budesonide in patients with mild asthma. *N Engl J Med* 331: 700–705

48 Selroos O, Backman R, Forsen KO, Löfroos AB, Niemistö M, Nyberg P, Nyholm JE, Pietinalho A, Riska H (1994) The effect of inhaled corticosteroids in asthma is related to the duration of pretreatment symptoms. *Am J Respir Crit Care Med* 149: A211

49 Bel EH, Timers MC, Zwinderman AH, Dijkman JH, Sterk PJ (1991) The effect of inhaled corticosteroids on the maximal degree of airway narrowing to methacholine. *Am Rev Respir Dis* 143: 109–113

50 Pedersen S, Hansen OR (1995) Budesonide treatment of moderate and severe asthma in children. A dose response study. *J Allerg Clin Immunol* 1: 29–33

51 Pedersen S, O'Byrne P (1997) A comparison of the efficacy and safety of inhaled corticosteroids in asthma. *Allergy* 52: 1–34

52 Shapiro GG (1992) Childhood asthma: update. Pediatr Rev 13: 403–412

53 Marshall L, Francis P, Khafagi F (1994) Aerosol deposition in cystic fibrosis using an aerosol conservation device and a conventional nebuliser. *J Pediatr Child Health* 30: 65–67

54 Agertoft L, Pedersen S (1997) A randomized, doubleblind dose reduction study to compare the minimal effective dose of budesonide Turbuhaler and fluticasone propionate Diskhaler. *J Allerg Clin Immunol* 99: 773–780

55 Fuglsang G, VikreJørgensen J, Agertoft L, Pedersen S (1998) Influence of salmeterol treatment upon Nitric Oxide level in exhaled air and bronchodilator response to terbutaline in children with mild asthma. *Pediat Pulmonol; in press*

56 Waalkens HJ, van Essen Zandvliet EE, Gerritsen J, Duiverman EJ, Kerrebijn KF, Knol K (1993) The effect of an inhaled corticosteroid (budesonide) on exercise induced asthma in children. Dutch CNSLD Study Group. *Eur Respir J* 6: 652–656

57 Henriksen JM, Dahl R (1983) Effects of inhaled budesonide alone and in combination with lowdose terbutaline in children with exerciseinduced asthma. *Am Rev Respir Dis* 128: 993–997

58 Henriksen JM (1985) Effect of inhalation of corticosteroids on exerciseinduced asthma: Randomised double blind crossover study of budesonide in asthmatic children. *Br Med J* 291: 248–249

59 Hummel S, Lehtonen L (1992) Comparison of oralsteroid sparing by highdose and lowdose inhaled steroid in maintenance treatment of severe asthma. *Lancet* 340: 1483–1487

60 Boe J, Rosenhall L, Alton M et al (1989) Comparison of dose response effects of inhaled beclomethasone dipropionate and budesonide in the management of asthma. *Allergy* 44: 349–355

61 Dahl R, Lundback B, Malo J et al (1993) A dose ranging study of fluticasone propionate in adult

patients with moderate asthma. *Chest* 5: 1352–1358

62 Youngchaiyud P, Permpikul C, Suthamsmai T, Wong E (1995) A doubleblind comparison of inhaled budesonide, a longacting theophylline and their combination in the treatment of nocturnal asthma. *Allergy* 50: 28–33

63 Simons FER (1997) A comparison of beclomethasone, salmeterol, and placebo in children with asthma. *N Engl J Med* 337: 1665

64 Østergaard P, Pedersen S (1982) Bronchial hyperreactivity in children with perennial extrinsic asthma. *In*: S Oseid, AM Edwards (eds): *The asthmatic child in play and sport*. Pitman Books Ltd., London, 326–331

65 Fuglsang G, Agertoft L, VikreJørgensen J, Pedersen S (1995) Influence of Budesonide on the response to inhaled Terbutaline in children with mild asthma. *Pediatr Allergy Immunol* 6: 103–108

66 Suzuki N, Kobayashi N, Kudu K (1997) Early start of inhaled corticosteroid therapy is important for the improvement of bronchial hyperresponsiveness. *J Aerosol Med* 10(3): 277

67 Overbeek SE, Kerstjens HA, Bogaard JM, Mulder PG, Postma DS (1996) Is delayed introduction of inhaled corticosteroids harmful in patients with obstructive airways disease (asthma and COPD)? *Chest* 1: 335–341

68 Selroos O, Pietinalho A, Lofroos AB, Riska H (1995) Effect of early vs late intervention with inhaled corticosteroids in asthma. *Chest* 108: 1228–1234

69 Panhuysen CI, Vonk JM, Koeter GH, Schouten JP, van Altena R, Bleecker ER, Postma DS (1997) Adult patients may outgrow their asthma: a 25year followup study. *Am J Respir Crit Care Med* 155: 1267–1272

70 Sont JK, Willems LNA, Evertse CE, Vanderbroucke JP, Sterk PJ (1997) Longterm management of asthma: is it worth to treat bronchial hyperresponsiveness (BHR) beyond clinical symptoms and lung function. *Am J Respir Crit Care Med* 155: A203

71 Ruttenvan Mölken M, Van Doorslaer EK, Jansen MC, Van EssenZandvliet EE, Rutten FF (1993) Cost effectiveness of inhaled corticosteroid plus bronchodilator therapy *versus* bronchodilator monotherapy in children with asthma. *PharmacoEconomics* 4: 257–270

72 Agertoft L, Pedersen S (1997) Costeffectiveness of inhaled budesonide in children with chronic asthma. *Am J Respir Crit Care Med* 155: A351

73 Booth PC, Wells NE, Morrison AK (1996) A comparison of the cost effectiveness of alternative prophylactic therapies in childhood asthma. *PharmacoEconomics* 10: 262–268

74 Soferman R, Sapir N, Spirer Z, Golander A (1995) Urinary growth hormone (UGH) in asthmatic children. *Eur Respir J* 8 (suppl 19): 470

75 Martinati LC, Sette L, Chiocca E, Zaninotto M, Plebani M, Boner AL (1993) Effect of beclomethasone dipropionate nasal aerosol on serum markers of bone metabolism in children with seasonal allergic rhinitis. *Clin Exp Allergy* 23: 986–991

76 Ghigo E, Valetto MR, Gaggero L, Visca A, Valente FE (1993) Therapeutic doses of salbutamol inhibit the somatotropic responsiveness to growth hormonereleasing hormone in asthmatic children. *J Endocrinol Invest* 16: 271–275

77 Zeitlin S, Wood P, Evans A, Radford M (1993) Overnight urine growth hormone, cortisol and adenosine3' 5'cyclic monophosphate excretion in children with chronic asthma treated with inhaled beclomethasone dipropionate. *Respir Med* 87: 445–448

78 Pedersen S (1996) Inhalers and Nebulizers, which to choose and why. *Respir Med* 90: 69–77

79 Falcoz C, Mackie AE, Moss J, Horton J, Ventresca GP, Brown A, Field E, Harding SM, Wire P, Bye A (1997) Pharmacokinetics of fluticasone propionate inhaled from the Diskhaler® and the Diskus® after repeat doses in healthy subjects and asthmatic patients. *J Allerg Clin Immunol* 99: S505

80 Barnes PJ, Pedersen S (1993) Efficacy and safety of inhaled corticosteroids in asthma. *Am Rev Respir Dis* 148: 126

81 Pedersen S (1996) Efficiacy and safety of Inhaled Corticosteroids in Children. *In*: R Schleimer, W Busse, P O'Byrne (eds): *Topical glucocorticoids in asthma mechanisms and clinical actions*. Marcel Dekker, New York, 551–560

82 Marshall W (1971) Evaluation of growth rate in height over periods of less than one year. *Arch Dis Child* 46: 414–420

83 Butler GE, McKie M, Ratcliffe SG (1990) The cyclical nature of prepubertal growth. *Ann Hum Biol* 17: 177–198

84 Voss LD, Wilkin TJ, Balley BJR, Betts PR (1991) The reliability of height and height velocity in

the assessment of growth (the Wessex Growth Study). *Arch Dis Child* 66: 833–837
85 Karlberg J, Gelander L, AlbertssonWikland K (1993) Distinctions between short and longterm human growth studies. *Acta Paediat* 82: 631–634
86 Karlberg J, Low L, Yeung CY (1994) On the dynamics of the growth process. *Acta Paediat* 83: 777–778
87 Balfour Lynn L (1987) Effect of asthma on growth and puberty. *Pediatrician* 14: 237–241
88 Agertoft L, Pedersen S (1998) Final height in children treated for several years with high dose inhaled budesonide. *Am J Respir Crit Care Med*; *in press*
89 Allen DB, Mullen ML, Mullen B (1994) A metaanalysis of the effect of oral and inhaled corticosteroids on growth. *J Allerg Clin Immunol* 93: 967–976
90 Doull IJ, Freezer NJ, Holgate ST (1995) Growth of prepubertal children with mild asthma treated with inhaled beclomethasone dipropionate. *Am J Respir Crit Care Med* 151: 1715–1719
91 Merkus PJ, van Essen Zandvliet EE, Duiverman EJ, van Houwelingen HC, Kerrebijn KF, Quanjer PH (1993) Longterm effect of inhaled corticosteroids on growth rate in adolescents with asthma. *Pediatrics* 91: 1121–1126
92 König P, Ford L, Galant S, Lawrence M, Lemanske R, Mendelson L, Pearlman R, Wyatt R, Allen D, Baker K et al (1996) A 1year comparison of the effects of inhaled fluticasone propionate (FP) and placebo on growth in prepubescent children with asthma. *Eur Respir J* 9: 294
93 Wolthers O, Juul A, Hansen M, Müller J, Pedersen S (1995) The insulinlike growth factor axis and collagen turnover in asthmatic children treated with inhaled budesonide. *Acta Paediat* 84: 393–397
94 König P, Hillman G, Cervantes Ce (1993) Bone metabolism in children with asthma treated with inhaled beclomethasone dipropionate. *J Pediat* 122: 219–226
95 Wolthers O, Kaspersen Nielsen H, Pedersen S (1993) Bone turnover in asthmatic children treated with dry powder inhaled fluticasone propionate and beclomethasone dipropionate. European Paediatric Respiratory Society Oslo: 86
96 Pedersen S (1989) Safety of inhaled glucocorticosteroids. *Excerpta Medica* 40–51
97 Wolthers OD, Juel Riis B, Pedersen S (1993) Bone turnover in asthmatic children treated with oral prednisolone or inhaled budesonide. *Pediat Pulmonol* 16: 341–346
98 Wolthers O, Juul A, Hansen M, Müller J, Pedersen S (1993) Growth factors and collagen markers in asthmatic children treated with inhaled budesonide. *Eur Respir J* 6(suppl 17): 261
99 Sorva R, Turpeinen M, JuntunenBackman K, Karonen SL, Sorva A (1992) Effects of inhaled budesonide on serum markers of bone metabolism in children with asthma. *J Allerg Clin Immunol* 90: 808–815
100 Birkebaek NH, Esberg G, Andersen K, Wolthers O, Hassager C (1995) Bone and collagen turnover during treatment with inhaled dry powder budesonide and beclomethasone dipropionate. *Arch Dis Child* 73: 524–527
101 Agertoft L, Pedersen S (1998) Bone mineral density in children with asthma receiving longterm treatment with inhaled budesonide. *Am J Respir Crit Care Med* 157: 1–6
102 Kinberg KA, Hopp RJ, Biven RE, Gallagher JC (1994) Bone mineral density in normal and asthmatic children. *J Allerg Clin Immunol* 94: 490–497
103 Martinati LC, Bertoldo F, Gasperi E, Micelli S, Boner AL (1996) Effect on cortical and trabecular bone mass of different antiinflammatory treatments in preadolescent children with chronic asthma. *Am J Respir Crit Care Med* 153: 232–236
104 Hopp RJ, Degan JA, Phelan J, Lappe J, Gallagher GC (1995) Cross-sectional study of bone density in asthmatic children. *Pediat Pulmonol* 20(3): 189–192
105 Baraldi E, Bollini MC, De Marchi A, Zacchello F (1994) Effect of beclomethasone dipropionate on bone mineral content assessed by Xray densitometry in asthmatic children: a longitudinal evaluation. *Eur Respir J* 7: 710–714
106 Hopp RJ, Degan JA, Biven RE, Kinberg K, Gallagher GC (1995) Longitudinal assessment of bone mineral density in children with chronic asthma. *Ann Allergy Asthma Immunol* 75: 143–148
107 Agertoft L, Pedersen S (1997) Posterior subcapsular cataracts, bruises and hoarseness in children with asthma receiving longterm treatment with inhaled budesonide. *Eur Respir J*; *in press*
108 Abuekteish F, Kirkpatrick JN, Russell G (1995) Posterior subcapsular cataract and inhaled corticosteroid therapy. *Thorax* 50: 674–676
109 Toogood JH, Markov AE, Baskerville J, Dyson C (1993) Association of ocular cataracts with inhaled and oral steroid therapy during longterm treatment of asthma. *J Allerg Clin Immunol* 91: 571–579

110 Simons FER, Persaud MP, Gillespie CA, Cheang M, Shuckett EP (1993) Abscence of posterior subcapsular cataracts in young patients treated with inhaled glucocorticoids. *Lancet* 342: 776–778
111 Sevel D, Weinberg EG, van Niekerk CH (1977) Lenticular complications of longterm steroid therapy in children with asthma and eczema. *J Allergy* 60: 215–217
112 Nassif E, Weinberger M, Sherman EA (1987) Extrapulmonary effects of maintenance corticosteroid therapy with alternateday prednisone and inhaled beclomethasone in children with chronic asthma. *J Allerg Clin Immunol* 80: 518–529

CHAPTER 6
Treatment of Asthma in Children: the Case Against Inhaled Corticosteroids as First Line Agents

Peter König

Department of Child Health, University of Missouri, Columbia, MO 65212, USA

1. Introduction

With the increasing awareness of the importance of inflammation in the pathogenesis of asthma even in relatively mild patients [1], more and more emphasis is being put on anti-inflammatory approaches to treatment.

The place of anti-inflammatory drugs is defined by the latest international guidelines (The Global Initiative for Asthma: GINA) as starting with patients with mild persistent asthma, who have symptoms more frequently than 1 day per week [2].

Anti-inflammatory drugs can be divided into oral and inhaled steroidal, and inhaled non-steroidal (cromolyn sodium and nedocromil sodium). The choice between steroidal and non-steroidal drugs needs to be made, based on a risk/benefit assessment. The safety record of cromolyn sodium and nedocromil sodium is excellent [3–5]. Most of the side-effects due to cromolyn sodium are attributable to a local irritant effect, mainly with dry powder administration, resulting in transient cough or wheezing. More serious adverse effects are rare and were described in 2% of patients in one study, manifesting as dermatitis, myositis, and gastro-enteritis [6]. There are only a few published cases of anaphylaxis to cromolyn sodium [7–9].

The safety record of nedocromil sodium is also very good [10]. Unpleasant taste has been described as the most frequent unwanted event, but its occurrence varied between 0% [11, 12], 6% [13] and 13% [14].

2. The Side-Effects of Inhaled Corticosteroids are Both Topical and Systemic

2.1. Topical Side-Effects

Oral candidiasis has been described with an incidence varying between 5 and 77% [15], but the incidence is less in children [16, 17].

Dysphonia seems to be more frequent than candidiasis, and has been described in 30–50% of cases [18, 19]. Cough and throat irritation are also fairly common [19]. Oral blood blisters have been found in adults treated with large doses of inhaled corticosteroids [20]. A few children have developed stridor on inhaled beclomethasone dipropionate [21]. Linder et al. reported on three premature infants who developed hypertrophy of the tongue while being treated with nebulized beclomethasone 200–400 µg/day. Discontinuation of the steroid resulted in reversal of the hypertrophy [22].

2.2. Systemic Side-Effects

Systemic unwanted effects are influenced by: a) dose, b) pharmacokinetics, c) delivery system, d) individual sensitivity, and e) asthma severity. The first two are self-explanatory. Relevant pharmacokinetic factors may include lung *versus* oral bioavailability (the latter from the swallowed portion); half-life; receptor affinity; and lipophilicity.

2.2.1. Delivery Systems: Delivery systems are important because of differences in the dose delivered to the lungs, from which absorption freely occurs. Thus Thorsson and associates showed that the same dose of budesonide given as dry powder, produced 50% more systemic bioavailability than as an MDI, because of greater delivery of steroid to the lungs [23].

2.2.2. Individual Sensitivity: Individual sensitivity to the systemic effects of inhaled corticosteroids varies substantially between patients. In addition to rare case reports of so-called idiosyncratic reactions such as obesity, hirsutism, growth retardation and adrenal suppression at regular doses [24], in some studies where the group mean results justified the conclusion of no unwanted event, a few individual patients can be found who do show side-effects. Thus, Godfrey and König [25] showed no growth suppression for the whole group of pediatric asthmatics treated with beclomethasone dipropionate, but five of the 26 children grew at a rate slower than expected.

2.2.3. Asthma Severity: Asthma severity is not a widely recognized factor affecting systemic side-effects of inhaled corticosteroids, but there is increasing evidence that it does. In a study on adult asthmatics, fluticasone propionate 2000 µg/day caused more adrenal suppression in milder patients than in severe ones [26]. This could be due to greater lung deposition and absorption in the less obstructed mild patients. Numerous studies have shown no growth suppression in severe patients treated with beclomethasone dipropionate in regular doses [25, 27]. More recently, two studies performed in mild-to-moderate patients showed significant growth suppression with beclomethasone dipropionate at a low dose of 400 µg/day [28, 29] (Fig 1).

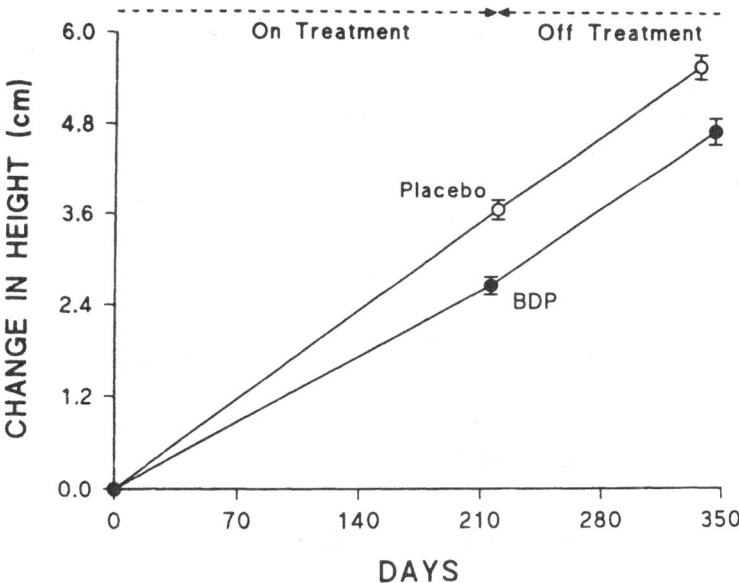

Figure 1. Change in height from baseline of children receiving BDP (closed circles) and those receiving placebo (open circles). From: Doull et al. Am J Respir Crit Care Med 1995; 151: 1715–1719 (reference [29]).

Why should there be more growth suppression reported in milder disease? Ninan and Russell [30] found that poorly controlled asthma itself results in growth suppression. In severe asthma, the introduction of inhaled corticosteroids results in a marked improvement in asthma control. In addition, severe patients often need short or more prolonged courses of systemic steroids which have a powerful growth-suppressive effect. The introduction of inhaled steroids in such patients greatly reduces or eliminates the need for systemic steroids. Thus, in severe patients inhaled corticosteroids have two beneficial effects on growth which will balance out any negative effect and the end result is no growth suppression or even accelerated growth. In mild patients, the introduction of inhaled corticosteroids has a less dramatic effect on asthma control and these patients rarely need systemic steroids. Therefore, in mild

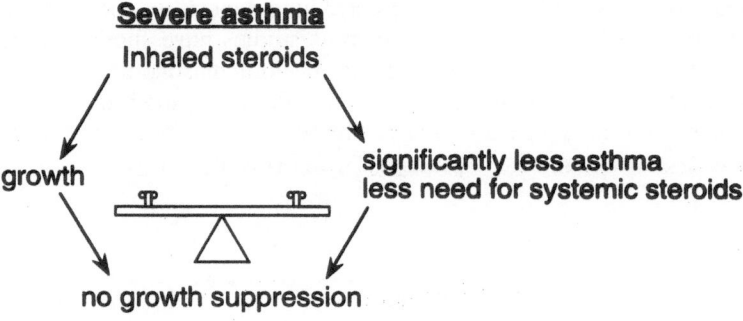

Severe asthma
Inhaled steroids

growth

significantly less asthma
less need for systemic steroids

no growth suppression

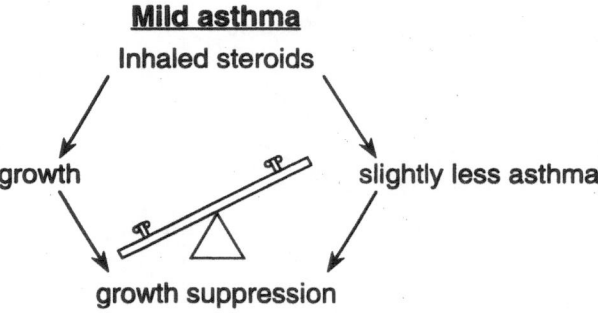

Mild asthma
Inhaled steroids

growth

slightly less asthma

growth suppression

Figure 2. Growth suppression with inhaled corticosteroids in severe versus mild asthma.

patients the two beneficial effects on growth are much less important and the negative effect predominates, resulting in growth suppression (Fig 2).

The systemic undesirable effects of inhaled corticosteroids at regular doses can be classified into: 1) Rare, idiosyncratic reactions; 2) Statistically significant changes in biochemical levels with unclear clinical significance; 3) Side-effects affecting only certain severity groups, such as growth suppression in mild-to-moderate asthmatic children [28, 29]; 4) Side-effects demonstrated in adults but not studied in children; and 5) Theoretically possible side-effects which were not yet clinically studied, such as increased IgE synthesis and decreased lung growth.

Idiosyncratic reactions: The exact prevalence of such cases is hard to establish because not all cases are diagnosed or published. Thomas and associates [31] described six patients with growth suppression on beclomethasone dipropionate 300–800 µg, but they did not state how large was the original group treated with beclomethasone

Statistically significant changes with unclear clinical significance: Tabachnik and Zadik [32] found that treatment with beclomethasone dipropionate 400 µg/day in children with asthma caused a 63% suppression of nocturnal cortisol production

There is no evidence that this adrenal suppression entails a risk for life threatening adrenal insufficiency [33, 34]. However, there is some evidence that suppression of nocturnal endogenous cortisol production increases late allergic reactions in the skin [35] and may have a role in nocturnal asthma [36]. The clinical significance, if any, of this finding in asthma remains to be established.

Studies on bone metabolism have yielded somewhat contradictory results. In children, Sorva and associates in a longitudinal study, reported significant reduction in osteocalcin and procollagen I (markers of osteoblastic activity) with budesonide 400 µg/day [37]. Our own cross-sectional study showed no effect on osteocalcin or on bone mineral density with beclomethasone 300–800 µg/day [38] and one longitudinal study showed no effect on bone mineral content with beclomethasone 300–400 µg/day [39].

In adults, with larger doses of inhaled corticosteroids (800–2000 µg/day) both osteocalcin [40] and bone mineral density [40, 41] were found to be significantly reduced and at these doses the changes are probably clinically significant.

Side-effects affecting only certain severity groups: This has been shown in terms of adrenal suppression in adults [26] and of growth suppression which is more common in milder patients than in more severe patients [28, 29]

In a retrospective study of 201 children Saha and associates [42] reported growth retardation from treatment with beclomethasone or budesonide 100–2500 µg/day and they concluded that growth suppression was more pronounced in severe patients. However, their severity classification was very different from the more widely accepted classifications, such as those in the GINA [2] or other international guidelines. The authors used a severity score based on four criteria, two of which (use of steroids for allergic rhinitis and "difficulty in cooperation") are not used in other classifications. Therefore, their results cannot be compared (in terms of the effect of the severity of disease) with other studies based on more conventional severity classifications. Nevertheless, it does show growth suppression with an average dose of 500 µg/m^2 body surface area, which is not an excessively high dose.

Many studies enroll patients already on some prophylactic drug regime (non-steroidal or steroidal) and the severity classification is based on frequency of symptoms and/or pulmonary function, which creates confusion between degree of control and disease severity [43]. This makes it difficult to analyze the effect of disease severity on steroid side-effects.

Side-effects shown in adults, but not studied in children: These are mostly side-effects affecting the skin, resulting from treatment with inhaled corticosteroids, in most cases with large doses. Autio et al. [44] studied skin collagen synthesis. They concluded that budesonide either 400 µg/day or 1600 µg/day, significantly reduced type I and type III procollagen propeptides compared to a control group treated with nedocromil sodium. This confirms an earlier study by Capewell and associates [45] who demonstrated skin thinning in adults on high doses of beclomethasone (1000–2250 µg/day) but not on low doses (200–800 µg/day)

Skin bruising has been reported in 47–48% of adult patients taking large doses of inhaled corticosteroids [41, 46]. It was more pronounced among females, older patients, and among patients with adrenal suppression, and it correlated with the dose of inhaled corticosteroids.

Theoretically possible side-effects, which were not studied clinically: Zieg and associates [48], in a group of adult asthmatics treated with oral prednisone, showed a significant increase in total IgE. In a study in children with atopic dermatitis, Hiratsuka et al., compared beclomethasone with cromolyn sodium, both drugs by topical application [49]. IgE production by peripheral blood B cells was significantly increased by beclomethasone dipropionate, but significantly decreased by cromolyn sodium. *In vitro* studies confirm the fact that glucocorticosteroids increase IgE synthesis [50] and cromolyn sodium inhibits it [51]. Studies have not investigated the effect of inhaled corticosteroids on IgE synthesis

Systemic corticosteroids given to rat fetuses cause profound pulmonary hypoplasia [52], and in newborn rats they partly suppress the outgrowth of new interalveolar septa, resulting in larger and fewer air spaces [53]. It is not known if this occurs in humans and if inhaled corticosteroids might have the same effect.

3. Corticosteroids *versus* Cromolyn Sodium

In terms of efficacy, several studies have compared cromolyn sodium with inhaled corticosteroids in children. The outcome of these studies depends very much on the severity of the patient population. As one would expect, in severe patients, inhaled corticosteroids are more efficacious than cromolyn sodium [54–56].

However, studies performed on mild-to-moderately severe children have yielded very mixed results. Of the five published studies, only two [57, 58] (one of them not a controlled study) [58] showed a superiority for inhaled corticosteroids over cromolyn, while three others showed equal efficacy [59–61]. Thus, there is no conclusive evidence that inhaled corticosteroids are more efficacious than cromolyn sodium in mild to moderate asthmatics. It is in these same mild-to-moderate patients that inhaled corticosteroids are more likely to produce systemic side-effects than in patients with severe disease [26, 28, 29]. Therefore the risk/benefit ratio of inhaled corticosteroids is excellent in severe asthma but not as favorable as the inhaled non-steroidal agents in mild-to-moderate asthma.

For many years this was the widely accepted philosophy behind a stepwise approach to treatment, in which inhaled non-steroidal anti-inflammatory drugs such as cromolyn sodium were tried first in mild to moderate patients, and inhaled corticosteroids were reserved for severe asthmatics, who failed to be controlled by the nonsteroidal agents [62–64].

More recently, this approach has been questioned by some investigators, who have raised the possibility that delay in starting inhaled corticosteroids may result in irreversible airway obstruction [65]. This postulate was based on a study by Agertoft and Pedersen [65], in which one group of children was treated with budesonide for 6 years and a control group was treated with other antiasthmatic agents, including cromolyn sodium in some. The authors found a greater increase in FEV_1 in patients with a shorter delay in starting budesonide. The study, however, was not designed to evaluate irreversible airway obstruction. The published spirometry results are only prebronchodilator values with no postbronchodilator values given and there was no attempt made to reverse airway obstruction with a short course of systemic steroids. Thus, it cannot be said that the obstruction was truly irreversible. Another shortcoming in this study is that the control group was not chosen on a random basis, but was comprised of patients or parents who refused to take inhaled corticosteroids. The patients were also treated with maintenance adrenergic agonists. Some studies have shown that maintenance adrenergic agonist therapy can cause less effective asthma control [66], increased bronchial hyperreactivity [67] and an increase in the late asthmatic response to allergen [68].

We performed a retrospective study specifically designed to examine the hypothesis that delay in starting inhaled corticosteroids might cause irreversible airway obstruction [69]. The patients were classified as mild, moderate and severe as defined by Warner et al. [62] and treated with "as needed" adrenergic agents, cromolyn sodium, or inhaled corticosteroids, respectively. If the clinical control, based on symptoms and pulmonary function tests, changed for the better or worse, the treatment was stepped up or down accordingly. Both groups treated originally with inhaled anti-inflammatory drugs (cromolyn sodium or inhaled corticosteroids) had better pulmonary function tests at the end of follow-up (a mean of 8.4 years) than at the start, and the only group that showed worsening was those started on bronchodilators alone. Postbronchodilator values in the group started on cromolyn sodium were quite normal (FVC 104%; FEV_1 100%, FEF_{25-75} 94%). (Fig. 3). Final pulmonary function tests showed a significant negative correlation with delay in starting cromolyn sodium in terms of FVC pre- and postbronchodilator values, but delay in starting inhaled corticosteroids had no effect on any of the pulmonary function tests. Thus it seems that the crucial step is the start of anti-inflammatory treatment, but not necessarily with inhaled corticosteroids.

A cross-sectional study from Finland [70] examined pulmonary function tests in a group of children treated according to the same asthma guidelines

Final pulmonary function test

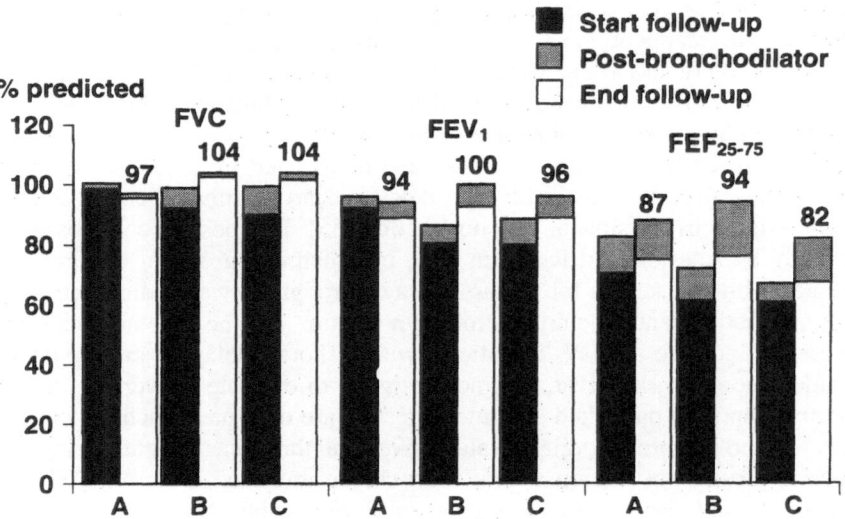

Figure 3. Pulmonary function tests at start and end of follow-up. (A) Mild asthma (p.r.n. bron-chodilators). (B) Moderately severe asthma (cromolyn sodium). (C) Severe asthma (inhaled corticos-teroids). (Modified from König, Shaffer; *J Allergy Clin Immunol* 1996; 98: 1101–1111; reference [69]).

[62]. Their moderately severe group was treated with cromolyn sodium or nedocromil sodium. The conclusions of their study were very similar to ours [69], namely that inhaled non-steroidal agents (cromolyn sodium or nedocromil sodium) resulted in very good pulmonary function tests and should be started earlier than the recommendations of the guidelines [62] (patients with symptoms more than 3 days/week). Their results are almost identical with the pulmonary function tests observed in our study [69].

Oswald and associates [71] conducted a longitudinal study with a 28-year follow-up. They concluded that patients with relatively mild asthma who were not treated with inhaled corticosteroids did not have a negative outcome in terms of lung function tests.

Thus, three studies [69–71] have shown no evidence that moderately severe patients treated with inhaled non-steroidal anti-inflammatory agents develop irreversible airways obstruction. Of course, if control with these drugs is unsat-isfactory, the treatment needs to be stepped up to inhaled corticosteroids, a step that was not possible in most patients of the control group in the Agertoft and Pedersen study [65], who refused steroid therapy.

In conclusion, in mild to moderately severe asthma in children, non-steroidal inhaled anti-inflammatory drugs such as cromolyn sodium and nedocromil sodium have comparable efficacy and better overall safety than inhaled corticosteroids. The milder the patient's illness, the less readily we should accept the risk of side-effects. In severe patients, the superiority of inhaled corticosteroids is clear and in those patients the risk/benefit ratio of these drugs is excellent.

Therefore, a stepwise approach, as recommended by various guidelines [62–64], is still the best approach. The latest set of guidelines, incorporated in GINA [2], is further improved by recommending earlier introduction of inhaled non-steroidal agents than the previous guidelines [62–64] (in patients symptomatic more than 1 day/week, as opposed to the previously recommended more than 3 days/week).

References

1   Beasley R, Roche WR, Roberts JA, Holgate ST (1989) Cellular events in the bronchi in mild asthma and after bronchial provocation. *Am Rev Respir Dis* 139: 806–817

2   National Institutes of Health Publication No 95-3659, January (1995) Global initiative for asthma: Global strategy for asthma management and prevention NHLBI/WHO workshop report

3   Morrison-Smith J, Pizarro YA (1972) Observations on the safety of disodium cromoglycate in long-term use in children. *Clin Allergy* 2: 143–151

4   Kuzemko JA (1977) Long-term experiences in the use of sodium cromoglycate (SCG) in young children with asthma. *Acta Allergol Suppl* 13: 28–33

5   König P, Shapiro GG (1985) Cromolyn sodium: A review. *Pharmacotherapy* 5: 156–170

6   Settipane GA, Klein DE, Boyd GK, Sturam JH, Freye HB, Weltman JK (1979) Adverse reactions to cromolyn. *JAMA* 23: 811–813

7   Sheffer AL, Rocklin RE, Goetzl EJ (1975) Immunologic components of hypersensitivity reactions to cromolyn sodium. *N Engl J Med* 293: 1220–1224

8   Brown LA, Kaplan RA, Benjamin PA, Loffman LS, Shearer WT (1981) Immunoglobulin E-mediated anaphylaxis with inhaled cromolyn sodium. *J Allerg Clin Immunol* 68: 416–420

9   Ibanez MD, Laso MT, Martinez-San Irineo M, Alonso E (1996) Anaphylaxis to disodium cromoglycate. *Ann Allergy Asthma Immunol* 77: 185–186

10 Brogden RN, Sorkin EM (1993) Nedocromil sodium: An updated review of its pharmacological properties and therapeutic efficacy in asthma. *Drugs* 45(5): 693–713

11 Businco L, Cantani A, Di Fazio A, Bernardini L (1990) A double-blind, placebo-controlled study to assess the efficacy of nedocromil sodium in the management of childhood grass-pollen asthma. *Clin Exp Allergy* 20: 683–688

12 Armenio L, Baldini G, Bardare M, Boner A, Burgio R, Cavagni G et al (1993) Double blind, placebo controlled study of nedocromil sodium in asthma. *Arch Dis Child* 8: 193–197

13 König P, Eigen H, Ellis MH, Ellis E, Blake K, Geller D et al (1995) The effect of nedocromil sodium on childhood asthma during the viral season. *Am J Respir Crit Care Med* 152: 1879–1886

14 Evans R (1996) Safety of nedocromil sodium, 4 inhalations, bid, in children. *Ann Allergy Asthma Immunol* 76: 99

15 Barnes PJ, Pedersen S (1993) Efficacy and safety of inhaled corticosteroids in asthma. *Am Rev Respir Dis* 148: S1–S26

16 Brogden RN, McTavish D (1992) Budesonide. An updated review of its pharmacological properties and therapeutic efficacy in asthma and rhinitis. *Drugs* 44: 375–407

17 Brogden RN, Heel RC, Speight TM, Avery GS (1992) Beclomethasone dipropionate. A reappraisal of its pharmacodynamic properties and therapeutic efficacy after a decade of use in asthma and rhinitis. *Drugs* 28: 99–126

18 Toogood JA, Jennings B, Greenway RW, Chung L (1980) Candidiasis and dysphonia complicating beclomethasone treatment of asthma. *J Allerg Clin Immunol* 65: 145–153

19 Williamson I, Matusiewicz S, Brown PH, Crompton GK, Greening AP (1991) Frequency of voice problems and cough in patients using aerosol preparations. *Thorax* 46: 769P

20 High AS, Main DMG (1988) Angina bullosa haemorrhagica: a complication of long-term steroid inhaler use. *Br Dent J* 165: 176–179
21 Storr J, Tranter R, Lenney W (1988) Stridor in childhood asthma. *Br J Dis Chest* 82: 197–199
22 Linder N, Kuint J, German B, Lubin D, Loewenthal R (1995) Hypertrophy of the tongue associated with inhaled corticosteroid therapy in premature infants. *J Pediat* 127: 651–653
23 Thorsson L, Edsbäcker S, Conradson T-B (1994) Lung deposition of budesonide from Turbuhaler® is twice that from a pressurized metered-dose inhaler P-MDI. *Eur Respir J* 7: 1839–1844
24 Hollman GA, Allen DB (1988) Overt glucocorticoid excess due to inhaled corticosteroid therapy. *Pediatrics* 81: 452–455
25 Godfrey S, König P (1974) Treatment of childhood asthma for 13 months and longer with beclomethasone dipropionate aerosol. *Arch Dis Child* 49: 591–596
26 Harris TAJ, Fuller RW (1996) High dose fluticasone propionate (FP) and its effect on serum cortisol (sCORT) in patients with asthma. *Eur Respir J* 9 (suppl 23): 163S–164S
27 Allen DB, Mullen M, Mullen B (1994) A meta-analysis of the effect of oral and inhaled corticosteroids on growth. *J Allerg Clin Immunol* 93: 967–976
28 Tinkelman DG, Reed CE, Nelson HS, Offord KP (1993) Aerosol beclomethasone dipropionate compared with theophylline as primary treatment of chronic, mild to moderately severe asthma in children. *Pediatrics* 92: 64–77
29 Doull IJM, Freezer MJ, Holgate ST (1995) Growth of prepubertal children with mild asthma treated with inhaled beclomethasone dipropionate. *Am J Respir Crit Care Med* 151: 1715–1719
30 Ninan TK, Russell G (1992) Asthma, inhaled corticosteroid treatment, and growth. *Arch Dis Child* 67: 703–705
31 Thomas BC, Stanhope R, Grant DB (1994) Impaired growth in children with asthma during treatment with conventional doses of inhaled corticosteroids. *Acta Pædiat* 83: 196–199
32 Tabachnik E, Zadik Z (1991) Diurnal cortisol secretion during therapy with inhaled beclomethasone dipropionate in children with asthma. *J Pediat* 118: 294–297
33 Smith MJ, Hodson ME (1983) Effects of long term inhaled high-dose beclomethasone dipropionate on adrenal function. *Thorax* 38: 676–681
34 Toogood JH, Jennings B, Baskerville J, Lefcoe NM (1984) Personal observations on the use of inhaled corticosteroid drugs for chronic asthma. *Eur J Respir Dis* 65: 321–338
35 Herrscher RF, Kasper C, Sullivan TJ (1992) Endogenous cortisol regulates immunoglobulin E-dependent late phase reactions. *J Clin Invest* 90: 596–603
36 Kallenbach JM, Panz VR, Joffe BI, Jankelow D, Anderson R, Haitas B, Seftel HC (1988) Nocturnal events related to "morning dipping" in bronchial asthma. *Chest* 93: 751–757
37 Sorva R, Turpeinen M, Juntunen-Backman K, Karonen S-L, Sorva A (1992) Effects of inhaled budesonide on serum markers of bone metabolism in children with asthma. *J Allerg Clin Immunol* 90: 808–815
38 König P, Hillman L, Cervantes C, Levine C, Maloney C, Douglass B et al (1993) Bone metabolism in children with asthma treated with inhaled beclomethasone dipropionate. *J Pediat* 122: 219–226
39 Baraldi E, Bollini MC, De Marchi A, Zacchello F (1994) Effects of beclomethasone dipropionate on bone mineral content assessed by X-ray densitometry in asthmatic children: a longitudinal evaluation. *Eur Respir J* 7: 710–714
40 Hanania NA, Chapman KR, Sturtridge WC, Szalai JP, Kesten S (1995) Dose-related decrease in bone density among asthmatic patients treated with inhaled corticosteroids. *J Allerg Clin Immunol* 96: 571–579
41 Packe GE, Robb O, Robins SP, Reid DM, Douglas JG (1996) Bone density in asthmatic patients taking inhaled corticosteroids: comparison of budesonide and beclomethasone dipropionate. *J Roy Coll Phys Lond* 30: 128–132
42 Saha M-T, Laippala P, Lenko HL (1997) Growth of asthmatic children is slower during than before treatment with inhaled glucocorticoids. *Acta Paediat* 86: 138–142
43 Cockroft DW, Swystun VA (1996) Asthma control *versus* asthma severity. *J Allerg Clin Immunol* 98: 1016–1018
44 Autio P, Karjalainen J, Risteli L, Risteli J, Kiistala U, Oikarinen A (1996) Effects of an inhaled steroid (budesonide) on skin collagen systhesis of asthma patients *In Vivo*. *Am J Respir Crit Care Med* 153: 1172–1175
45 Capewell S, Reynolds S, Shuttleworth D, Edwards C, Finlay AY (1990) Purpura and dermal thin-

ning associated with high dose inhaled corticosteroids. *Br Med J* 300: 1548–1551
46 Mak VHF, Melchor R, Spiro SG (1992) Easy bruising as a side-effect of inhaled corticosteroids. *Eur Respir J* 5: 1068–1074
47 Roy A, Leblanc C, Paquette L, Ghezzo H, Côté J, Cartier A, Malo J-L (1996) Skin bruising in asthmatic subjects treated with high doses of inhaled steroids: frequency and association with adrenal function. *Eur Respir J* 9: 226–231
48 Zieg G, Lack G, Harbeck RJ, Gelfand EW, Leung DYM (1994) *In vivo* effects of glucocorticoids on IgE production. *J Allerg Clin Immunol* 94: 222–230
49 Hiratsuka S, Yoshida A, Ishioka C, Kimata H (1996) Enhancement of *in vitro* spontaneous IgE production by topical steroids in patients with atopic dermatitis. *J Allerg Clin Immunol* 98: 107–113
50 Nüsslein HG, Weber G, Kalden JR (1994) Synthetic glucocorticoids potentiate IgE synthesis. *Allergy* 49: 365–370
51 Kimata H, Yoshida A, Ishioka C, Mikawa H (1992) Disodium cromoglycate (DSCG) selectively inhibits IgE production and enhances IgG4 production by human B cells *in vitro*. *Clin Exp Immunol* 84: 395–399
52 Rotschild A, Solimano A, Sekhon HS, Massoud EAS, Thurlbeck WM (1997) Effect of triamcinolone acetonide on the development of the pulmonary airways in the fetal rat. *Pediat Pulmonol* 23: 76–86
53 Tschanz SA, Damke BM, Burri PH (1995) Influence of postnatally administered glucocorticoids on rat lung growth. *Biol Neonate* 68: 229–245
54 Francis RS, McEnery G (1984) Disodium cromoglycate compared with beclomethasone dipropionate in juvenile asthma. *Clin Allergy* 14: 537–540
55 Sarsfield JK, Sugden E (1977) A comparative study of betamethasone valerate aerosol and sodium cromoglycate in children with severe asthma. *Practitioner* 218: 128–132
56 Hiller EJ, Milner AD (1975) Betamethasone 17 valerate aerosol and disodium cromoglycate in severe childhood asthma. *Br J Dis Chest* 69: 103–106
57 Ng SH, Dash CH, Savage SJ (1977) Betamethasone valerate compared with sodium cromoglycate in asthmatic children. *Postgrad Med J* 53: 315–320
58 Price JF, Weller PH (1995) Comparison of fluticasone propionate and sodium cromoglycate for the treatment of childhood asthma (an open parallel group study). *Resp Med* 89: 363–368
59 Mitchell I, Paterson IC, Cameron SJ, Grant IWB (1976) Treatment of childhood asthma with sodium cromoglycate and beclomethasone dipropionate aerosol singly and in combination. *Br Med J* 2: 457–458
60 Shapiro GG, Sharpe M, DeRouen TA, Pierson WE, Furukawa CT, Virant FS et al (1991) Cromolyn *versus* triamcinolone acetonide for youngsters with moderate asthma. *J Allerg Clin Immunol* 88: 742–748
61 Petersen W, Daugbjerg P, Fog E, Friis B, Howitz P, Pedersen FK, Nielsen F (1993) Sodium cromoglycate (10 mg, tds) together with terbutaline (0.5 mg, tds) can replace inhaled steroids (200 µg) in childhood asthma. *Eur Respir J* 6 (Suppl 17): 356S
62 Warner JO, Götz M, Landau LI, Levison H, Milner AD, Pedersen S et al (1989) Management of asthma: a consensus statement. *Arch Dis Child* 64: 1065–1079
63 Hargreave FE, Dolovich J, Newhouse MT (1990) The assessment and treatment of asthma: a conference report. *J Allerg Clin Immunol* 85: 1098–1111
64 National Heart Lung, Blood Institute, National Institutes of Health, Bethesda Maryland (1992) International Consensus Report on Diagnosis and Management of Asthma. NIH publication no. 92-3091
65 Agertoft L, Pedersen S (1994) Effects of long-term treatment with an inhaled corticosteroid on growth and pulmonary function in asthmatic children. *Respir Med* 88: 373–381
66 Sears MR, Taylor DR, Print CG, Lake DC, Li Q, Flannery EM et al (1990) Regular inhaled beta-agonist treatment in bronchial asthma. *Lancet* 336: 1391–1396
67 Kerrebijn KF, van Essen-Zandvliet EEM, Neijens HJ (1987) Effects of long-term treatment with inhaled corticosteroids and beta-agonists on the bronchial responsiveness in children with asthma. *J Allerg Clin Immunol* 79: 653–659
68 Cockroft DW, O'Byrne PM, Swystun V, Bhagat R (1995) Regular use of inhaled albuterol and the allergen-induced late asthmatic response. *J Allerg Clin Immunol* 96: 44–49
69 König P, Shaffer J (1996) The effect of drug therapy on long-term outcome of childhood asthma: A possible preview of the international guidelines. *J Allerg Clin Immunol* 98: 1103–1111

70 Korppi M, Remes K (1996) Asthma treatment in schoolchildren: lung function in different ther-
    apeutic groups. *Acta Paediat* 85: 190–194
71 Oswald H, Phelan PD, Lanigan A, Hibbert M, Carlin JB, Bowes G, Olinsky A (1977) Childhood
    asthma and lung function in mid-adult life. *Pediat Pulmonol* 23: 14–20

CHAPTER 7
Future Trends in the Use of Corticosteroids in Asthma

Paul M. O'Byrne

Asthma Research Group and Department of Medicine, McMaster University, Hamilton, Ontario, Canada L8N 3Z5

1. Introduction

Corticosteroids have been used to treat a variety of airway diseases since the early 1950s, following an initial study of Carryer et al. [1], who reported the benefits of oral cortisone on ragweed pollen-induced hay fever and asthma. This was followed by a report by Gelfand [2], demonstrating clinical benefit from inhaled cortisone in a small group of patients with both allergic or non-allergic asthma. Subsequently, a multicenter trial run by the Medical Research Council in the United Kingdom in 1956 demonstrated improvement in acute severe asthma in a placebo controlled trial [3], and reports at that time described benefit in chronic asthma [4], demonstrating the unequivocal benefit of corticosteroids in asthma. Subsequently, both oral and inhaled corticosteroids have evolved into the most important and useful drugs currently available to treat asthma.

The initial studies evaluating the efficacy of inhaled corticosteroids in asthma were performed on patients with moderate to severe disease. At the time of their introduction to clinical practice in the early 1970s, and for many years thereafter, their use was mainly limited to patients who had persisting symptoms despite aggressive oral or inhaled bronchodilator use. The increased appreciation, in the mid 1980s, of the central role of airway inflammation in the pathogenesis of all asthma [5–7], provided a rationale for the earlier introduction of inhaled corticosteroids, particularly as the ability of inhaled corticosteroids to reduce airway inflammation [8] and improve some of the airway structural abnormalities associated with asthma was being identified. This has led to a reappraisal of how inhaled corticosteroids may be best used in the current and future management of asthma.

2. Clinical Use of Inhaled Corticosteroids

Asthma is a disease characterized by the presence of symptoms such as dyspnea, wheezing, chest tightness, and cough. These symptoms are usually caused by airflow obstruction, which is characteristically variable. Asthmatics are also known to have airway hyperresponsiveness to a variety of chemical bronchoconstrictor stimuli and physical stimuli such as exercise and hyperventilation of cold dry air. It is now accepted that asthma symptoms, variable airflow obstruction and airway hyperresponsiveness occur as a consequence of a characteristic form of cellular inflammation and structural changes in the airway wall [9]. The inflammation consists of the presence of activated eosinophils, lymphocytes, and an increased number of mast cells, which have been described both in bronchoalveolar lavage and airway biopsies from patients with mild stable asthma [6, 7, 10], as well as asthmatic subjects with much more severe disease [9]. Also, there are characteristic structural changes described in asthmatic airways, which appear to be characteristic of the disease

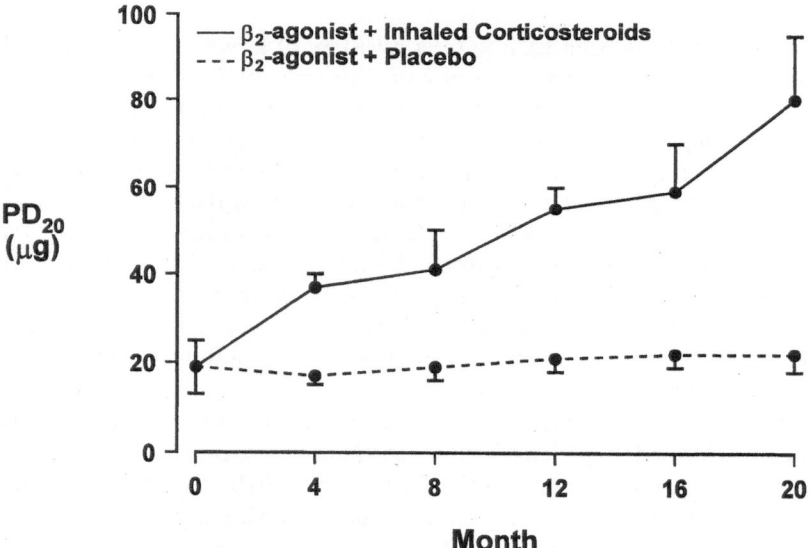

Figure 1. Effect of 22 months' treatment with an inhaled corticosteroid plus an inhaled β_2-agonist or placebo plus an inhaled β_2-agonist on methacholine airway responsiveness in asthmatic children. The inhaled corticosteroid progressively improved methacholine airway responsiveness over time. (Reproduced with permission from [15]).

and which are likely caused by persisting airway inflammation [9]. These changes include patchy desquamation of the airway epithelium [11]; thickening of the reticular collagen layer of the basement membrane [12]; and increased volume of airway smooth muscle [9].

It has been only with this increased appreciation of the pivotal role of airway inflammation in asthma, that an emphasis been placed on treating airway inflammation rather than the consequences of the inflammation, which are bronchoconstriction and asthma symptoms. The only anti-asthma medications which have been demonstrated to improve airway inflammation [8, 13], airway hyperresponsiveness [14, 15] (Fig. 1), airflow obstruction and symptoms in asthmatics are inhaled corticosteroids. This evidence has been used as a rationale for using inhaled corticosteroids much earlier in the treatment of asthma than was previously the case, when they were suggested to be reserved as third- or fourth-line therapy for asthma, and only when bronchodilators were not providing control of asthma [16].

3. Objectives of Asthma Management

There have been many published consensus statements from a variety of countries on asthma management [17, 18]. While the consensus statements have differed in some regards, they have been remarkably consistent in identifying the goals and objectives of asthma treatment. These are:
1. To minimize or eliminate asthma symptoms;
2. to achieve the best possible lung function;
3. to prevent asthma exacerbations;
4. to do the above with the lowest number possible medications;
5. to educate the patient about the disease and the goals of management.

One objective which is implied, but not explicitly stated, is the prevention of the decline in lung function and the development of fixed airflow obstruction which occurs in some asthmatic patients.

In addition to these goals and objectives, each of these documents has described what is meant by the term "asthma control". This includes the above objectives of minimal or no symptoms and best lung function, but also includes minimizing the need for rescue medications, such as inhaled β_2-agonists to less than daily use, minimizing the variability of flow rates that is characteristic of asthma, as well as having normal activities of daily living. Achieving this level of asthma control should be an objective from the very first visit of the patient to the treating physician. Unfortunately, many studies suggest that this does not happen. This may be, in part, because the patient has learned to live with daily asthma symptoms and limitations in his daily activities, and minimizes these to the physician. Alternatively, the idea of asthma control may not be widely accepted or understood by many physicians who see patients with asthma. This means that many (perhaps even most) patients with diagnosed asthma are not optimally controlled.

These concepts have resulted in a much lower threshold than previously for intervening with inhaled corticosteroids in asthma. This "early intervention" with an effective anti-inflammatory medication in asthma has scientific rationale, and is now being supported by clinical studies which have been completed or are underway.

4. Reasons for Early Intervention with Inhaled Corticosteroids

Early intervention with inhaled corticosteroids in asthma means beginning this treatment as the first regular treatment used after a diagnosis is established. An argument for early intervention with inhaled corticosteroids could be made if one or more of the following conditions were met:
1. Inhaled corticosteroids were *more effective* than other regular treatment to achieve optimal asthma control and meet the other treatment objectives;
2. inhaled corticosteroids prevented the decline in lung function over time that occurs in asthmatics;
3. inhaled corticosteroids were safer than an *equally effective* treatment modality;
4. inhaled corticosteroids were cost beneficial as an initial treatment of asthma, as measured by a benefit to the patient and/or to society by reducing the morbidity of asthma, which was not available by using any other medication.

Studies using inhaled corticosteroids have addressed all of these issues and these will be considered below.

5. Efficacy of Early Intervention with Inhaled Corticosteroids

There is little debate in the literature that corticosteroids are the most effective treatment for asthma [19, 20], and that the inhaled route is preferable to minimize unwanted effects. There is, however, considerable debate over the early use of inhaled corticosteroids in asthmatic patient considered to have mild asthma [21]. These patients are usually treated with regular inhaled β_2-agonists, or with drugs considered to be less clinically effective than inhaled corticosteroids, such as cromoglycate or nedocromil sodium. In a study of newly diagnosed asthmatics seen in speciality clinics, early intervention with the inhaled corticosteroid, budesonide, was shown to be an effective first-line treatment, when compared with an inhaled β_2-agonist, as indicated by reduced symptoms, improvements in lung function, and improvements in methacholine airway hyperresponsiveness [22]. However, many patients considered to have mild asthma are not seen in speciality clinics but are managed in primary care practices. It is possible that these patients are, in fact, ideally controlled without the use of inhaled corticosteroids. To address this issue, one study has examined the efficacy and cost-benefit of inhaled corticosteroids, supplemented with bronchodilators as needed, compared to bronchodilators alone, as first-line treatment of asthma in primary care practice [23]. This double blind study compared budesonide 400 μg/day, budesonide 800 μg/day, and placebo in patients considered by their primary care physician to have such mild asthma that they would not derive any clinical benefit from inhaled corticosteroids. In this patient population, in whom self-reported symptoms were mild at the start of the study, 40–70% of the patients were experiencing nocturnal or early morning symptoms in the month before entering the study (Fig. 2). These symptoms suggest that asthma control was not optimal. The study demonstrated that inhaled budesonide 400 μg/day provided better asthma control and is cost-beneficial when compared to bronchodilators alone in the management of these patients with mild asthma and that no differences could be demonstrated between 400 μg/day and 800 μg/day of budesonide; however, the study had insufficient power to detect differences between dosages, had they been present. The percentages of patients experiencing daily symptoms fell to less than 10% over the course of the study in the budesonide treatment groups (Fig. 2). Also, there was a mean 60–70 l/min increase in morning and evening peak expired flow rates (Fig. 3), and an elimination of exacerbations of asthma requiring emergency room management, indicating that a clinically useful improvement was achieved in this patient population with a dose of budes-

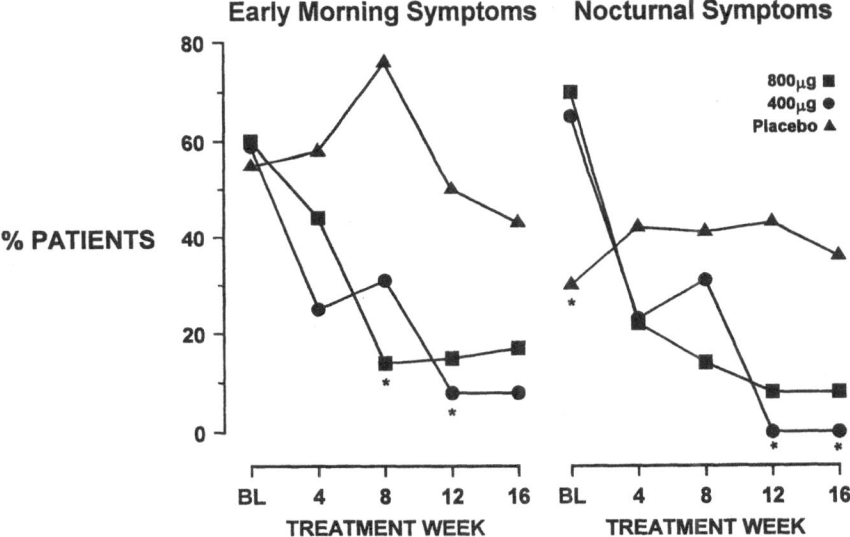

Figure 2. Proportion of patients considered by their family physician as having mild asthma, experiencing early morning symptoms or nocturnal symptoms in the month prior to evaluation at baseline, and after treatment with inhaled budesonide at treatment weeks 4 to 16 for patients on placebo (open circles), budesonide 400 μg/day (closed circles) and 800 μg/day (closed squares). $^* p < 0.05$, $^{**} p < 0.01$, $^{***} p < 0.001$. (Reproduced with permission from [23])

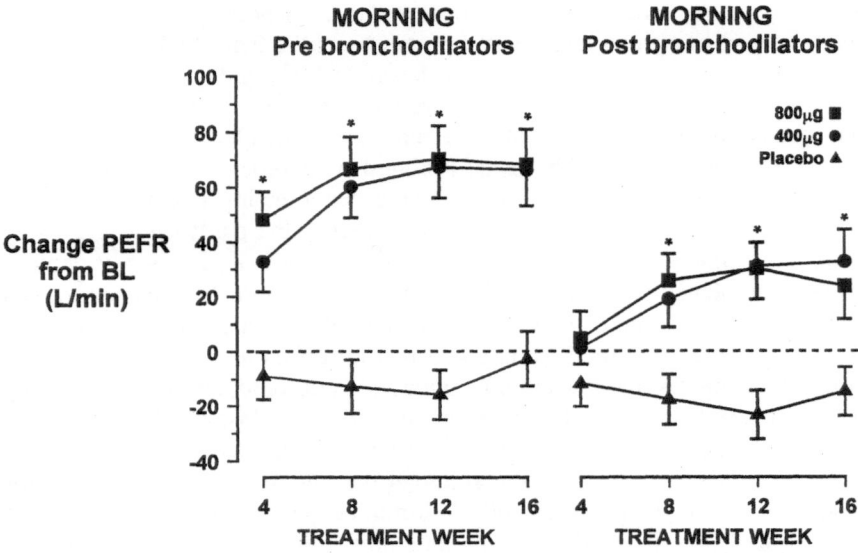

Figure 3. Changes in PEFR from baseline measured in the morning upon waking in patients considered by their family physician as having mild asthma, both before and after inhaled bronchodilator, after treatment with inhaled budesonide for treatment weeks 4 to 16 for patients on placebo (open circles), budesonide 400 μg/day (closed circles) and 800 μg/day (closed squares). ** $p < 0.01$, *** $p < 0.001$. (Reproduced with permission from [23].)

onide as low as 400 μg/day. This study supports the early intervention with inhaled corticosteroids for adult patients with regular daily symptoms of asthma, and suggests that low doses (budesonide 400 μg/day or possibly less) are effective in the management of asthmatic patients with mild to moderate asthma. In addition, the study reinforced the need to strive for optimal control of asthma, and once control is achieved, to identify the minimum amounts of medication needed to maintain control. Lastly, this study demonstrated that inhaled corticosteroid treatment is more cost-beneficial than asthma therapy with bronchodilators alone.

Another reason for recommending low doses of inhaled corticosteroids as first-line therapy for asthma, is the recent concern about the safety of regular short acting inhaled β_2-agonists. Sears et al. [24] have demonstrated deterioration in a number of parameters of asthma control, and reduced the time to an asthma exacerbation [25] when the short acting inhaled β_2-agonist fenoterol was used on a regular rather than intermittent basis. A subsequent study of the regular use of the short acting inhaled β_2-agonist, salbutamol, in milder asthmatics, showed an overall trend towards deterioration in a number of asthma outcomes, although none were statistically significant [26]. Also, retrospective studies have associated increased risk of asthma mortality with the overuse of the β_2-agonist fenoterol [27, 28], and salbutamol [28]. Regular use of inhaled

β_2-agonists has been demonstrated to increase airway responsiveness in asthmatics [29, 30], and to result in loss of functional antagonism to the bronchoconstrictor effects of inhaled methacholine [31], and adenosine monophosphate (AMP) [32].

6. Effects of Inhaled Corticosteroids on Lung Function over Time

Asthmatics lose lung function more rapidly than nonasthmatics [33], although less rapidly than cigarette smokers. In occasional asthmatics, this leads to severe, permanent, fixed airflow obstruction, with all of the attendant disability and handicap associated with this condition. A number of recent studies in both adults and children have demonstrated that inhaled steroids provide a protective effect against the deterioration in lung function seen with prolonged regular use of inhaled bronchodilator therapy alone. In one study, patients with asthma and patients with chronic obstructive pulmonary disease, previously treated with regular inhaled bronchodilators, were treated with inhaled beclomethasone 800 µg/day or placebo for 2 years [34]. Prior to the addition of inhaled corticosteroids, the forced expired volume in 1 s (FEV_1) had been declining at a rate of 160 ml/year. In the first 6 months of corticosteroid therapy, the FEV_1 *increased* by 460 ml and then continued to decline at a rate of 100 ml/year (significantly less than with bronchodilators alone). This protective effect of inhaled corticosteroids was most marked in the asthmatic patients, and was associated with significant improvement in methacholine airway hyperresponsiveness in the asthmatic patients only, and with decreased asthma symptoms and exacerbations.

A second study [35], has addressed this issue in a different way. These investigators had previously reported that the treatment of newly diagnosed asthmatics with inhaled budesonide 1200 µg/day for 2 years improved asthma control as indicated by reduced symptoms, improvements in lung function, and improvements in methacholine airway hyperresponsiveness, when compared to inhaled β_2-agonists [22]. The subjects receiving budesonide were subsequently randomly allocated to continuing for a third year on a lower dose of inhaled budesonide (400 µg/day) or placebo. The improvements in all parameters were maintained on the lower dose of budesonide, but were lost on placebo. The subjects who had previously been treated with inhaled β_2-agonists only were treated with the higher dose of inhaled budesonide for the third year, and while they improved in all parameters when compared to the first 2 years of treatment, the improvement in lung function (Fig. 4) or methacholine airway hyperresponsiveness was significantly less than that achieved by the subjects treated for the first year of the study with inhaled budesonide. This suggests that these asthmatics had lost lung function which might have been preserved with the early use of inhaled corticosteroids.

A study in asthmatic children has been reported by Agertoft and Pedersen [36], who have studied two cohorts for up to 7 years. One cohort had been

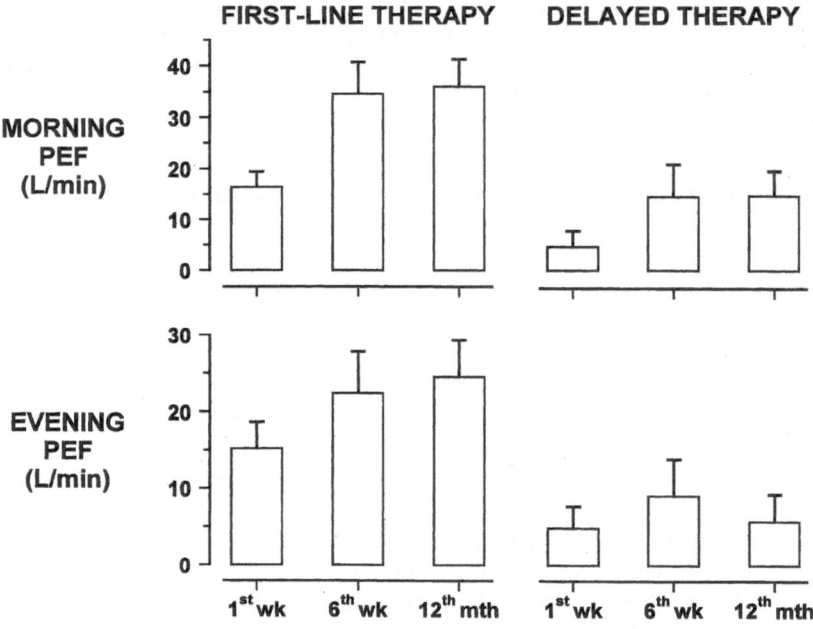

Figure 4. Comparison of the improvements in peak expired flow rates in patients treated with budes-onide as first line therapy within 1 year of diagnosis of asthma, and patients treated more than 2 years after diagnosis. (Redrawn and reproduced with permission from [35])

treated with inhaled corticosteroids shortly after diagnosis, while the other had received a variety of other antiasthma medications, including cromones, theo-phylline and regular inhaled β_2-agonists, but not inhaled corticosteroids. Some children in the second cohort were converted to inhaled corticosteroids, but on average 5 years after an initial diagnosis. These children in whom treatment with inhaled corticosteroids was started later did not achieve the level of lung function of the children treated early, even after 3 years of treatment with inhaled corticosteroids. The study also measured growth velocity in these chil-dren and concluded that doses of inhaled budesonide up to 400 µg/day was not associated with a reduction in growth velocity. A subsequent study in adult asthmatics, has confirmed these observations [37].

These studies, taken together, suggest that inhaled corticosteroids can diminish the decline in lung function that occurs in asthmatics, and that early intervention with inhaled corticosteroids can optimize lung function in asth-matics. Each of these studies, however, has limitations, mainly in that none were explicitly designed to address this issue in a prospective fashion. Therefore, while the results are consistent between the studies, the results are not conclusive. This has lead to the development of a very large, multination-al, prospective, randomized and placebo controlled study of the effects of early intervention with inhaled corticosteroids in both childhood and adult asthma. This study, known as the START (Steroid Therapy As Regular Treatment) trial, will evaluate the potential beneficial effects of inhaled corticosteroids treatment started within the first 2 years of the development of asthma, in patients with very mild disease.

7. Cost Benefit of Inhaled Corticosteroids in Asthma

Until recently, few studies have examined the cost benefit of early intervention with inhaled corticosteroids. However, several recent studies have demonstrated that inhaled corticosteroids are cost beneficial when compared to other anti-asthma treatments. For example, Adelroth and Thompson [38], have shown that the costs to the Swedish health care system declined when patients were treated with inhaled corticosteroids because of a reduction in hospital utilization and physician visits, when asthma control was optimized. Also, in the Canadian study already discussed [23], a cost-effectiveness analysis of the use of inhaled corticosteroids in patients thought to have very mild asthma treated in primary care practice, demonstrated an advantage with inhaled corticosteroids (again, mainly by keeping patients out of hospital emergency rooms), as asthma control is improved.

8. Future Trends in Inhaled Corticosteroid Use

The studies described above suggest that low doses of inhaled cotricosteroids will be used earlier in the onset of asthma and in patients with milder disease. The impact of earlier treatment on the progression of the disease is a critical issue which needs to be evaluated in future studies. It is plausible that, by preventing the airway structural abnormalities associated with asthma, the development of fixed airflow obstruction and more severe disease can be prevented. Also, it is clear from the studies which have evaluated this, that the severity of asthma is often underappreciated by both patients and physicians. This leads to undertreatment, less than ideal asthma control, and the attendant effects on patients' quality of life and increased costs to society. The only way to ensure that this does not happen, is to offer optimal treatment to all patients with established asthma, and this would most often be a therapeutic trial of inhaled corticosteroids.

9. Conclusions

Inhaled corticosteroids are the most effective medications currently available to treat symptomatic asthma, and are, fortunately, free of clinically relevant unwanted effects, when used in the doses needed to provide optimal control in most asthmatics. Inhaled corticosteroids also improve the physiological abnormalities of variable airflow obstruction and airway hyperresponsiveness that characterised asthma, as well as reducing the decline in lung function over time that occurs in asthmatics. Inhaled corticosteroids are also cost-beneficial when compared to other treatments, even in patients with milder asthma treated in primary care. For these reasons, inhaled corticosteroids are now being considered the first-line therapy for patients with regular, daily asthma symptoms, and should be started early after a diagnosis is made, rather than delaying until all other treatment options have been tried and have not provided optimal control of asthma.

There are, however, several issues about the early intervention with inhaled corticosteroids that have not yet been resolved. One such issue, already discussed, is whether inhaled corticosteroids should be used in all asthmatic patients, including those who have very mild and infrequent symptoms, or who develop symptoms only after being exposed to an inciting stimulus, such as exercise or cold air, and who have normal airway caliber most of the time. The current consensus statements do not recommend regular treatment in such patients, and this recommendation should probably be adhered to until more information is available about the natural history of asthma in such patients. These asthmatics do have evidence of airway inflammation and structural changes in airway biopsies; however, we do not yet know whether they lose lung function more rapidly than nonasthmatics, or whether the morbidity of having very mild asthma warrants the use of regular treatment. This information may be available when the results of the START trial are available. Also, not enough is yet known about the long-term effects of even low doses of inhaled corticosteroids. Although the studies of Agertoft and Pedersen [36] have provided details of up to 7 years of treatment on some of the potential unwanted effects in children, these studies will need to be more long-term before the concerns and fears of using inhaled corticosteroids very early in asthma will be allayed.

References

1 Carryer HM, Koelshe GA, Prickman LE et al (1950) The effect of cortisone on bronchial asthma and hay fever occurring in subjects sensitive to ragweed pollen. *J Allergy* 21: 282–7
2 Gelfand ML (1951) Administration of cortisone by the aerosol method in the treatment of bronchial asthma. *N Engl J Med* 245: 293–4
3 Medical Research Council (1956) Controlled trial of effects of cortisone acetate in status asthmaticus. *Lancet* 2: 803–6
4 Foulds GS, Greaves DP, Herxheimer H, Kingdom LG (1955) Hydrocortisone in treatment of allergic conjunctivitis, allergic rhinitis, and bronchial asthma. *Lancet* 1: 234–5
5 O'Byrne PM (1986) Airway inflammation and airway hyperresponsiveness. *Chest* 90: 575–7
6 Kirby JG, Hargreave FE, Gleich GJ, O'Byrne PM (1987) Bronchoalveolar cell profiles of asthmatic and nonasthmatic subjects. *Am Rev Respir Dis* 136: 379–83
7 Beasley R, Roche WR, Roberts JA, Holgate ST (1989) Cellular events in the bronchi in mild asthma and after bronchial provocation. *Am Rev Respir Dis* 139: 806–17

8 Jeffery PK, Godfrey RW, Adelroth E, Nelson F, Rogers A, Johansson SA (1992) Effects of treatment on airway inflammation and thickening of basement membrane reticular collagen in asthma. A quantitative light and electron microscopic study. *Am Rev Respir Dis* 145: 890–9

9 Drazen JM (1986) Inhalation challenge with sulfidopeptide leukotrienes in human subjects. *Chest* 89: 414–9

10 Jeffery PK, Wardlaw AJ, Nelson FC, Collins JV, Kay AB (1989) Bronchial biopsies in asthma. An ultrastructural, quantitative study and correlation with hyperreactivity. *Am Rev Respir Dis* 140: 1745–53

11 Laitinen LA, Heino M, Laitinen A, Kava T, Haahtela T (1985) Damage of the airway epithelium and bronchial reactivity in patients with asthma. *Am Rev Respir Dis* 131: 599–606

12 Roche WR, Beasley R, Williams JH, Holgate ST (1989) Subepithelial fibrosis in the bronchi of asthmatics. *Lancet* 1: 520–4

13 Adelroth E, Rosenhall L, Johansson SA, Linden M, Venge P (1990) Inflammatory cells and eosinophilic activity in asthmatics investigated by bronchoalveolar lavage. The effects of anti-asthmatic treatment with budesonide or terbutaline. *Am Rev Respir Dis* 142: 91–9

14 Juniper EF, Kline PA, Vanzieleghem MA, Ramsdale EH, O'Byrne PM, Hargreave FE (1990) Effect of long-term treatment with an inhaled corticosteroid (budesonide) on airway hyperresponsiveness and clinical asthma in nonsteroid-dependent asthmatics. *Am Rev Respir Dis* 142: 832–6

15 van Essen-Zandvliet EE, Hughes MD, Waalkens HJ, Duiverman EJ, Pocock SJ, Kerrebijn KF (1992) Effect of 22 months of treatment with inhaled corticosteroids and/or β_2-agonists on lung function, airway responsiveness and symptoms in patients with asthma. *Am Rev Respir Dis* 146: 547–54

16 Rebuck AS, Chapman KR (1987) Asthma: Trends on pharmacological therapy. *Can Med Assn J* 136: 483–8

17 National Heart LaBINIoH (1991) Guidelines for the diagnosis and management of asthma. US Department of Health Services Publication #91-3042:

18 Sheffer AL, Bartal M, Bousquet J, Carrasco E et al (1995) Global strategy for asthma management and prevention. National Institutes of Health 95-3659: 70–114

19 Barnes PJ, Pedersen S (1993) Efficacy and safety of inhaled corticosteroids in asthma. *Am Rev Respir Dis* 148:S1–S26

20 Pedersen S, O'Byrne PM (1997) A comparison of the efficacy and safety of inhaled corticosteroids in asthma. *Allergy* 52: 1–34

21 Drazen J, Israel E (1994) Treating mild asthma, when are inhaled steroids indicated? *N Engl J Med* 331: 737–8

22 Haahtela T, Jarvinen M, Tuomo K (1991) Comparison of a β_2-antagonist, terbutaline, with an inhaled corticosteroid, budesonide, in newly detected asthma. *N Engl J Med* 325: 388–92

23 O'Byrne PM, Cuddy L, Taylor DW, Birch S, Morris J, Syrotiuk J (1996) The clinical efficacy and cost benefit of inhaled corticosteroids as therapy in patients with mild asthma in primary care practice. *Cancer Res* 3: 169–75

24 Sears MR, Taylor DR, Print CG et al (1990) Regular inhaled beta-agonist treatment in bronchial asthma. *Lancet* 336: 1391–6

25 Taylor DR, Sears MR, Herbison GP et al (1993) Regular inhaled β-agonists in asthma: effects on exacerbations and lung function. *Thorax* 48: 134–8

26 Drazen JM, Israel E, Boushey HA et al (1996) Comparison of regularly scheduled with as-needed use of albuterol in mild asthma. *N Engl J Med* 335: 841–7

27 Crane J, Pearce N, Flatt A et al (1989) Prescribed fenoterol and death from asthma in New Zealand, 1981–83: case-control study. *Lancet* 1: 917–22

28 Spitzer WO, Suissa S, Ernst P et al (1992) The use of beta-agonists and the risk of death and near death from asthma. *N Engl J Med* 326: 501–6

29 Krahn J, Koeter GH, van der mark TW, Sluiter HJ, De Vries K (1985) Changes in bronchial hyperactivity induced by 4 weeks of treatment with anti-asthmatic drugs in patients with asthma: a comparison between budesonide and terbutaline. *J Allerg Clin Immunol* 76: 628–36

30 Vathenen AS, Knox AJ, Higgins BG, Britton JR, Tattersfield AE (1988) Rebound increase in bronchial responsiveness after treatment with inhaled terbutaline. *Lancet* 1: 554–8

31 Cheung D, Timmers MC, Zwinderman AH, Bel EH, Dijkman JH, Sterk PJ (1992) Long-term effects of a long-acting β_2-adrenoceptor agonist, salmeterol, on airway hyperresponsiveness in patients with mild asthma. *N Engl J Med* 327: 1198–203

32 O'Connor BJ, Aikman SL, Barnes PJ (1992) Tolerance to the nonbronchodilating effects of inhaled β_2-agonists in asthma. *N Engl J Med* 327: 1204–8

33 Peat JK, Woolcock AJ, Cullen K (1987) Rate of decline of lung function in subjects with asthma. *Eur J Respir Dis* 70: 171–9

34 Dompeling E, van Schayck CP, van Grunsven PM et al (1993) Slowing the deterioration of asthma and chronic obstructive pulmonary disease during bronchodilator therapy by adding inhaled corticosteroids. *Ann Intern Med* 1993: 770–8

35 Haahtela T, Jarvinen M, Kava T et al (1994) Effects of reducing or discontinuing inhaled budesonide in patients with mild asthma. *N Engl J Med* 331: 700–5

36 Agertoft L, Pedersen S (1994) Effects of long-term treatment with an inhaled corticosteroid on growth and pulmonary function in asthmatic children. *Respir Med* 88: 373–81

37 Selroos O, Pietinalho A, Lofroos AB, Riska H (1995) Effect of early vs late intervention with inhaled corticosteroids in asthma. *Chest* 108: 1228–34

38 Adelroth E, Thompson S (1988) Advantages of high dose budesonide. *Lancet* 1: 476

CHAPTER 8
Steroid Sparing Therapies in Asthma

David J. Evans and Duncan M. Geddes

Royal Brompton Hospital, Sydney Street, London SW3 6NP, UK

1. Introduction

The recognition that asthma is a consequence of airway inflammation has focused treatment goals towards anti-inflammatory agents. Inhaled and systemic corticosteroids are of proven benefit and inhaled steroids are so effective that systemic corticosteroids are usually reserved for acute exacerbations of the condition.

However there is a group of asthmatic patients who continue to have symptoms despite high doses of inhaled steroid and who require maintenance treatment with oral corticosteroid. Whilst these patients are a relative minority of the asthmatic population, in the order of 1–2%, this subset constitute a significant number and consume a considerable fraction of the available health care resources. Furthermore these patients are at risk from the unwanted effects of long-term treatment with systemic corticosteroid. These include osteoporosis, diabetes, cataracts, hypertension, and neuropsychiatric disturbances as well as growth retardation in children. Therefore, despite their efficacy in the treatment of asthma, there is a need to manage patients on the lowest dose of corticosteroid possible.

A structured approach to management of patients with steroid dependent asthma should be adopted. Firstly the diagnosis of asthma should be carefully examined. Chronic obstructive pulmonary disease (COPD) is common and a number of patients fall into this diagnostic category rather than asthma. Airway tumours, vocal cord dysfunction, connective tissue diseases, and hyperventilation syndrome should all be excluded. In addition psychological morbidity should be considered and appropriately treated as this may contribute to poor asthma control. Review of inhaled treatments for both dose and delivery is essential and patient compliance should be confirmed. Bronchodilator therapy with long-acting β_2-agonists and theophylline should be optimised. Avoidance of relevant allergens and occupational exposures remain central to asthma management and are especially important in this group of patients.

When asthma remains uncontrolled in spite of optimisation of both standard therapeutic and non-therapeutic management then alternative steroid sparing approaches should be considered. Various "second line" immunosuppressant drugs have been used including methotrexate, gold and cyclosporin. A number of trials have been done examining their usefulness in the treatment of asthma and the evidence for their use as steroid sparing agents is the subject of this review.

2. Design of Trials for Steroid Sparing Treatments in Asthma

Although some of the earlier trials examined immunosuppressants in isolation, the current treatment guidelines rely on the use of inhaled and systemic corticosteroids prior to the use of these "second line" agents. Therefore most of the trials published examine the effects of these drugs in addition to systemic corticosteroids. This rationale is based on the established benefits of corticosteroids in the treatment of asthma. In this context the fundamental issue is the risk/benefit ratio of systemic corticosteroids alone or in combination with a steroid sparing drug.

The trials looking at steroid sparing therapies have shown mixed results. There are a number of problems concerning patient selection and/or study design that should be highlighted prior to reviewing the evidence and reaching conclusions.

With the exception of methotrexate and cyclosporin, the literature is flawed by a lack of randomised, blinded, placebo-controlled studies. Many trials are either open studies or case reports providing merely anecdotal evidence for the use of these drugs. Further problems arise from those studies utilising a crossover design. The lengthy duration of effects of many of the drugs introduces bias in favour of placebo consequent upon carry-over effects—a consideration that has been overlooked in many of the trials in question.

Secondly the issue of steroid sparing effects is not strictly the same as efficacy. Various commentators argue that a drug that allows reduction in the dose of steroid dose without loss of asthma control must be efficacious. This is not in fact the case as improvement in control was neither sought nor often properly measured within the design of those studies. This is an important difference as comparison of those trials looking at steroid sparing effects and those showing efficacy becomes difficult.

Patient characteristics need to be carefully defined. It should be clearly shown that study patients are truly steroid dependent. The minimum dose of systemic corticosteroid should be established to allow possible steroid sparing effects of second line agents to be manifest. A good illustration of this point is seen in those studies showing marked steroid reduction in the placebo limb. A graphic expression of the importance of corticosteroid reductions ("steroid tapering") prior to trials is shown in Figure 1. A prerequisite for study entry should be that all subjects are on maximal doses of inhaled steroid (beclomethasone/budesonide 2 mg daily, or equivalent), appropriate adjunctive treatments, the lowest dose of systemic corticosteroid and despite these treatments remain symptomatic. Many of the trials to date have not clearly shown the steroid dependence of the study subjects and also show a heterogeneous population in terms of steroid requirements at baseline.

The question of steroid resistance is rarely addressed. Ideally for future research, subjects should be both corticosteroid responsive and dependent.

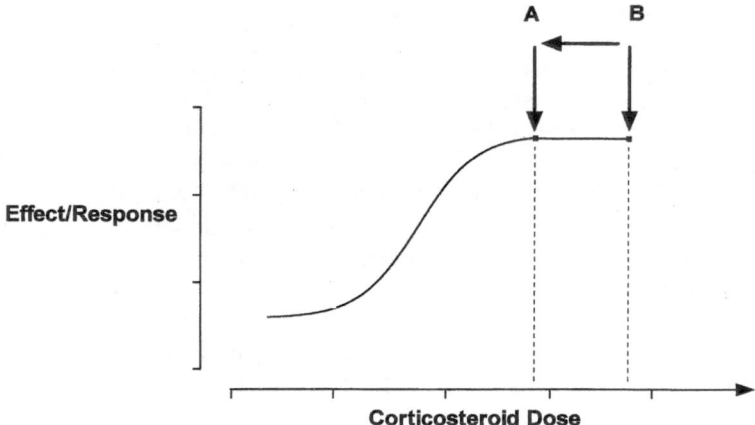

Figure 1. Illustration of dose/response for corticosteroids in the treatment of asthma. The importance of steroid dose tapering prior during run-in. Failure to use the lowest possible dose of corticosteroid (Dose A) during the treatment phase will allow reductions in corticosteroid use without loss of control, independent of other treatment. Reductions during tapering from maintenance dose B, to dose A will allow a true demonstration of steroid sparing effects of added treatments as further reductions would otherwise result in loss of asthma control.

For each drug reviewed below the evidence for steroid sparing effects (or lack of them) will be presented in addition to a brief synopsis of relevant side-effects and safety data.

3. Drugs

3.1. Methotrexate

3.1.1. Mode of Action: Methotrexate is the most widely studied non-steroidal immunosuppressant agent in the treatment of asthma. Methotrexate has been used in the treatment of malignant diseases for over 50 years and more recently for inflammatory disease of the joints and skin [1, 2].

The mechanism of action of methotrexate in asthma and other inflammatory conditions is thought to be different from its effects in malignancy. Whilst it is a potent inhibitor of the enzyme dihydrofolate reductase causing inhibition of thymidine synthesis and thus blocking nucleic acid synthesis in dividing cells, methotrexate probably also acts *via* direct inhibition of immune cell function. Blockade of granulocyte chemotaxis and the effects of interleukin-1 (IL-1), as well as inhibition of histamine release by basophils have all been demonstrated following *in vitro* experiments with the drug [3–5]. As methotrexate does not seem to cause leucopaenia in the doses used for the treatment of asthma, nor is its effect in inflammatory conditions lost following concomitant medication with folinic acid, the actions directed against immune cell function are thought to be more relevant to airway inflammation.

3.1.2. Clinical Trials: The possible benefits of methotrexate in asthma followed from the observation by Mullarkey that a patient with psoriasis and steroid dependent asthma was able to discontinue systemic corticosteroid treatment following the institution of methotrexate for her psoriatic arthropathy [6]. Alongside the index case the authors reported a further five patients in whom steroid reduction was possible without loss of asthma control. Further randomised, double-blind, placebo-controlled trials examining the effects of methotrexate over 24-week treatment periods endorsed the initial report showing steroid sparing effects of the drug [7, 8]. In the first of these trials, also reported by Mullarkey, 14 patients with a mean daily prednisolone dose of 25 mg were prescribed Methotrexate 15 mg/week or placebo using a cross-over study design. In these patients there was a 36.5% reduction in steroid requirements in the methotrexate limb compared to placebo without change in lung function [7]. This result clearly shows benefit for methotrexate treatment but does not give adequate details of concomitant asthma treatment nor inhaled steroid treatment, thus raising doubt about the steroid dependence of the patients. Furthermore, details of the eight patients who failed to complete the study are not reported. Shiner conducted a similar study using a parallel group design. This study presented evaluable data on 60 patients and more clearly defined steroid dependence. Both placebo and methotrexate patients were on high-dose inhaled steroid and at least 7.5 mg systemic corticosteroid for no less than 1 year previously. At the end of the study there were significantly greater reductions in the dose of steroid in the methotrexate group compared to placebo (50% vs 14%). In support of the anti-inflammatory effects of methotrexate there were significant fewer exacerbations in the active treatment group compared to placebo, although no changes in PEFR, PEFR variability, nor symptom scores [8].

Subsequently there have been three further blinded, placebo-controlled trials showing a steroid sparing effect of methotrexate. Dyer studied 12 patients, 10 of whom completed the trial, and showed a 30% greater reduction in steroid dose during treatment with methotrexate compared to placebo over a 12-week treatment period [9]. No changes in lung function, rescue medication use or symptoms were reported. This study is endorsed by both its requirement for steroid dependence of at least 7.5 mg a day and a steroid tapering period prior to run-in. Stewart showed significantly greater reductions in steroid dose on methotrexate compared to placebo and associated improvements in symptom scores [10]. Twelve patients studied by Hedman et al. showed a significant reduction of 38% during methotrexate treatment with no change in lung function. These patients were also subjected to steroid tapering regimens prior to run-in [11]. The mean daily prednisolone dose at baseline for these studies was 13 mg, 23 mg and 10 mg respectively [9–11].

In contrast to these trials there are five double-blind, placebo-controlled trials that fail to show steroid sparing effects of methotrexate. The first of these trials was conducted by Erzurum. Following a 12-week treatment period studying 19 patients using a parallel group design there were significant reductions in steroid dose in both placebo and methotrexate 15 mg/week groups but no difference between treatments. The average dose of steroids at baseline was 20 mg and there was an adequate steroid tapering regimen prior to randomisation [12]. This study may have failed to identify a benefit of methotrexate due to an inadequate treatment period in keeping with the delayed response seen by Shiner [8]. Against this hypothesis are the results from the studies published by Mullarkey and Dyer that did show earlier effects [7, 9].

A further negative study examining data from nine patients has been reported by Taylor. In favour of this study the treatment period was 24 weeks in length—although the authors do not give details of the washout period between treatments and did not undertake a steroid tapering phase prior to randomisation. Nevertheless no difference was seen between methotrexate at a dose of 15 mg/week and placebo in patients with an initial mean dose of systemic corticosteroid of 16 mg [13]. Trigg showed similar results amongst nine patients who were diagnosed as steroid dependent on a median dose of prednisolone of 17.5 mg/day. This study was conducted over two 12-week treatment periods (although using a cross-over design), and in common with the work of Taylor, there was no washout period notwithstanding the fact that only the data from the last 8 weeks of each treatment limb were analysed. The dose of methotrexate in this trial was 30 mg/week and the authors report no reduction in steroid dose compared to placebo [14]. Coffey, studying 11 patients using 15 mg/week in a crossover design [15] and Kanzow, using a parallel design with 21 patients [16], both failed to show a significant steroid sparing effect of methotrexate. In the latter study there was reduction in steroid dose of 24% in the active treatment limb compared to a 5% reduction with placebo, although this change was not sustained during a subsequent 8 week run-out period. The baseline prednisolone doses were 30 mg (following steroid tapering) in both these trials. A subsequent efficacy study looking at the effects of methotrexate and triamcinolone compared to placebo in a small group of severe asthmatics showed no benefits for methotrexate for lung function, symptom control or airway responsiveness. No attempts to reduce steroids was made in this study [17]. A summary of the findings of the placebo controlled trials for methotrexate is shown in Table 1.

For those trials showing a steroid sparing benefit of methotrexate, the question remains as to whether this effect is maintained in the longer term. The evidence from early follow-up data suggested that this was not the case [8, 16]. In contrast however four subsequent open trials have addressed this issue with follow-up periods of between 12 and 28 months. Mullarkey demonstrated a significant reduction in steroid dose with 15 out of 31 patients discontinuing systemic corticosteroid treatment over approximately 2 years [18]. Shiner showed similar results with 13 out of 21 patients weaning altogether during the

Table 1. Placebo controlled trials for methotrexate

Author	Year	Study design	Patients	Treatment duration	Baseline steroid dose/day	Steroid reduction on methotrexate	Efficacy/other outcomes
Mullarkey [7]	1988	Cross-over	14	12 weeks	25 mg	36.5% greater than placebo	-
Shiner [8]*	1990	Parallel	60	24 weeks	approx 15 mg	MTX 50%, Placebo 14%	Less exacerbations on MTX ($p < 0.05$)
Dyer [9]*	1991	Cross-over	10	12 weeks	8–12 mg	30% greater than placebo	-
Erzurum [12]*	1991	Parallel	18	13 weeks	20 mg	40% reduction for both MTX and Placebo	Increases in eosinophil counts
Trigg [14]	1993	Cross-over	12	12 weeks	median 17.5 mg	No difference between MTX and Placebo	Small improvements FEV_1 favouring MTX ($p < 0.05$)
Taylor [13]	1993	Cross-over	9	24 weeks	16 mg	16% MTX, 30% Placebo (NS)	-
Stewart [10]	1994	Cross-over	21	9 weeks	23 mg	14% reduction in MTX, no change Placebo	-
Hedman [11]	1994	Cross-over	12	12 weeks	10 mg	38% reduction on MTX ($p < 0.05$)	Significant improvements in symptoms and β-agonists
Coffey [15]*	1994	Cross-over	11	12 weeks	30 mg	20% reduction both MTX and Placebo	-
Kanzow [16]*	1995	Parallel	21	16 weeks	approx 30 mg	24% MTX, 5% Placebo (NS)	-

Definition of abbreviations; MTX, Methotrexate: FEV_1, forced expiratory volume in 1 s:
* Steroid tapering during run-in. six uncontrolled trials [18–21, 23, 24] are not detailed above.

long-term review [19]. Even more striking reductions were recorded by Stanziola during the follow-up of 13 patients over periods ranging from 54 to 72 weeks. In this group there was a mean reduction of 87% in steroid dose with nine patients stopping prednisolone therapy completely [20]. Clearly these open studies are difficult to interpret, nevertheless the magnitude of change implies a real effect. Contrary to these reports, Becquart failed to demonstrate reduction in systemic corticosteroid dose or improvements in lung function in a group of 10 patients over a 14-month methotrexate treatment period and a further 7-month post treatment follow-up [21].

The experience with methotrexate in the treatment of children is limited. A small number of case reports and open studies reported to date show possible steroid sparing effects and improvements in lung function [22–24]. However the number of subjects is small and, with the exception of the study of Stempel [22], are of too short duration to draw conclusions about benefits or safety.

3.1.3. Adverse Effects: All the trials to date show a high incidence of nausea, and abdominal discomfort and this symptom has a variously reported incidence of between 28 and 75% [25]. Other common side-effects include mucocutaneous ulceration, stomatitis, and alopecia. Abnormalities of liver enzymes occur with low dose treatment with methotrexate although these are usually mild and recover on discontinuation of the drug. Twelve patients in the study reported by Shiner, three of whom were withdrawn, showed increases in serum transaminases, although all with no subsequent untoward consequences [8]. Although no serious or permanent hepatic side-effects have been reported in these asthma trials, the risk of liver fibrosis during long-term treatment with methotrexate for psoriasis and rheumatoid arthritis has led to one group recommending liver biopsy after a cumulative dose of 1.5 g. Evidence showing that this approach reduces morbidity has not been published. A history of diabetes, obesity, and alcohol excesses are all relative contra-indications to the use of this drug as these factors have been shown to increase the likelihood of this complication [26]. Mild impairment of renal function, macrocytosis (although it is unusual for the doses relevant to asthma to cause haematological suppression) and hypogammaglobulinaemia have been recognised as possible side-effects of methotrexate and therefore careful monitoring of these parameters is important during treatment. There are anecdotal reports that methotrexate may actually precipitate asthma [27].

Drug-induced pulmonary complications of methotrexate are potentially severe. An idiosyncratic pneumonitis has been reported and is usually reversible on stopping the drug [28]. In contrast an insidious pulmonary fibrosis may occur and despite withdrawal may be irreversible [29]. Careful monitoring of both radiology and lung function are important to monitor for this possible adverse effect. There are reports of *Pneumocystis carinii* pneumonia amongst patients on methotrexate [30–32] and there is probably increased incidence of pulmonary and extra-pulmonary infections including reactivation of latent herpetic infection [33]. Trigg reported two cases of pneumonia (warranting withdrawal from the trial) and one zoster infection in patients receiving methotrexate 30 mg/week [14].

Methotrexate is a teratogen and should be avoided in individuals who do not use adequate contraception. Sulphonamides, non-steroidal anti-inflammatory drugs, and diuretics should be avoided in patients prescribed methotrexate [34].

3.1.4. Conclusion: Comparing the various studies, particularly with respect to the different patient populations, is very complex. A recent meta-analysis of the randomised trials has failed to conclusively support this agent as a steroid sparing treatment. There was however a small effect in favour of methotrexate in the parallel group designs endorsing the possibility of carryover effects for the crossover studies [35]. Given the lack of data showing efficacy and the side-effect profile of this drug there are no clear indications for the use of methotrexate in the treatment of asthma. In those instances where it is prescribed careful monitoring of liver, renal and lung function are mandatory.

3.2. Cyclosporin A

3.2.1. Mode of Action: Cyclosporin is a cyclic undecapeptide metabolite extracted from the fungus *Tolypocyladium inflatum*. It is used for the prevention of allograft rejection and has been found to be effective in the treatment of a variety of inflammatory disorders such as rheumatoid arthritis [36], psoriasis [37], lichen planus [38] and nephrotic syndrome [39]. Cyclosporin acts either directly or indirectly to inhibit lymphocytes, eosinophils, mast cells, and basophils.

At a cellular level cyclosporin diffuses easily into cells and binds cytosolic proteins, for example cycophilin, whose roles include regulation of protein kinases, phospholipase A_2 and post-translational protein folding [40]. It also binds to pro-inflammatory transcription factors inclusive of activator protein 3 (AP_3) [41], and nuclear factor κB ($NF\kappa B$) [42]. Additionally cyclosporin blocks the membrane receptor for interleukin-1 (IL-1) [43]. Through these effects, and relevant to allergic inflammation, cyclosporin has been shown to inhibit 1) mast cell and basophil secretion of leukotriene C_4 (LTC_4), platelet activating factor (PAF), and histamine [44], 2) lymphocyte synthesis of cytokines, for example IL-2, IL-3, IL-4, IL-5, GM-CSF [45], 3) B cell IL-4 stimulated IgE synthesis [46], 4) eosinophil function [47], and 5) macrophage respiratory burst oxidase and IL-1 production [48].

The drug is well tolerated by the oral route and is given at a dose range of between 3 and 7.5 mg/kg body weight. Cyclosporin treatment should be monitored and maintained at drug levels of 80–150 ng/mL to give optimal anti-inflammatory effects and minimal side-effects.

3.2.2. Clinical Trials: In view of the experience with other inflammatory states and the *in vitro* evidence for mechanisms of action it is not suprising there has been considerable interest in the possibility that this compound may have benefits in the treatment of asthma. The first randomised trial was reported by Alexander [49]. Thirty patients with a mean systemic corticosteroid dose of 8.5 mg a day received cyclosporin in a placebo controlled cross-over study. The treatment period was 12 weeks and the mean cyclosporin levels was 152 ng/mL. This efficacy study showed significant improvements compared to placebo in lung function, PEFR, and PEFR variability but no differences in symptom scores or rescue medication use. Analysis of an 11-week run-out period showed the mean morning PEFR remained significantly higher compared to baseline following cyclosporin treatment.

A subsequent study by Nizankowska examined both the efficacy and possible steroid sparing effects of cyclosporin in 32 patients [50]. These individuals were steroid dependent as demonstrated by failed attempts to taper systemic corticosteroid in the 6 months prior to study entry. The mean dose of prednisolone in this group of patients was 16 mg a day. In this study the mean cyclosporin level was 120 ng/mL. No benefits were recorded for lung function, PEFR, or PEFR variability in the efficacy treatment phase of 12 weeks although there were significant differences in symptom scores and rescue medication use in favour of the cyclosporin patients. During the steroid sparing phase (22 weeks) no differences were seen between the two groups for steroid reduction or exacerbation rates. The authors concluded no benefits following the introduction of cyclosporin.

Lock studied the steroid sparing effects of cyclosporin using a placebo controlled parallel study design [51]. Thirty-nine patients were studied and all were established steroid dependent asthmatics with a mean daily prednisolone dose of 12 mg. Contrary to the reports of Nizankowska, this study showed significantly greater steroid reduction in cyclosporin treated patients of 25% compared to placebo for "lowest dose" steroid during the 36-week treatment phase (i.e. not necessarily at the end of treatment periods). However over the whole duration of treatment there was no statistically significant difference between treatment groups despite the fact that the within group steroid reduction for cyclosporin was significant. Despite reductions in steroid treatment the cyclosporin patients showed significant increases in PEFR, although no change in other parameters of lung function, PEFR variability, or symptom scores. The mean cyclosporin level during this study was 144 ng/mL. The details of these trials are shown in Table 2.

Two further open studies by Szczeklik [52] and Mungan [53] showed steroid reduction in studies of 3 and 9 months duration respectively. Neither were placebo controlled and there were six nonresponders in the first trial and evaluable data from only seven individuals in the second. The mean cyclosporin levels for these studies were 105 ng/mL and 77 ng/mL respectively.

3.2.3. Side-Effects: The effects of cyclosporin on blood pressure and renal function are established and require careful monitoring. In the studies report-

Table 2. Placebo controlled trials for cyclosporin A

Author	Year	Study design	Patients	Cyclosporin level ng/ml	Treatment duration	Baseline steroid dose/day	Steroid reduction on CsA	Efficacy/other outcomes
Alexander [49]	1988	Cross-over	30	152	12 weeks	8.5 mg	Not documented	Significant improvements for PEFR, FEV_1, and exaberations
Nizankowska [50]*	1995	Parallel	32	120	34 weeks (2 phases; 12 weeks efficacy, 22 weeks steroid reduction)	16 mg	Similar reductions in Placebo and CsA groups symptoms in favour of CsA	No benefit for lung function during efficacy phase, significant improvements in β-agonist use and
Lock [51]*	1996	Parallel	39	144	36 weeks	12 mg	25% greater reduction in median steroid dose on CsA compared to placebo	Mean PEFR a.m. and p.m. improved with CsA ($p < 0.05$). No increases in FEV_1 or symptom scores compared to placebo

Definition of abbreviations; CsA, Cyclosporin A: FEV_1, forced expiratory volume in 1 s:
* Steroid tapering: uncontrolled trials [52, 53] are not detailed above.

ed above there were a number of patients who either developed hypertension or had worsening of pre-existing hypertension. Blood pressure was significantly higher in the cyclosporin treated patients in the studies reported by Alexander [49] and Lock [51]. These two trials also showed significant worsening of renal function during treatment with the GFR remaining decreased after the run-out phase, perhaps indicating lasting damage to the kidney [51].

Other side-effects include elevations in liver enzymes, increased risk of infection, hypertrichosis, neuropathy/paraesthesia and gastrointestinal disturbances.

3.2.4. Conclusion: The trial data does not support the routine use of cyclosporin in the treatment of asthma. In view of its potentially serious side-effect profile it should only be used by physicians with experience of it, and careful monitoring is essential. The development of inhaled cyclosporin may allow the drug to be given more safely. The evidence to date at best predicts a role in only a subgroup of patients.

3.3. Gold

3.3.1. Mechanism of Action: Gold sodium thiomalate, gold thioglucose and auranofin are the agents used as gold therapy. The latter is a synthetic compound that, unlike the other two parenteral compounds, is lipid soluble and therefore administered by mouth. In addition to its route of administration, there are other pharmacokinetic differences between the formulations of gold that strongly favour auranofin. Not least of these relates to the doses of the various agents required to give a similar clinical effect, these being significantly less for the oral compound. This is particularily relevant in the light of the cumulative toxicity of gold treatments [54].

The mechanism of action of gold is not well understood. Furthermore the action of parenteral gold differs from auranofin [55]. The possible anti-inflammatory effects of these agents is summarised in Table 3.

Gold is usually prescribed at a dose of 25–50 mg a week and taken either orally or by intramuscular injection.

3.3.2. Clinical Trials: Elemental gold has been used as a treatment of various ailments for hundreds of years, although its use in inflammatory conditions such as rheumatoid arthritis was not fully recognised until 1929 [56]. Subsequently the use of gold in the treatment of arthritic conditions has been extensively examined and the benefits in some patients are proven. Studies in asthma have been attempted for over 50 years, the earliest work in Europe [57–59] and thereafter most of the interest in this treatment has been in Japan [60–62]. These uncontrolled studies, evaluating parenteral gold, showed promising results for efficacy and suggested that gradual reductions in bronchodilator and corticosteroid treatments was possible.

Table 3. Mechanisms of action of gold

Mechanism	Parenteral gold	Auranofin
Inhibition of lymphocyte responses to mitogen	✔	✔
Inhibition of prostaglandin synthesis	✔	
Inhibition of lysozymes	✔	✔
Inhibition of mast cell/basophil mediator release		✔
Inhibition of chemotaxis		✔
Inhibition of antibody synthesis		✔
Inhibition of IL-1 and IL-2 release		✔
Inhibition of allergen-induced contraction of guinea pig trachea		✔

(Parenteral gold; Gold sodium thiomalate, gold thioglucose)

Given the various possible mechanisms of action and established differences in pharmacolgical profiles between auranofin and parenteral gold, comparisons of steroid sparing effects and efficacy are difficult. Nevertheless for the purpose of review the studies reported for both oral and parenteral gold will be summarised together.

The first blinded, placebo-controlled trial looking at the benefits of parenteral gold was published by Muranaka [63]. Sixty-four steroid dependent asthmatic patients whose systemic corticosteroid requirements were approximately 5 mg a day were studied over a 30-week treatment period. The analysis of the data constituted a physician's evaluation of rescue medication consumption and responses to questions concerning asthma control. In this way the authors reported a significant improvement in asthma control in the gold treated patients compared to the placebo group.

In an open trial examining the effects of auranofin, over 24 weeks in 20 steroid dependent asthmatics (mean daily prednisolone 15 mg), Bernstein showed non-significant improvements in asthma symptoms and exacerbations but did demonstrate significant reductions in IgE mediated immune responses during *ex vivo* peripheral blood studies [64].

Subsequently further placebo-controlled, double-blind trials have been published [65–68], the first of which examined the effects of parenteral gold [67], the remainder concentrating on oral auranofin. All these trials adopted a steroid tapering phase prior to run-in. However the patients in these studies represent a wide spectrum of severity with half of one study population on inhaled corticosteroids (the remaining half steroid naïve) [65] to groups requiring 7–9 mg [66] and others dependent on 20–25 mg prednisolone a day [67, 68]. With the exception of the trial by Honma (which succeeded in its design to show a bronchoprotective effect of oral gold) all these studies demonstrated significant steroid sparing effects of gold. Only the study by Nierop showed significant improvements in lung function in addition to reductions in systemic corticosteroid requirements [66]. The details of these trials are shown in Table 4.

Table 4. Clinical trials for gold

Author	Agent	Study design	Patients	Duration	Baseline steroid dose/day	Steroid reduction on gold	Efficacy/other outcomes
Muranaka [63]	parenteral gold	DBPCT	64	30 weeks	approx 5 mg	Not documented	Physician's assessment favoured gold($p < 0.05$)
Bernstein [64]	auranofin	Open	20	24 weeks	15 mg	34% (NS)	Half doubling dose reduction in PC_{20} (NS)Reduced ex vivo IgE stimulated mediator release ($p < 0.05$)
Honma [65]	auranofin	DBPCT	25	12 weeks	inhaled/nil*		reduction PC_{20} auranofin vs placebo
Nierop [66]	auranofin	DBPCT	28	26 weeks	7–9 mg	33% auranofin vs 0% placebo	Improved exacerbation rates and FEV_1 ($p < 0.05$)
Klaustermeyer [67]	parenteral gold	DBPCT	8	22 weeks	approx 23 mg	5/8 patients significantly	decreased steroid
Bernstein [68]	auranofin	DBPCT	157	8 months	66% 15–20, 35% >20 mg	60% auranofin vs 32% placebo achieved more than 50% reduction ($p < 0.05$)	Mean serum IgE reduced on auranofin ($p < 0.05$), no change lung function cf. placebo
McNeill [69] improvements	auranofin	Open	9	7–17 months	30–40 mg	approx 50% reduction	Non-significant in lung function

Definition of abbreviations; DBPCT, double-blind placebo-controlled trial: FEV_1, forced expiratory volume in 1 s: PC_{20} provocative concentration of agonist causing a 20% fall in FEV_1

One open report looking at the effects of auranofin in salicylate-sensitive steroid dependent asthmatics has shown significant reductions in systemic corticosteroid requirements, without any improvement in lung function over 7–17 months of therapy [69].

3.3.3. Adverse Effects: Auranofin and parenteral gold cause proteinuria in a minority of patients. Two patients became nephrotic and were withdrawn in one study [65], while three had lesser degrees of proteinuria in another [61]. The authors reporting the latter study documented that the renal abnormality recovered on discontinuation of the drug but no details concerning resolution are given for the other patients. Gastrointestinal problems including nausea and diarrhoea are common side-effects of gold and Bernstein attributes intestinal perforation in two patients and haemorrhage in two other patients to the use of gold [66]. Eczema, either *de novo* or worsening of pre-existing disease, frequently occurs and caused a patient withdrawal in one study [64]. Blood dyscrasias, liver enzyme abnormalities and pulmonary infiltrates are less common complications of gold therapy.

3.3.4. Conclusion: The data for gold suggest steroid sparing effects although the study populations are very mixed and the size of the reduction between the studies is variable. Furthermore the inconsistent use of inhaled steroids makes the clinical relvance difficult to judge. The experience with rheumatoid arthritis is that treatment usually has to be discontinued after a period due to side-effects. As many of these are potentially serious the likelihood of gold becoming an established treatment for asthma is low.

3.4. Immunoglobulin

3.4.1. Mechanism of Action: Intravenous immunoglobulin (IVIG) may have broad based immunomodulatory actions that account for its effects in a variety of diseases. Clearly it may be valuable in the protection against infection in those individuals with hypogammaglobulinaemia. However in the majority of patients there are no immunodeficiencies and in these patients the mechanism of action is complex and under debate. It may act *via* interference with the Fc gamma receptor mediated clearance of IgG coated particles which, although relevant to thrombocytopaenia, is probably not relevant to actions in asthma. An interesting hypothesis for IVIG involves the concept of anti-idiotype effects. In these circumstances the IVIG may act to block the effects of IgE in allergic responses. Other possibilities include the inhibition of mononuclear cell responses in particular the differentiation of B cells into antibody secreting cells [70].

3.4.2. Clinical Trials: IVIG has been used in the treatment of immunologically mediated diseases, for example immune thrombocytopaenias and polyneuropathy. Interest in the possibility that IVIG may be of benefit in the treatment of asthma has emerged in the light of increasing knowledge about the pathogenesis of the airway inflammation seen in asthma and the various successes of this modality in the treatment of the other conditions.

The literature on the evidence for IVIG in asthma goes back over 30 years although it is very difficult to arrive at a consensus about either efficacy or possible steroid sparing properties. The reasons for this are threefold. Firstly the indications for therapy vary. In the earlier trials the rationale for therapy was based on a need to limit infection in the asthmatic patients, indeed some studies concentrated only on patients who were hypogammaglobulinaemic [71]. Secondly the doses used vary greatly both in those trials looking at immunomodulatory effects of the treatment and those using IVIG as a protection against infection. Finally there is considerable variation in study design and end-points, in particular many of the reports are not blinded or placebo controlled. The studies concentrate on children and adolescents.

Abernathy in 1958 [72] and Brown in 1960 [73] were the first authors to undertake formal trials using IVIG in the treatment of asthma following on from initial abstract reports of successful control of sinopulmonary infection in asthmatic subjects. Abernathy evaluated 22 asthmatic children using a double-blind, placebo-controlled design and found no evidence in terms of exacerbations, treatment requirements or infection rates to support IVIG. In contrast Brown found evidence for an effect in 23 of 29 of study patients, although this trial gave limited details of other treatments and was conducted in an open fashion. These trials were both low-dose IVIG—approximately 300 mg/kg. Soon after these papers Fontana published the results of a double-blind, placebo-controlled trial with low dose IVIG looking at 41 patients with recurrent episodes of asthma related to infection [74]. As with the other studies previously reported these individuals were immunocompetent. This study concluded no benefit for the treatment.

Subsequently Page [71], in five children with immunoglobulin sub-class deficiency, and Smith [75], in 50 subjects with chronic infection, have reported clinical improvements in symptoms although they failed to show any immunological parameters to support anything other than added protection against infection. The issue of steroid sparing properties was not examined in theses studies.

Two studies focus on an immunomodulatory mechanism and selected patients with asthma and atopy contrary to the previous work where history of infection was central to recruitment. Mazer conducted a comprehensive study looking at clinical and immunological markers of asthma control, albeit in an open design amongst eight steroid dependent children. In this study, despite a steroid tapering run-in over 3 months, the mean steroid requirements of the subjects was 32.5 mg alternate days. The run-in was followed by 6 monthly IVIG treatments. The results show a threefold reduction in maintenance steroid requirements and reduced doses of steroids during exacerbations and improvements in PEFR and symptom scores. There were diminished skin prick responses to aero-allergens and in parallel to this significant reductions in total IgE levels, but no change in airway responsiveness to methacholine challenges. This study used higher doses of IVIG, 2 g/kg, distinguishing it from the previous lower dose trials [76]. Jackobsson repeated the study in a group of less severe asthmatics whose mean daily steroid dose requirement was only 720 μg of inhaled steroid using an IVIG dose of 800 mg/kg monthly for 5 treatments. The authors report significant reductions in steroid consumption but no difference from controls in terms of rescue medication use or symptom scores [77]. As for the patients studied by Mazer there were no changes in airway responsiveness.

3.4.3. Adverse Effects: IVIG is well tolerated although headache is commonly experienced by patients during the infusion and there are reports of aseptic meningitis occurring following this therapy [78]. The other concern for IVIG is the occurrence of acute allergic reactions to the infusions and anaphylaxis has been reported.

3.4.4. Conclusion: The evidence for a steroid sparing effect for IVIG is limited. Furthermore there are no data to strongly support efficacy beyond those effects attributable to infection protection. In addition IVIG is an expensive and inconvenient treatment. IVIG cannot be recommended for routine use in asthma. Carefully controlled placebo trials are required, although the data to hand do not predict useful immunomodulatory effects for asthmatic patients.

3.5. Troleandomycin

3.5.1. Mechanism of Action: Troleandomycin (TAO) is a macrolide antibiotic with established benefits in the treatment of infections. The most likely relevant mechanism of action relates to the clearance of methylprednisolone. Studies in both humans [79] and animals [80] show definite effects in keeping with inhibition of methylprednisolone clearance with consequent increases in half-life. Interestingly this effect seems to be specific to methylprednisolone. However there is some *in vitro* work showing reductions in neutrophil chemotaxis [81], inhibitory effects on mitogen-stimulated lymphocytic responses [82], reductions in basophil histamine release [83] and airway mucous secretion [84]. Overall the evidence supports steroid related actions more than immunomodulatory effects for this drug.

3.5.2. Clinical Trials: Celmer prepared a derivative of oleandomycin, formerly named triacetyloleandomycin, in 1957 [85]. This drug was shown to have superior antibiotic efficacy to its parent compound and was adopted as an antibiotic in the treatment of Gram positive infection. As a consequence of this use it became clear that asthmatic patients with infective exacerbations, treated with TAO, fared better than might be expected compared to individuals treated with other appropriate antibiotics [86, 87]. These reports stimulated the first controlled trials of this compound examining the effects in asthma in the late 1960s and early 1970s [88, 89]. Since these trials there have been a considerable number of further studies looking at the possible benefits of TAO as a steroid sparing agent, the results of which are summarised in Table 5. Initial impressions of these studies would suggest an impressive effect for this drug although there are few placebo controlled trials and no attempts to define independent anti-inflammatory mechanisms have been made.

In common with many of the other compounds with reputed steroid sparing effects, the literature for TAO is flawed by a failure to either examine for steroid sparing effects or efficacy, and not tapering the dose of steroid in the run-in periods. Scrutiny of the data for TAO shows significant placebo effects in the placebo controlled studies.

In addition, and specific to TAO, there are further problems in the reported studies: too small sample sizes, various arbitrary end-points (in particular issues surrounding infection and sputum production), short treatment periods, and a mixture of reports looking at children and adults. In fact, only two of the placebo-controlled studies had adequate numbers of patients [89, 97]. Nelson reported neither steroid sparing effects nor efficacy [97] and Spector did not randomize treatment sequence [89]. Given the questions surrounding mechanism for this drug, namely the inhibition of methylprednisolone clearance, it is not suprising that the consensus is that the effects seen are merely a consequence of increased effective doses of steroid.

There are two arguments in favour of TAO as a steroid sparing agent. Rosenburg reported the case of a patient whose asthma improved despite not receiving systemic glucocorticoids (in particular methlyprednisolone) [99]. However this patient remained on inhaled flunisolide and there is now evidence that TAO also inhibits clearance of this steroid. Secondly the proponents of TAO claim that the effects seen are in excess of the improvements expected from the relative increases in effective steroid dose. This has to be countered by the observation that many patients, despite tapering the dose of methylprednisolone, develop Cushingoid side-effects on TAO. Furthermore there appear to be no benefits for those patients on TAO who use prednisolone or other systemic corticosteroids.

3.5.3. Side-Effects: Almost without exception the studies reported show evidence of steroid related side-effects, inclusive of cataracts and abnormal glucose intolerance. TAO is an established cause of deranged liver function in addition to the problems often associated with macrolides such as gastrointestinal upset. Care should be exercised with the concomitant use of theophylline as TAO inhibits its hepatic metabolism which can result in toxicity.

3.5.4. Conclusion: Despite many trials showing reductions in the dose of steroid and efficacy, there is no parallel data showing a mechanism for these effects. The incidence of steroid related side-effects weigh heavily in favour of

Table 5. Clinical trials for troleandomycin

Reference	Year	Patients	Study design	Duration	Steroid sparing	Efficacy	Steroid side-effects	TAO side effects
Itkin [88]	1969	12 Adults	DBPCT	8 weeks	Not examined	↑FEV$_1$ by 22% (Placebo ↑7.4%)	x	✓
Spector [89]	1974	74 Adults	DBPCT	4–8 weeks	67% pts dose ↓ by >50%	↑FEV$_1$ by 0.42L, (Placebo ↓0.16L)	✓	✓
Zieger [*90]	1980	16 Adults	Open	4–18 months	MP 29 mg o.d. to 11 mg alt days	↑FEV$_1$ by 39%	✓	✓
Eitches [*91]	1985	11 Children	Open	12–38 months	MP 21.5 mg o.d. to 3.4 mg o.d.	↑FEV$_1$ by 81%	✓	✓
Wald [*92]	1985	15 Adults	Open	12 months	MP 38.9 mg o.d. to 12.6 mg o.d.	↑FEV$_1$ 1.76 to 2.18L at 3 weeks	x	✓
Ball [*93]	1990	15 Children (3 groups of 5)	DBPCT	2 weeks	50% reduction with MP, Pred and Placebo	↑FEV$_1$ (% predicted) 73% to 88%; Placebo 83 to 91)	x	✓
Menz [94]	1990	16	Open	4–21 months	Yes,?degree	11 responders arbitrarily defined	?	✓
Kamada [*95]	1991	18 Children (3 groups of 6)	DBPCT	12 weeks	Reductions, TAO/MP 80%, MP 44%	FEV$_1$ (% predicted) 80 to 75% i.e. worse (NS)	✓	✓
Flotte [*96]	1991	9 Children	Open	4–34 months	MP 15 mg o.d. to 1.4 mg o.d.	x	✓	x
Nelson [97]	1993	75 Adults	DBPCT	2 years	Significant & similar reductions in TAO and Pl	Not examined	✓	x
Siracusa [*98]	1993	14 Adults	Open	14 months	MP dose reduction by 20%	↑FEV$_1$ (% predicted) 60% to 68% (NS)	x	✓

Definitions of abbreviations; TAO, troleandomycin: DBPCT, double-blind, placebo-controlled trial: FEV, forced expiratory volume in 1 s: MP, methylprednisolone: Pl, placebo: Pred, prednisolone: * studies with pre-treatment steroid tapering: Steroid side-effects on TAO.

a mechanism dependent on methylprednisolone. Beneficial effects relating to theophylline metabolism also cannot be discounted. As there are side-effects of TAO, independent of the systemic steroid, there would appear to be no indication for this drug in the treatment of asthma.

3.6. Anti-Malarials

3.6.1. Mechanism of Action: Chloroquine and hydroxychloroquine both exert anti-inflammatory effects *via* the inhibition of phospholipase A_2, an enzyme responsible for the mobilisation of membrane phospholipid in the synthesis of leukotrienes and prostaglandins [100]. Both these families of mediators have been implicated in the aetiology of inflammation as well as airway smooth muscle spasm in the lung.

3.6.2. Clinical Trials: The antimalarial drugs chloroquine and hydroxy-chloroquine have been used in the treatment of connective tissue disease and rheumatoid arthritis for many years. The potential value of anti-malarial agents in asthma has been noted in anecdotal reports for well over 30 years [101, 102]. In these papers the authors claim response rates of 75%. Subsequent uncontrolled open studies endorsed this earlier data [103, 104]. Tennebaum showed delayed improvements in symptom control and exercise tolerance approximately after 10 weeks amongst four subjects—three of whom discontinued steroid treatment over the subsequent 6 months [104].

Following from this work there have been three further publications reporting contrasting results for the steroid sparing role of chloroquine. Roberts published the results of a double-blind placebo controlled cross-over trial examining hydroxychloroquine 400 mg/day in nine steroid dependent asthmatics over 2 months. The mean steroid requirements of the subjects at the start of the trial was 11.6 mg/day. Neither hydroxychloroquine nor placebo limbs resulted in change in steroid dose nor lung function. The authors concluded that hydroxychloroquine was of no benefit in the treatment of asthma [105].

In contrast, Charous has reported two open trials showing improvements in both steroid requirements and asthma control. The first 11 asthmatics treated over 28 weeks showed increases in lung function of the order of 15%, and the 7 steroid dependent patients were able to reduce their mean monthly prednisolone doses from 383 mg to 191 mg. Of interest the authors also report significant reductions in the levels of total serum IgE [106]. The second report showed sustained improvements amongst 10 patients in asthma control and reduced steroid doses over a 22 month follow-up period [107].

3.6.3. Side-Effects: The most serious side-effects of chloroquine relate to ocular and central nervous system toxicity. Whilst the retinopathy associated with this drug is rare at the doses used in the treatment of inflammatory disease it can be irreversible. Regular eye examinations should be undertaken whilst on

Table 6. Clinical trials for Azathioprine

Author	Year	Study design	Patients	Duration	Baseline steroid dose/day	Steroid reduction on azothioprine	Efficacy/other outcomes
Kaiser [110]	1966	SBPCT	3	16 weeks	All on steroid, dose not disclosed	No effect	No improvement lung function or symptoms
Arkins [111] improvement	1966	DBPCT	10	3 weeks	Not all receiving steroid, details not disclosed	No effect	No effect on lung function. Non significant in symptoms in both groups
Hodges [112] productive	1971	DBPCT	20	7 weeks	Three patients not taking steroid, mean dose of remainder 12 mg	Not evaluated	Two patients with cough showed marked improvement. No change lung function
Asmundsson [113]	1971	Open	11	12 weeks	Only six had previously taken steroids. Doses not disclosed	Prednisolone reduced in three patients	Five patients characterised by short duration of asthma improved

Definition of abbreviations; SBPCT, single-blind placebo-controlled trial: DBPCT, double-blind placebo-controlled trial.

therapy. Chloroquine should be avoided in epileptics, and patients with renal and hepatic impairment. Non-specific gastrointestinal side-effects and rashes can occur but are usually well tolerated. Neither Roberts or Charous reported side-effects in their respective studies [105–107].

3.6.4. Conclusion: The data in favour of anti-malarial treatments in asthma is derived from open trials with relatively small numbers of patients. The only placebo controlled trial, albeit with equally small numbers of patients, was strikingly negative. Until studies of this design are done with adequate numbers of patients, the use of chloroquine for either steroid sparing effects or efficacy cannot be recommended. In the event of such data, carefully monitored treatment should not present safety problems given the side-effect profiles reported to date.

3.7. Azathioprine

3.7.1. Mode of Action: Antimetabolite drugs have been used in the treatment of inflammatory disease for many years. Initially 6-mercaptopurine was used although this has been superseded by azathioprine, a less toxic derivative. Both agents are incorporated into DNA and prevent cell division. The mechanism by which this action results in immunosuppression is poorly understood but the evidence from organ transplantation and in conditions such as rheumatoid arthritis have endorsed this conclusion.

3.7.2. Clinical Trials: Following anecdotal case reports with azathioprine [108] and the earlier experience with antimetabolites and alkylating agents in asthma [109] interest in the possible use of azathioprine developed. Four trials have been reported [110–113], three of which were placebo controlled. There are minor flaws in design in each, such as lack of washout periods [111, 112], failure to randomise sequence [110], and in common with many of the other reports already discussed, no steroid tapering during run-in. In fact in only one of the trials were all the patients on steroids [110]. The numbers of subjects studied was small (ranging from four to 13) and the treatment periods were inadequate perhaps with the exception of the 12 week open trial reported by Asmundssen [113]. Notwithstanding these problems the results of all the trials universally show neither efficacy or steroid sparing effects for azathioprine/6-mercaptopurine although Hodges observed improvement in a subgroup of patients who previously expectorated large volumes of sputum [112]. No mechanism for this effect has been forthcoming.

3.7.3. Side-Effects: Azathioprine is an established cause of bone marrow suppression and increased susceptibility to infections. Hepatotoxicity has also been reported. Amongst the trial data there were a number of patients who sustained considerable gastrointestinal upset and in one case this necessitated withdrawal from treatment [110].

3.7.4. Conclusion: Despite the problems with design all the trials have failed to support the use of azathioprine in the treatment of asthma.

3.8. Colchicine

3.8.1. Mechanism of Action: Colchicine has also been used in various inflammatory disorders to good effect. In particular colchicine is central to the treatment of gout. Its anti-inflammatory mechanism has not been fully elucidated although it is probably multi-factorial and complex. Colchicine has been shown both *in vivo* and *in vitro* to correct deficiency of Concanavalin-A induced suppressor cell function seen in patients with both familial Mediterranean fever and primary biliary cirrhosis [114]. As colchicine remains effective treatment in these conditions—it has been postulated that this mechanism of action may underlie an anti-inflammatory effect. The discovery that patients with asthma also have a deficiency in Concanavalin-A induced suppressor cell function has led investigators to examine the possibility of treating the condition with colchicine [115]. Interestingly theophylline also corrects this defect and the combination of theophylline and colchicine is additive with respect to this deficiency. The exact pathway through which colchicine achieves this is unknown.

Colchicine has also been shown to inhibit neutrophil functions [116] and block the release of leukotrienes and IL-1 from lymphocytes [117] as well increasing intracellular levels of cyclic AMP [118]. These effects that may be mediated by the binding of the drug to microtubules within the cell.

3.8.2. Clinical Trials: Despite the experience with other inflammatory conditions there have only been three trials looking at the effects of colchicine in asthma. Furthermore the issue of steroid sparing effects for oral treatment has not been examined at all. In the first study reported by Schwartz, the use of colchicine resulted in improvements in symptom scores and rescue medication use compared with placebo but there were no differences in lung function between the two treatment limbs amongst 10 steroid naïve patients [119]. Another trial looked at the effect of treatment on 30 children all of whom were taking theophylline. Only nine were on inhaled steroids and none was taking oral corticosteroids. The results were identical to the previous study with marginal benefits for symptom scores and no differences in lung function [120]. Newman looked at the steroid sparing effect of colchicine in 20 patients maintained on inhaled treatment (1600 μg a day) over 4 months. No effect was seen and no benefits for asthma control were found [121].

3.8.3. Side-Effects: Colchicine is a safe drug, although diarrhoea is relatively common. There are rare reports of myopathy and neuropathy and these remain the only severe risks of treatment.

3.8.4. Conclusion: Appropriate studies looking at colchicine as a steroid sparing agent in asthma have not been done although the data currently available suggest that this drug will not have a role to play despite the attractive concept of impaired suppressor T cell immune responses in asthma.

3.9. Dapsone

3.9.1. Mechanism of Action: Dapsone (4,4'-diaminodiphenyl sulfone) is established as a treatment for leprosy and rheumatological conditions. The rationale for the use of dapsone in asthma is based on the assumption that the neutrophil is an important cell type in the pathogenesis of airway inflammation. Clearly the evidence for this is limited despite the data from allergen challenge studies in both human [122, 123] and animal [124] subjects. Dapsone inhibits neutrophil functions, inclusive of respiratory burst [125] and chemotaxis [126]. If the neutrophil were crucial to airway inflammation in asthma these effects might limit tissue injury.

3.9.2. Clinical Trials: There is only one trial looking at the possible steroid sparing effects of dapsone. Berlow studied 10 patients in an open trial for between 3 and 20 months. The dose of dapsone was 100 mg twice daily. The mean monthly prednisolone dose was reduced from 428 mg to 82 mg. Five of the patients were able to discontinue steroid treatment within 6 months.

Apart from the open design of this study (amongst a small number of subjects), there was no steroid tapering phase and the group were heterogeneous with steroid requirements at baseline ranging from 5 mg to 60 mg daily. In addition, three other patients were withdrawn during the study and the data from these patients were not included in the analysis [127].

3.9.3. Adverse Effects: Dapsone has a diverse and potentially serious side-effect profile. Complications include haemolytic anaemia (contraindicated in glucose-6-phosphate dehydrogenase deficiency), methaemoglobinaemia, agranulocytosis, gastrointestinal upset, hepatitis, neuropsychiatric reactions, and skin rashes.

3.9.4. Conclusion: The study reported for dapsone shows impressive reductions in corticosteroid requirements. Given the *in vitro* data for dapsone and its effects on the neutrophil this result has interesting implications from a mechanistic point of view. With respect to clinical use of this drug, further controlled studies are necessary before this agent can be considered in the treatment of asthma.

4. Summary

To date there is no conclusive evidence to support the widespread use of any "second-line agents" in the treatment of asthma. With a few notable exceptions the trials show faults in design that preclude definite conclusions. The experience of the reported studies has given a clear guide to appropriate design in the examination of possible steroid sparing drugs. Meticulous observation of appropriate methodology in future work will allow more confident assessments. The use of these agents should be restricted to controlled trials until their roles are more clearly defined.

References

1 Gubner R, August S, Ginsberg V (1951) Therapeutic suppression of tissue reactivity. II. Effect of aminopterin in rheumatoid arthritis and psoriasis. *Am J Med* 221: 176–182
2 Weinblatt ME, Coblyn JS, Fox DA, Fraser PA (1985) Efficacy of low dose methotrexate in rheumatoid arthritis. *N Engl J Med* 312: 818–822
3 O'Callaghan JW, Forrest MJ, Brooks PM (1988) Inhibition of neutrophil chemotaxis in methotrexate treated rheumatoid arthritis patients. *Rheumatol Int* 8: 41–45
4 Segal R, Mozes E, Yaron M, Tartakovsky B (1989) The effects of methotrexate on the production and activity of interleukin-1. *Arthritis Rheum* 32: 370–377
5 Nolte H, Skov PS (1988) Inhibition of basophil histamine release by methotrexate. *Actions Agents* 23: 173–176
6 Mullarkey MF, Webb R, Pardee NE (1986) Methotrexate in the treatment of steroid-dependent asthma. *Ann Allergy* 65: 347–50
7 Mullarkey MF, Blumenstein BA, Andrade WP, Bailey GA, Olason I, Wetzel CE (1988) Methotrexate in the treatment of steroid-dependent asthma. A double blind crossover study. *N Engl J Med* 318: 603–7
8 Shiner RJ, Nunn AJ, Chung KF, Geddes DM (1990) Randomised, double-blind placebo-controlled trial of methotrexate in steroid-dependent asthma. *Lancet* 336: 137–40
9 Dyer PD, Vaughan TR, Weber RW (1991) Methotrexate in the treatment of steroid-dependent asthma. *J Allerg Clin Immunol* 88: 208–12
10 Stewart GE, Diaz JD, Lockey RF, Seleznick MJ, Trudeau WL, Ledford DK (1994) Comparison of oral pulse methotrexate with placebo in the treatment of severe corticosteroid-dependent asthma. *J Allerg Clin Immunol* 94: 482–89
11 Hedman J, Seideman P, Albertioni F, Stenius-Aarniala B (1996) Controlled trial of methotrexate in patients with severe chronic asthma. *Eur J Clin Pharmacol* 49: 347–49
12 Erzurum SC, Leff JA, Cochran JE, Ackerson LM, Szefler SJ, Martin RJ, Cott GR (1991) Lack of benefit of methotrexate in severe, steroid-dependent asthma. *Ann Intern Med* 114: 353–60
13 Taylor DR, Flannery EM, Herbison GP (1993) Methotrexate in the management of severe steroid-dependent asthma. *N Z Med J* 106: 409–11
14 Trigg CJ, Davies RJ (1993) Comparison of 30 mg methotrexate per week with placebo in chronic steroid-dependent asthma: a 12-week double-blind, crossover study. *Respir Med* 87: 211–216
15 Coffey MJ, Sanders G, Eschenbacher WL, Tsien A, Ramash S, Weber RW, Toews GB, McCune WJ (1994) The role of methotrexate in the management of steroid-dependent asthma. *Chest* 105: 117–21
16 Kanzow G, Nowak D, Magnussen H (1995) Short term effect of methotrexate in severe steroid-dependent asthma. *Lung* 173: 223–231
17 Ogirala RG, Sturm TM, Aldrich TK, Meller FF, Pacia EB, Keane AM, Finkel RI (1995) Single high dose intramuscular triamcinolone acetonide *versus* weekly oral methotrexate in life threatening asthma: a double-blind study. *Am J Respir Crit Care Med* 152: 1461–66
18 Mullarkey MF, Lammert JK, Blumenstein BA (1990) Long term methotrexate treatment in corticosteroid-dependent asthma. *Ann Intern Med* 112: 577–81

19 Shiner RJ, Katz I, Shulimzon T, Silkoff P, Benzaray S (1994) Methotrexate in steroid-dependent asthma: long term results. *Allergy* 49: 565–68

20 Stanziola A, Sofia M, Mormile M, Molino A, Carratu L (1995) Long term treatment with methotrexate in patients with corticosteroid-dependent bronchial asthma. *Monaldi Arch Chest Dis* 50(2): 109–13

21 Becquart LA, Wallaert B, Lassalle P, Guene-Ribassin C, Tonnel AB (1994) Le methotrexate dans le traitement de l'asthme. *Rev Mal Respir* 11: 565–71

22 Stempel DA, Lammert J, Mullarkey MF (1991) Use of methotrexate in the treatment of steroid-dependent adolescent asthmatics. *Ann Allergy* 67: 346–48

23 Sole D, Costa-Carvalho BT, Soares FJP, Rullo VV, Naspitz CK (1996) Methotrexate in the treatment of corticodependent asthmatic children. *J Invest Allerg Clin Immunol* 6(2): 126–30

24 Guss S, Portnoy J (1992) Methotrexate treatment of severe asthma in children. *Pediatrics* 89: 635–39

25 Wilkie WS, Calabrase LH, Segal AM (1982) Incidence of untoward reactions in patients with rheumatoid arthritis treated with methotrexate. *Arthritis Rheum* 26:S56A

26 Lewis JH, Schiff E (1988) Methotrexate induced chronic liver injury: guidelines for detection and prevention. *Am J Gastroenterol* 88: 1337–45

27 Jones G, Mierins E, Karsha J (1991) Methotrexate induced asthma. *Am Rev Respir Dis* 143: 179–81

28 Tsai JJ, Shin JF, Chen CH, Wang SR (1993) Methotrexate pneumonitis in bronchial asthma. *Int Arch Allergy Appl Immunol* 100: 287–90

29 Cannon GW, Ward JR, Clegg DO (1983) Acute lung disease associated with low-dose pulse methotrexate therapy in patients with rheumatoid arthritis. *Arthritis Rheum* 26: 1269–74

30 Vallerand H, Cossart C, Milsevic D, Lavaud F, Leone J (1992) Fatal pneumocystis pneumonia in an asthmatic patient treated with methotrexate. *Lancet* 339: 1551–52

31 Kuitert LM, Harrison AC (1991) Pneumocystis carinii pneumonia as a complication of methotrexate treatment in asthma. *Thorax* 46: 936–37

32 Wollner A, Mohle-Boetani J, Lambert RE, Perruquet JL, Raffin TA, McGuire JL (1991) Pneumocystis carinii pneumonia complicating low dose treatment with methotrexate for rheumatoid arthritis. *Ann Rheum Dis* 48: 247–49

33 Reid DJ, Segars LW (1993) Methotrexate for the treatment of chronic corticosteroid-dependent asthma. *Clin Pharmacy* 12: 762–67

34 Bardin PG, Fraenkel DJ, Beasley RW (1993) Methotrexate in asthma; A safety perspective. *Drug Safety* 9(3): 151–55

35 Wong E, Lacasse Y, Guyatt GH, Sears MR, Cook DJ (1997) Is methotrexate effective as a steroid sparing agent in steroid-dependent asthmatics? A meta-analysis. *Am J Respir Crit Care Med* 152: 801A

36 Tugwell P, Bombardier C, Gent M, Bennett KJ, Carette S, Chalmers A, Esdaile JM, Klinkoff AV, Kraag GR (1990) Low-dose cyclosporin *versus* placebo in patients with rheumatoid arthritis. *Lancet* 335: 1051–55

37 Heule F, Meinardi MM, van Joost T, Bos JD (1988) Low-dose cyclosporin is effective in severe psoriasis: a double blind study. *Transplant Proc* 20(suppl): 32–41

38 Eisen D, Ellis EA, Duell CE (1990) Effect of topical cyclosporin rinse on oral lichen planus—a double-blind analysis. *N Engl J Med* 323: 290–94

39 Garim EH, Orak JK, Hiott KL, Sutherland SE (1988) Cyclosporin therapy for steroid-resistant nephrotic syndrome: a controlled study. *Am J Dis Child* 142: 985–88

40 Takahashi N, Hayano T, Suzuki M (1989) Peptidyl-prolyl *cis-trans* isomerase is the cyclosporin A-binding protein cyclophilin. *Nature* 337: 473–75

41 Emmel EA, Verweij CL, Durand BD, Higgins KM, Lacy E, Crabtree GR (1989) Cyclosporin specifically inhibits function of nuclear proteins involved in T cell activation. *Science* 246: 1617–20

42 Shimizu H, Mitomo K, Watanabe T, Okamoto S, Yamamoto K (1990) Involvement of a NFκB-like transcription factor in the activation of the interleukin-6 gene by inflammatory lymphokines. *Mol Cell Biol* 10: 561–68

43 Bendtzen K, Dinarello CA (1984) Mechanism of action of cyclosporin A. Effect on T cell binding of interleukin-1 and antagonising effect on insulin. *Scand J Immunol* 20: 43–51

44 Cirillo R, Triggiani M, Sri L, Ciccarelli A, Pettit GR, Condorelli M, Marone G (1990) Cyclosporin A rapidly inhibits mediator release from human basophils presumably by interact-

ing with cyclophilin. *J Immunol* 144: 3891–97
45 Pereira GM, Miller JF, Shevach EM, (1990) Mechanism of action of cyclosporin A *in vivo*. *J Immunol* 144: 2109–16
46 Renz H, Mazer BD, Gelfand EW (1990) Differential inhibition of T and B cell function in IL-4-dependent IgE by cyclosporin A and methylprednisolone. *J Immunol* 145: 3641–46
47 Thomson AW, Milton JI, Aldridge RD (1986) Inhibition of drug-induced eosinophilia by cyclosporin A. *Scand J Immunol* 24: 163–70
48 Palay DA, Cluff CW, Wentworth PA, Ziegler HK (1986) Cyclosporin inhibits macrophage-mediated antigen presentation. *J Immunol* 136: 4348–53
49 Alexander AG, Barnes NC, Kay AB (1992) Trial of cyclosporin in cortico-dependent chronic severe asthma. *Lancet* 339: 324–28
50 Nizankowska E, Soja J, Pinis G, Bochanak G, Sladek K, Domagala B, Pajak A, Szczeklik A (1995) Treatment of steroid-dependent bronchial asthma with cyclosporin. *Eur Respir J* 8: 1091–99
51 Lock SH, Kay AB, Barnes NC (1996) Double-blind placebo-controlled trial of cyclosporin A as a corticosteroid-sparing agent in cortico-dependent asthma. *Am J Respir Crit Care Med* 153: 509–514
52 Szczeklik A, Nizankowksa E, Dworski R, Domagala B, Pinis G (1991) Cyclosporin for steroid-dependent asthma. *Allergy* 46: 312–15
53 Mungan D, Misirligil Z, Sin B, Kaya A, Demirel Y, Gurbuz L (1995) Cyclosporin in steroid-dependent asthma. *Allergol Immunopathol* 23(5): 202–6
54 Blodgett RC (1983) Auranofin; the experience to date. *Am J Med* 30: 86–89
55 Bernstein DI, Bernstein IL (1991) Use of gold in the severe asthmatic patient. *Immunol Allergy Clin N Am* 11: 81–90
56 Rodnan GP, Benedek TG (1970) The early history of anti-rheumatic drugs. *Arthritis Rheum* 13: 145–59
57 Dudan A (1932) Vingt cas d'asthma bronchique traites par la sanocrysine. *Schweiz Med Wochenschr* 4: 96–100
58 Montagna CP, Rimoldi AA (1936) Die goldebehandlung des kindlichem asthmas. *Deut Med Wochenschr* 50: 2055–58
59 Von Lebinski (1936) Beitrag zur Goldtherapie. *Ther Ggw* 77: 564–67
60 Ishizaki T, Muranaki M, Araki H, Katsuta Y, Miyamoto T, Makino S, Kajino M, Ohtsuka M (1965) Clinical study on the effect of aurothioglucose on patients with bronchial asthma. *Diagnosis Treatment* 53: 750–55
61 Araki H (1969) Clinical study on the effect of sodium aurothiomalate in bronchial asthma. *Jpn J Allergy* 18: 106–9
62 Okatani Y (1970) Gold salt therapy on bronchial asthma. *Jpn Med J* 2432: 17–21
63 Muranaka M, Miyamoto T, Shida T, Kabe J, Makino S, Okumura H, Takeda K, Suzuki S, Horiuchi Y (1978) Gold salt in the treatment of bronchial asthma—a double-blind study. *Ann Allergy* 40: 132–37
64 Bernstein DI, Bernstein IL, Bodenheimer SS, Pietrusko RG (1988) An open study of auranofin in the treatment of steroid-dependent asthma. *J Allerg Clin Immunol* 81: 6–16
65 Honma M, Tamura G, Shirato K, Tkishima T (1994) Effect of an oral gold compound, auranofin, on non-specific bronchial hyperresponsiveness in mild asthma. *Thorax* 49: 649–51
66 Nierop G, Gijzel WP, Bel EH, Zwinderman AH, Dijkman JH (1992) Auranofin in the treatment of steroid-dependent asthma. *Thorax* 47: 349–54
67 Klaustermeyer WB, Noritake DT, Kwong FK (1987) Chrysotherapy in the treatment of corticosteroid-dependent asthma. *J Allerg Clin Immunol* 79: 720–25
68 Bernstein IL, Bernstein DI, Dubb JW, Faiferman I, Wallin B, participants of the auranofin multicenter drug trial (1996) A placebo-controlled multicenter study of auranofin in the treatment of patients with corticosteroid-dependent asthma. *J Allerg Clin Immunol* 98: 317–24
69 McNeill DL (1990) Oral gold therapy in steroid-dependent asthma, nasal polyposis, and aspirin hypersensitivity. *Ann Allergy* 65: 288–90
70 Levinson AL, Wheatley LM (1991) Intravenous immunoglobulin: A new therapeutic approach in steroid-dependent asthma? *J Allerg Clin Immunol* 88: 552–54
71 Page R, Friday G, Stillwagon P, Skoner D, Calguiri L, Fireman P (1988) Asthma and selective immunoglobulin deficiency: improvement after immunoglobulin replacement therapy. *J Pediat* 112: 127–31

72 Abernathy RS, Strem EL, Good RA (1958) Chronic asthma in childhood: double-blind controlled study of treatment with gamma-globulin. *Pediatrics* 21: 908–93
73 Brown EB, Botstein A (1960) The effect of gamma globulin in asthmatic children. *N Y State J Med* 109:.2539–45
74 Fontana VJ, Kuttner AG, Wittig HJ, Moreno F (1963) The treatment of infectious asthma in children with gamma globulin. *J Pediat* 62: 80–84
75 Smith TF, Muldoon MF, Bain RP, Wells EL, Tiller TL, Kutner MH, Schiffman G, Pandley JP (1988) Clinical results of a prospective double-blind placebo-controlled trial of intravenous γ-globulin in children with chronic chest symptoms. *Monogr Allergy* 23: 168–76
76 Mazer BD, Gelfand EW (1991) An open-label study of high-dose intravenous immunoglobulin in severe childhood asthma. *J Allerg Clin Immunol* 87: 976–83,
77 Jakobssen T, Croner S, Kjellman N-IM, Petterson A, Vassella C, Bjorksten B (1994) Slight steroid-sparing effect of intravenous immunoglobulin in children and adolescents with moderately severe bronchial asthma. *Allergy* 49: 413–20
78 Sekul EA, Cupler EJ, Dalakas MC (1994) Aseptic meningitis associated with high-dose intravenous immunoglobulin therapy: frequency and risk factors. *Ann Intern Med* 121: 259–62
79 Selenke WM, Leung GW, Townley RG (1980) Non antibiotic effects of the oleandomycin-erythromycin group with special reference to their steroid-sparing effects. *J Allerg Clin Immunol* 65: 454–64
80 Szefler SJ, Rose JQ, Ellis EF, Spector SL, Green AW, Jusko WJ (1980) The effect of troleandomycin on methylprednisolone elimination. *J Allerg Clin Immunol* 66: 447–51
81 Greos LS, Szefler SJ, Larsen GL, Irvin CG, Hill MR (1990) Troleandomycin reduces airways inflammation. *Am Rev Respir Dis* 141:A933
82 Ong KS, Grieco MH, Rosner W (1978) Enhancement by oleandomycin of the inhibitor effect of methylprednisolone on phytohaemagglutinin-stimulated lymphocytes. *J Allerg Clin Immunol* 62: 115–18
83 Mendoza GR, Eitches RW, Orner FB (1983) Direct effects of oleandomycin on histamine release in human basophils. *J Allerg Clin Immunol* 71: 135A
84 Goswami SK, Kivity S, Marom Z (1990) Erythromycin inhibits respiratory glyconjugate secretion from human airways *in vitro. Am Rev Respir Dis* 141: 72–78
85 Celmer WD, Els H, Murai K (1958) Oleandomycin derivatives; preparation and characterization. *In: Antibiotics annual, 1957–1958.* Interscience Publishers Inc., New York.
86 Kaplan MA, Goldin M (1959) The use of triacetyloleandomycin in chronic infectious asthma. *In: Antibiotics annual 1958–1959.* Interscience Publishers Inc., New York
87 Fox JL (1961) Infectious asthma treated with triacetyloleandomycin. *Penn Med J* 64: 634–38
88 Itkin IH, Menzel ML (1970) The use of macrolide antibiotic substances in the treatment of asthma. *J Allergy* 45: 146–62
89 Spector SL, Katz FH, Farr RS (1974) Troleandomycin: effectiveness in steroid-dependent asthma and bronchitis. *J Allerg Clin Immunol* 54: 367–79
90 Zieger RS, Schatz M, Sperling W, Simon RA, Stevenson DD (1980) Efficacy of troleandomycin in outpatients with severe, corticosteroid-dependent asthma. *J Allerg Clin Immunol* 66: 438–46
91 Eitches RW, Rachelefsky GS, Katz RM, Mendoza GR, Siegel SC (1985) Methylprednisolone and troleandomycin in treatment of steroid-dependent asthmatic children. *Am J Dis Child* 139: 264–68
92 Wald JA, Friedman BF, Farr RS (1985) An improved protocol for the use of troleandomycin (TAO) in the treatment of steroid-requiring asthma. *J Allerg Clin Immunol* 78: 36–43
93 Ball BD, Hill MR, Brenner M, Sanks R, Szefler SJ (1990) Effect of low-dose troleandomycin on glucocorticoid pharmacokinetics and airway hyperresponsiveness in severely asthmatic children. *Ann Allergy* 65: 37–45
94 Menz G, Rothe T, Schmitz M, Hauser F, Haack D, Virchow Chr (1990) Erfahrungen mit einer Kombinationtherapie von Methylprednisolon und Troleandomycin (TAO) bei schweren, hochkortoidbedurftigem Asthma bronchiale. *Pneumologie* 44: 238–40
95 Kamada AK, Hill MR, Ikle DN, Brenner M, Szefler SJ (1993) Efficacy and safety of low-dose troleandomycin in children with severe steroid-requiring asthma. *J Allerg Clin Immunol* 91: 873–82
96 FlooteTR, Loughlin GM (1991) Benefits and complications of troleandomycin (TAO) in young children with steroid-dependent asthma. *Pediat Pulmonol* 10: 178–82
97 Nelson HS, Hamilos DL, Corsello PR, Levesque NV, Buchmeier AD, Bucher BL (1993) A dou-

ble-blind study of troleandomycin and methylprednisolone in asthmatics who require daily corticosteroids. *Am Rev Respir Dis* 147: 398–404

98 Siracusa A, Brugnami G, Fiordi T, Areni S, Severini C, Marabini A (1993) Troleandomycin in the treatment of difficult asthma. *J Allerg Clin Immunol* 92: 677–82

99 Rosenburg SM, Gerhard H, Grunstein MM, Schramm CM (1991) Use of TAO without methylprednisolone in the treatment of severe asthma. *Chest* 100: 849–50

100 Kench JG, Seale JP, Temple DM, Tennant C (1985) The effect of non-steroidal inhibitors of phospholipase A_2 on leukotriene and histamine release from human and guinea pig lung. *Prostaglandins* 30: 199–208

101 Geshickter CF (1953) A new treatment for bronchial asthma. *Bull Georgetown U Med Ctr* 7: 39

102 Engeset A (1957) Therapeutic experiments with anti-malarials in the treatment of bronchial asthma. *Nord Med* 58: 1904

103 Goldstein JA (1983) Hydroxychloroquine for asthma. *Am Rev Respir Dis* 128: 1100–01

104 Tennebaum J, Smith R (1966) Anti-malarial therapy for resistant asthma. *Ann Allergy* 24: 37–40

105 Roberts JA, Gunneberg A, Elliott JA, Thompson NC (1988) Hydroxychloroquine in steroid-dependent asthma. *Pulm Pharmacol* 1: 59–61

106 Charous BL (1990) Open study of hydroxychloroquine in the treatment of severe symptomatic or corticosteroid-dependent asthma. *Ann Allergy* 65: 53–58

107 Charous BL. Effectiveness of long-term treatment of severe asthma with hydroxychloroquine (HCQ). *Ann N Y Acad Sci* 629: 432–33

108 Cohen EP, Petty TL, Szentivanyi A, Priest RE (1965) Clinical and pathological observations in fatal bronchial asthma. *Ann Intern Med* 62: 103–7

109 Waldblott GL (1952) Nitrogen mustard in the treament of bronchial asthma. *Ann Allergy* 10: 428–29

110 Kaiser HB, Beall GN (1966) Azathioprine (Imuran) in chronic asthma. *Ann Allergy* 24: 369–70

111 Arkins JA, Hirsch SR (1966) Clinical effectiveness of 6-mercaptopurine in bronchial asthma. *J Allergy* 37: 90–95

112 Hodges NG, Brewis AL, Howell JBL (1971) An evaluation of azothioprine in severe chronic asthma *Thorax* 26: 734–39

113 Asmundssen T, Kilburn KH, Laszio J, Krock CJ (1971) Immunosuppressive therapy of asthma. *J Allergy* 47: 136–47

114 Ilfield D, Theodor E, Delpre G, Kuperman O (1984) *In vitro* correction of a deficiency of Con A-induced suppressor cell function in primary biliary cirrhosis by a pharmacological concentration of colchicine. *Clin Exp Immunol* 57: 438–42

115 Hwang KC, Fikrig SM, Friedman HM, Gupta S (1985) Deficient concanavalin A-induced suppressor-cell activity in patients with bronchial asthma, allergic rhinitis, and atopic dermatitis. *Clin Allergy* 15: 67–72

116 Spilberg I, Mandell B, Mehta J, Simchowitz L, Rosenburg D (1979) Mechanism of action of colchicine in acute urate crystal-induced arthritis. *J Clin Invest* 64: 775–80

117 Kershenobich D, Alcocer J, Quiraga A, Rojkind M (1984) Effect of colchicine on immunoregulatory T-lymphocytes and monocytes in patients with primary biliary cirrhosis. *Clin Res* 32: 490A

118 Rudolph SA, Greengard P, Malawista SE (1977) Effects of colchicine on cyclic AMP levels in human leukocytes. *Proc Natl Acad Sci USA* 74: 3404–8

119 Schwartz YA, Kivity S, Ilfield DN, Schlesinger M, Greif J, Topilsky M, Garty MS (1990) A clinical and immunological study of colchicine in asthma. *J Allerg Clin Immunol* 85: 578–82

120 Adalioglu G, Turktas I, Saraclar Y, Tuncer A (1994) A clinical study of colchicine in childhood asthma. *J Asthma* 312: 361–66

121 Newman KB, Mason UG, Buchmeier A, Schmaling KB, Corsello P, Nelson HS (1997) Failure of colchicine to reduce inhaled triamcinolone dose in patients with asthma. *J Allerg Clin Immunol* 99: 176–78

122 Metzger WJ, Zavala D, Richerson HB (1987) Local allergen challenge and bronchoalveolar lavage of allergic asthmatic lungs. *Am Rev Respir Dis* 135: 433–40

123 Carroll M, Durham SR, Walsh G, Kay AB (1985) Activation of neutrophils and monocytes after allergen and histamine-induced bronchoconstriction. *J Allerg Clin Immunol* 75: 290–96

124 Murphy K, Wilson M, Irvine C (1986) The requirement of polymorphonuclear leukocytes in the late asthmatic response and heightened airways reactivity in an animal model. *Am Rev Respir Dis* 134: 62–68

125 Miyachi Y, Niwa Y (1982) Effects of potassium iodide, colchicine, and dapsone on the genera-
     tion of polymorphonuclear leukocyte-derived oxygen intermediates. *Br J Dermatol* 107: 209–14
126 Harvath L, Yancey K, Katz S (1986) Selective inhibition of human neutrophil chemotaxis to
     N-formyl-methionyl-leucyl-phenylalanine by sulfones. *J Immunol* 137: 1305–11
127 Berlow BA, Liehaber MI, Dyer Z, Spiegal TM (1991) The effect of dapsone on steroid-depend-
     ent asthma. *J Allerg Clin Immunol* 87: 710–15

Asthma: Epidemiology, Anti-Inflammatory Therapy and Future Trends
ed. by M. A. Giembycz and B. J. O'Connor
© 2000 Birkhäuser Verlag/Switzerland

CHAPTER 9
Leukotriene Receptor Antagonists and
5-Lipoxygenase Inhibitors in Asthma

K. Fan Chung

National Heart and Lung Institute, Imperial College School of Medicine and Royal Brompton Hospital, London SW3 6LY, UK

1. Introduction

Cysteinyl leukotrienes, leukotrienes C_4, D_4 and E_4, are important mediators of asthma derived from the oxidative 5-lipoxygenase pathway of archidonic acid metabolism, which were discovered by the late 1980s. Research programs within the pharmaceutical industry have led to the discovery of many molecules that are capable of inhibiting the effects of these mediators. These inhibitors have now become available for the treatment of asthma in the form of three cysteinyl leukotriene receptor antagonists, montelukast, zafirlukast and pranlukast, and one inhibitor of leukotriene synthesis, zileuton, which are available in many countries round the world.

2. Generation of Leukotrienes

Leukotrienes are synthesized from arachidonic acid, a normal constituent of the phospholipid bilayer, which is liberated by the action of phospholipases in responses to various stimuli. Leukotrienes are formed by the activation of 5-lipoxygenase (5-LO) enzyme on arachidonic acid to form an unstable intermediate, 5-hydroperoxy-eicosatetraenoic acid (5-HPETE) which is converted to epoxide leukotriene (LT)A_4 [1]. 5-LO is a member of a family of lipoxygenases and is an iron-containing enzyme consisting of 673 aminoacids which is dependent of Ca^{2+}, adenosine triphosphate and several cofactors for maximal activity [2]. 5-LO translocates from the cytosol to the nuclear cell membrane to initiate leukotriene biosynthesis. 5-HPETE is formed through the action of 5-LO and the 5-lipoxygenase-activating protein (FLAP), a nuclear membrane protein to which 5-LO binds to make a stable complex [3].

LTA$_4$ is the pivotal intermediate from which all other leukotrienes are synthesised. LTA$_4$ hydrolase is a zinc-containing cytosolic metalloproteinase possessing intrisic aminopeptidase activity [4], with considerable homology to aminopeptidase N family of enzymes. LTA$_4$ enzymatic activity can be inhibited by metallohydrolase inhibitors such as bestatin. LTA$_4$ is unstable and may either be hydrolysed to the dihydroxyacid LTB$_4$ by LTA$_4$ hydrolase, or glutathione is incorporated to form the peptido-leukotriene LTC$_4$ by the enzyme LTC$_4$ synthase. LTC$_4$ synthase is an 18-kDa integral microsomal membrane protein [5]. The nucleotide and deduced aminoacid sequences of its cDNA show no significant homology to glutathione S transferases but shares aminoacid identity with FLAP [5].

The subsequent conversion of LTC$_4$ to LTD$_4$, a cysteinyl glycinyl derivative, is through the action of α-glutamyl transpeptidase. LTD$_4$ is further metabolised to the cysteinyl derivative, LTE$_4$, by the action of a dipeptidase. Leukotrienes are rapidly metabolised and removed from the circulation. Peptidoleukotrienes undergo oxidation, resulting in biliary and urinary elimination of biologically less active and inactive metabolites. LTE$_4$ is an important urinary metabolite that can be used to monitor the production of leukotrienes in man [6, 7].

The location of leukotriene synthesis is determined by the cellular distribution of the enzymes controlling each step of the pathway. The distribution of 5-lipoxygenase is limited to myeloid cells including neutrophils, eosinophils, monocytes, macrophages, mast cells and basophils. LTC$_4$ synthase has been identified not only in mast cells and eosinophils but also in endothelial cells and platelets. LTA$_4$ hydrolase has been found in human plasma, human erythrocytes, inflammatory cells, bronchoalveolar lavage fluid and airway epithelial cells. Because these enzymes are distributed among different cell types, various inflammatory cells, in concert with noninflammatory cells such as endothelial cells or epithelial cells can participate in the transcellular synthesis of leukotrienes [8, 9].

A number of different cells can generate leukotrienes, including mast cells, basophils, eosinophils and macrophages. The predominant product of 5-lipoxygenase in eosinophils is LTC_4 rather than LTD_4, and cytokines such as IL-3, IL-5 and GM-CSF can enhance leukotriene synthesis [10, 11]. LTB_4 is preferentially produced by macrophages and neutrophils, whereas cysteinyl leukotrienes are produced predominantly by eosinophils, basophils and mast cells.

The cysteinyl LTD_4 and E_4 activate a $CysLT_1$ receptor on airways smooth muscle. This receptor has recently been cloned and shown to be highly expressed on airways smooth muscle. Another receptor, $CysLT_2$, may also be activated on pulmonary vascular smooth muscle. LTC_4-specific receptors have not been identified in human lung tissue. The bronchoconstrictor activity of LTC_4 may be derived from its conversion to LTD_4. LTB_4 acts on a different class of receptors, BLT receptors.

3. Inhibition of Leukotrienes

The role of leukotrienes in asthma can be investigated by using specific pharmacological agents that prevent their synthesis or receptor-mediated effects. The biosynthesis of leukotrienes can be inhibited directly by inhibitors of the 5-lipoxygenase enzyme such as zileuton, or indirectly by inhibitors of FLAP such as MK-886 or BAY-X-1005. Alternatively, a number of potent Cys LT_1 receptor antagonists have been developed including zafirlukast, pranlukast and montelukast. One potential advantage of leukotriene synthesis inhibitors over $CysLT_1$ receptor antagonists is that they also inhibit the formation of LTB_4. The contribution of LTB_4 in asthma is probably small.

4. Effects of Cysteinyl Leukotrienes

The cysteinyl LTs are very potent contractile agonists of human bronchi *in vitro*, being about 1000 times more potent than histamine [12]. This potent effect of cysteinyl leukotrienes can be demonstrated *in vivo* in normal subjects and in patients with asthma. In healthy subjects, LTD_4 displayed a 140-fold greater potency than histamine and LTE_4 was 14 times more potent [13, 14]. Although LTC_4 and LTD_4 are 100–150 times more potent than LTE_4 in producing airway bronchoconstriction in healthy subjects, they are only four to five times more potent in asthma patients, indicating a relative hyperresponsiveness to LTE_4 in asthmatic patients [15]. Inhaled LTD_4 is not only a more potent bronchoconstrictor than methacholine but it can also cause a greater degree of maximal airway narrowing [16]. LTE_4 can increase bronchial responsiveness to histamine in patients with asthma, an effect that can persist for 1 week [17]. LTB_4, by contrast, does not induce bronchoconstriction or bronchial hyperresponsiveness [18].

An important property of cysteinyl leukotrienes is their ability to increase airway microvascular permeability in the airways, thereby causing oedema and mucosal thickening, and providing also an additional source of secondary mediators such as the kinins derived from plasma. Leukotriene-induced airway microvascular leakage of fluorescein-labelled proteins into the extravascular space has been demonstrated in a hamster cheek pouch model. Leukotriene D_4 induced extravasation of Evans Blue dye at all levels of the airways of guinea pigs [19, 20]. In an experimental model using sensitised guinea pigs, inhibitors of the 5-lipoxygenase enzyme caused a dose-dependent inhibition of allergen-induced airway microvascular leakage at all airway levels [21]. Cysteinyl leukotrienes also increase mucus secretion, both by direct effects on goblet cells and by stimulating nerves and producing reflex secretion from submucosal glands [22–24].

Eosinophils have been identified as key inflammatory cells in the pathophysiology of asthma [25]. Both LTE_4 and allergen can induce the influx of eosinophils into the airways of sensitised guinea pigs and these effects can be blocked by a cysteinyl leukotriene receptor antagonist, zafirlukast [26]. Inhalation of LTE_4, but not of methacholine, by allergic asthmatic subjects also causes a significant increase in the number of eosinophils in bronchial biopsies [27]. Cysteinyl leukotrienes also facilitate the proliferative activity of growth factors such as epidermal growth factor on airway smooth muscle *in vitro* [28].

5. Release of Leukotrienes in Asthma

A number of studies measuring leukotrienes in bronchoalveolar lavage fluid, blood and urine have shown that leukotrienes are released during acute exacerbations of asthma. LTE_4 is the principal urinary metabolite of the cysteinyl leukotrienes and measurement of LTE_4 excretion in urine is a convenient method for examining leukotriene production *in vivo* [7]. For example, higher levels of LTE_4 in the urine of patients during acute severe asthma attacks when compared with those in a group of normal nonasthmatic individuals, or with those asthma patients whose lung function had returned to normal following treatment [29, 30]. Those presenting with acutely reversible airway narrowing had elevated LTE_4 in their urine. Cysteinyl leukotrienes have been recovered from urine during exercise-induced bronchoconstriction in some studies [31, 32], but not in others [33]. When atopic asthmatics were challenged with inhaled allergen, there was an increase in urinary LTE_4 excretion which parallels the bronchoconstriction and subsides with resolution of the airway response [29, 34]. Urinary LTE_4 levels are also increased after aspirin challenge of aspirin-sensitive asthmatic patients [35, 36]. Elevated levels of LTC_4 and E_4 have been measured in bronchoalveolar lavage fluid of atopic asthmatics following endobronchial allergen challenge [37–40].

6. Inhibitors of 5-Lipoxygenase

Inhibition of 5-lipoxygenase has been achieved in several ways including trapping of radical intermediates, chelation or reduction of iron, reversible binding at either an active or a regulatory site, as well as combinations of these mechanisms. Direct inhibition of 5-LO partly through an iron-catalysed redox mechanism has been possible with compounds such as benzofurans (L-670, 630 and L-650,224), hydroxamates (BWA4C), N-hydroxyurea derivatives (A-64077 or Zileuton) and indazolinones (ICI 207, 968) with good selectivity and potency [41]. ICI 207,968 and BWA4C, which are orally active, produce dose-dependent inhibition of the cysteinyl-leukotriene component of antigen-induced bronchoconstriction in sensitised guinea pigs [42]. BWA4C also exhibited *ex vivo* LTB$_4$ synthesis when dosed orally to volunteers. Zileuton has similar *in vitro* potency and selectivity to acetohydroxamates and inhibits leukotriene synthesis *ex vivo* [41]. Zileuton inhibits airway microvascular leakage and bronchoconstriction induced by inhaled allergen in the sensitised guinea-pig model [21], in addition to inhibiting leucocyte accumulation [21, 43]. Zileuton produces dose-dependent inhibition of leukotriene synthesis *ex vivo* following oral administration to volunteers, with a duration of action of 6 h at doses of 600–800 mg [44].

A new series of non-redox 5-lipoxygenase inhibitors devoid of iron-chelating properties, the methoxyalkyl-thiazoles, such as ICI D2138 are most potent and selective inhibitors of 5-lipoxygenase [45]. ICI D2138 exhibits prolonged inhibition of *ex vivo* leukotriene synthesis when administered orally to volunteers, with a half-life of around 12 h.

Inhibitors of FLAP such as MK-886 and MK-591 which is a structural analogue of MK-886, have no direct activity on 5-LO but antagonises FLAP thus preventing the translocation of the enzyme to the membrane [46]. MK 886 is a highly selective compound with no effects of prostaglandin synthesis. MK886 inhibits antigen-induced bronchoconstriction in *Ascaris*-sensitive squirrel monkeys [47, 48]. MK 591 inhibits LTB$_4$ synthesis *ex vivo* by up to 90% [49] and urinary LTE$_4$ by >80% at 24 h, with a half-life of 6 h [50]. Although FLAP antagonists REV5091 and WY50295 are active *in vitro* and in animals, they were inactive in inhibiting leukotriene synthesis in volunteers [51, 52]. BAY-X-1005 inhibits anti-IgE challenge in human airways *in vitro* [53].

To date, only one inhibitor of 5-lipoxygenase, zileuton, is now available for prescription in the USA.

7. Effects in Asthma

7.1. Inhibition of Bronchial Challenges

Zileuton has been most extensively evaluated in human studies. It inhibits bronchoconstriction induced by cold, dry air, exercise and by aspirin (in aspirin-sensitive asthma) [54–56]. Nasal, gastrointestinal and dermal reactions were also inhibited, together with urinary LTE_4 excretion [56]. ZD-2138 was also effective in inhibiting aspirin-induced asthma [57]. The effects of several 5-LO inhibitors on allergen-induced early and late responses have been more variable [58–62]. While zileuton and ZD-2138 did not inhibit early and late asthmatic responses [58, 60], MK-886, MK-0591 and BAY-X-1005, inhibit both responses [59, 61, 62]. MK-886 and MK-0591 protected against the late asthmatic response between 3–8 h, but this was lost afterwards [59, 61]. These compounds had no effect on allergen-induced airway hyperresponsiveness, despite effective blockade of LTB_4 biosynthesis and LTE_4 excretion at the time of measurement of airway responsiveness. A single oral dose of 800 mg zileuton caused an almost complete blockade of LTB_4 biosynthesis ex $vivo$, and a nearly 50% inhibition of urinary LTE_4 [58], while in the MK-886 studies, LTB_4 biosynthesis ex $vivo$ was reduced by 54% with an 80% reduction in LTE_4 urinary excretion at 3–9 h post challenge. Almost complete blockage of LTB_4 biosynthesis and LTE_4 urinary excretion were observed with MK-0591. Zileuton also reduced allergen-induced nasal congestion, and selectivity blocked leukotriene release in nasal lavage fluid in patients with allergic rhinitis [63].

Treatment with zileuton reduced the number of inflammatory cells recovered in bronchoalveolar lavage fluid from patients with the late asthmatic response after bronchopulmonary segmental allergen challenge [64].

7.2. Studies in Clinical Asthma

In a 4-week placebo-controlled trial in patients with mild to moderate asthma, it improved airway function and symptoms. At the highest dose of 2.4 gm/day, there were a mean increase in FEV_1 of 13.4%, a decrease in β-agonist usage by 24%, an improvement in morning peak expiratory flow rate of 10%, a decrease in overall symptom scores of 37% and a decrease in urinary leukotriene excretion by 39% [65]. There were no significant side-effects reported. In a longer clinical trials of up to six months, zileuton continued to maintain improvement in lung function with a peak improvement of the order of 20% for FEV_1, a decrease in symptoms and in the use of $β_2$-agonists, and lesser need for glucocorticoid rescue [66, 67]. The improvement in lung function after zileuton can be observed within 1 to 3 h [65–67]. The number of patients who required oral corticosteroid treatment for exacerbations of asthma was reduced by more than 60% [66, 67]. Zileuton was compared to twice-daily theophylline in a 3-month study in which theophylline doses were adjusted according to plasma drug concentrations. Similar increases in FEV_1 were observed with both, but theophylline caused a greater symptomatic improvement [68]. Zileuton gave additional benefits to aspirin-intolerant asthmatics already on conventional therapy [69].

8. Leukotriene Receptor Antagonists

The first leukotriene receptor antagonist of the hydroxyacetophenone class described was FPL-55712 [70], which exhibited poor bioavailability and a short half-life. Other compounds within the same class, e.g. LY 171883, L-649,923, and YM-16638 were synthesised, but did not possess sufficient potency to act effectively as an LTD_4 receptor antagonist. In addition to being inactive on allergen-induced responses, L-649,923 was poorly tolerated with a high incidence of gastrointestinal effects [71]. The newer generation of leukotriene antagonists such as ICI 204,219 (zafirlukast), the quinolones MK-571 and RG-12,525, ONO-1078 (prankulast) and SK&F 104,353 (pobilukast) were more potent. These compounds are at least 200-fold more potent than earlier LT antagonists in [^{3}H]-LTD_4 binding assays [72]. The efficacy and safety of potent LT receptor antagonists against leukotriene-induced bronchoconstriction in normals and asthmatics has been shown in several studies. Zafirlukast at a single oral dose of 40 mg shifted LTD_4-induced bronchoconstriction dose-response curve by 100-fold and provided significant antagonism for at least 24 h in normal subjects, with no apparent side-effects [34]. MK-571 provided a shift of greater than 88-fold in asthmatic patients [73]. MK-0476 (montelukast), now available for treating patients with asthma, also protects against LTD_4-induced bronchoconstriction, 20–24 h after administration, and is probably the antagonist with the longest duration of antagonist activity in man [74, 75].

8.1. Inhibition of Bronchial Challenges

Leukotriene receptor antagonists inhibit several bronchoconstrictor challenges such as exercise, allergen, and aspirin (Tab. 2). Exercise-induced asthma is partially inhibited by 50% to 80% [32, 76–81]. When administered before exercise, they shorten the time to recovery of normal lung function.

Both the early and late phase responses are partly inhibited by the leukotriene antagonists, zafirlukast and MK-571 [82–84]. Zafirlukast also inhibited airway hyperresponsiveness to histamine at 6 h after allergen challenge [82]. It inhibited the airway response to cumulative allergen challenge by 5.5-fold increase in allergen dose, associated with a shorter recovery time [85]. When administered by inhalation, zafirlukast [1.6 mg] reduced the early but not the late asthmatic response [86]. Inhaled L-648051 administered over 7 days attenuated the early and late responses to inhaled allergen [87]. Pretreatment with a combination of antihistamine, loratidine, and zafirlukast (80 mg bd) caused near complete abolition of the early and late phase response to allergen [88]. Zafirlukast can reduce cellular influx after allergen challenge in asthmatic patients [89]. Fourty-eight hours after segmental allergen challenge, the numbers of basophils, mast cells and lymphocytes, and the concentration of histamine and superoxide release from alveolar macrophages were

Table 1. Some clinical trials of leukotriene inhibitors in clinical asthma

Compound	Type of asthma	Effects	Reference.
Zileuton (2.4 mg/day) (1.6 mg/day)	Mild to moderate	↑ 13.4% FEV_1 ↓ 24% β-agonist use ↓ 10.9% FEV_1 ↓ 17% β-agonist use	Israel 1993 [65]
Zileuton (2.4 mg/day)	Baseline FEV1 = 62% ($n = 122$)	↑ 15% FEV_1 ↓ 30% β-agonist use ↓ 36% day-time symptoms	Liu 1996 [66]
Zafirlukast (5, 10 or 20 mg twice/day for 6 weeks)	Mild-to-moderate ($n = 276$)	At 40 mg/day: ↓ rescue β-agonist (30%) ↓ night waking (46%) ↓ day symptom (26%) ↑ FEV_1 (11%)	Spector 1994 [108]
Zafirlukast (20 mg twice daily)	Mild-to-moderate ($n = 762$)	As above	Fish 1997 [128]
MK-571 (75 mg TDS; 2 weeks, then 50 mg TDS for 4 weeks)	Mild-to-moderate ($n = 43$)	↑ 8–14% FEV_1 ↓ 30% symptom scores	Margolskee 1991 [105]
LY-171,883 600 mg twice/day (6 weeks)	mild-moderate ($n = 138$)	↑ Mean weekly FEV_1 of 4.5% ↓ use of β-agonist	Cloud 1989 [104]
Montelukast 10 mg/day	Mild to moderate Predicted FEV1 67% $n = 408$	↑ 13% FEV_1 ↓ β-agonist use ↑ morning PEFR ↓ day-time symptoms	Reiss 1998 [114]
Montelukast 5 mg/day	Asthmatic children Predicted FEV1 72%; 39% using inhaled steroids $n = 336$	↑ 8.2% FEV1 ↓ 16.8% β-agonist use ↓ 14.8% asthma symptoms	Knorr 1998 [111]
Pranlukast 337.5 mg twice daily	Mild-to-moderate Predicted FEV1 66% $n = 45$	↑ 11.5% FEV1 ↓ 28% night symptoms	Barnes and Pujet 1997 [110]

significantly reduced in bronchoalveolar lavage fluid after zafirlukast treatment.

Patients with aspirin-induced asthma have an increase in leukotriene C_4 synthase activity [90], which is associated with a mutation in the promoter region of the gene for this enzyme [91]. Pretreatment with pobilukast or MK-679 prevented the bronchoconstrictor response induced by lysine-aspirin [92, 93]. MK-679 also improves lung function in aspirin-sensitive patients with asthma [93]. In normal subjects, PAF-induced bronchoconstriction was inhibited by the LTD_4 leukotriene antagonist, zafirlukast [94] and pobilukast [95], in accord with the observation that PAF induces an increase in urinary LTE_4 excretion [96].

Prankulast (ONO-1078) after 1 week's treatment causes a small (half of one doubling dilution of methacholine PC_{20}) improvement in bronchial hyperresponsiveness in stable asthmatic patients [97]. Inhaled L-648051 also improved bronchial hyperresponsiveness by 1.5-doubling dilutions of methacholine after 9 days' treatment [87].

8.2. Studies in Clinical Asthma

8.2.1. Single Dosing: Leukotriene receptor antagonists similar to the synthesis inhibitors produce significant improvement in airways function, together with a reduction in symptoms (Tab. 1). In a study of ten patients with mild to moderate asthma, a single oral dose of zafirlukast induced significant bronchodilation, with a mean increase of 8% in FEV_1 (range: 2%–14%) [98]. However, inhaled zafirlukast (1600 μg dose) did not induce bronchodilatation [99], while pobilukast by inhalation was effective (5% mean increase in FEV_1) [100]. In 12 moderately severe asthmatics, infusion of MK-571 resulted in a mean 20% increase in FEV_1 noticed 20 min after the start of infusion, and persisted for the 5 hour observation period [101, 102]. The bronchodilator properties of LT antagonists and of the β_2-adrenergic agonist, salbutamol, appear to be additive. In addition, the degree of baseline airway obstruction was correlated with the degree of bronchodilation achieved with MK-571. Similarly, in eight patients with aspirin-sensitive asthma, MK-679, the (R)-enantiomer of MK-571, by oral administration, induced a 5–34% (mean 18%) improvement in FEV_1, lasting for at least 9 h [103]. Therefore, persistent activation of leukotriene receptor to increase airway tone is present in patients with chronic asthma. The bronchodilator response correlated strongly with the severity of asthma and with aspirin sensitivity. Leukotriene receptor antagonists do not induce bronchodilatation in normal volunteers [34, 73].

8.2.2. Multiple Dosing: The earlier relatively weak leukotriene receptor antagonist LY 171,883 (600 mg twice-daily for 6 weeks) caused a small improvement in basal lung function, with some reduction in the use of β_2-adrenergic agonist reliever medication [104]. MK-571 administered orally for 6 weeks resulted in a mean increase in FEV_1 of 8–14%, a decrease in daytime symptom scores by 30%, a decrease in β-agonist inhaler use by 30% and improved diurnal variation in peak expiratory flow rate [105]. Montelukast was dosed at 600 mg/day for 10 days and 200 mg for 6 weeks in asthmatics, causing similar degrees of bronchodilatation [106]. Further studies indicated that a dose-related improvement in patient-reported asthma end-points over the range 2–50 mg per day, with maximal beneficial effects using the 10 mg daily dosage in adult asthma [107]. In a 6-week study of zafirlukast (5, 10 or 20 mg twice daily) in patients with mild to moderate asthma, a dose-dependent improvement in symptoms was observed. The 40 mg/day dosage led to a significant improvement of evening peak expiratory flow, rescue β-agonist inhaler use (reduced by 30%), night-wakings (reduced by 46%), morning asthma symptoms and day-time symptoms (reduced by 26%) [108]. ICI 204,219 was more effective in subjects who had the lowest predicted FEV_1 at entry to the study and a linear response was observed with increasing doses of the antagonist [108]. Montelukast and pranlukast also caused similar sustained degrees of improvement in asthma with up to 11–13% increase in FEV_1, and decrease in symptoms in 12- and 4-week studies respectively [109, 110]. Dose-related improvements have been shown with montelukast [107]. In children, similar clinical beneficial effects are demonstrated for montelukast, including inhibition of exercise-induced asthma [111, 112].

9. Comparative Clinical Studies

In patients using inhaled corticosteroids (average 1,600 μg inhaled beclomethasone dipropionate per day), pranlukast allowed a reduction of 50% in inhaled dose of beclomethasone without loss of asthma control compared to placebo [113]. Indirect markers of inflammation such as exhaled nitric oxide and serum eosinophilic cationic protein levels increased in patients on placebo experiencing loss of asthma control. The bronchodilator effect of leukotriene antagonists is also present even in patients already on inhaled corticosteroid treatment [114–116]. In preliminary reports, addition of leukotriene antagonists to high doses of inhaled and often concomitant oral corticosteroid therapy in patients with severe disease can lead to additional clinical benefits with reduction in exacerbations [117]. Comparative studies with low dose inhaled corticosteroids in mild-to-moderate asthma have been published only in preliminary form and show that low dose inhaled corticosteroids (400 μg of beclomethasone per day) are more efficacious than the receptor antagonists, zafirlukast and montelukast [118, 119].

10. Anti-Inflammatory Effects of Leukotriene Receptor Antagonists

Treatment with the leukotriene receptor antagonist zafirlukast or the 5-lipoxygenase inhibitor zileuton reduced the number of inflammatory cells recovered in bronchoalveolar lavage fluid from patients with the late asthmatic response after bronchopulmonary segmental allergen challenge [64, 89]. Treatment of chronic asthmatics with pranlukast causes a reduction in the number of eosinophils and T-cells in the airways submucosa [120]. Montelukast caused a significant reduction in eosinophils in induced sputum of asthmatics [121], and in eosinophils in blood [107].

11. Safety of Leukotriene Receptor Antagonists and Inhibitors

In general, the leukotriene receptor antagonists and inhibitors are well tolerated in 6-month trials. In most studies, the incidence of reported adverse effects was similar to that reported in the placebo group [65, 104, 108]. No reports of unexpected adverse clinical or laboratory events have been reported with pranlukast since it was launched in Japan more than 2 years ago. In the montelukast phase 1–3 trials, adverse events and abnormal laboratory events were similar in both active and placebo groups. In a few patients treated with zafirlukast (and montelukast), Churg-Strauss syndrome that is characterised by marked circulating eosinophilia and eosinophilic vasculitis, has been reported [122]. It is likely that these are the result of reduction in oral corticosteroid dosage while these patients with unsuspected Churg-Strauss were being treated with these antagonists; however, an idiosyncratic effect of these new treatments cannot be entirely excluded.

Asymptomatic elevations of serum alanine amino-transferase concentrations by more than three-fold were observed in 4.6 patients receiving zileuton (600 mg four times per day) compared to 1.6 patients on placebo. Most elevations resolved after 3 months of either continuation or discontinuation of treatment. Doses of zafirlukast higher than 20 mg twice a day can cause elevation of liver enzymes.

12. Role in Asthma Management

Recent asthma guidelines for the management and treatment of chronic asthma recommend a stepwise approach for the pharmacological treatment of this disease [123, 124]. The selection of treatment is based upon the severity of the asthma and the number of medications and their dose and frequency titrated to the severity of disease. There is also emphasis on the early use of anti-inflammatory medication to gain early control of the disease. At present, inhaled corticosteroid therapy is considered to be the most effective and commonly used anti-inflammatory agents, with sodium cromoglycate and nedocromil sodium being less reliable and effective agents. Overall, the goals of management include the attainment of minimal or no symptoms, a decrease in the number of acute exacerbations, a reduction in the requirements for short-acting β_2-agonists, near normal lung function and a greater ability to participate in physical activities. Avoidance of known allergens or irritants and patient education are also important aspects of asthma management.

Where do the leukotriene inhibitors fit in the overall current management of asthma? Although studies are still being currently performed regarding the potential anti-inflammatory effects of leukotriene inhibitors, the limited data available indicate that these agents do possess anti-inflammatory effects, particularly in inhibiting eosinophil inflammation. These agents can therefore be considered as having anti-inflammatory properties in asthma. In the studies that have been reviewed above, these agents produce an overall modest improvement in lung function and symptom control, a reduction in the need for short-acting β_2-agonist therapy in patients with mild to moderate persistent asthma when compared to placebo, both in patients on or not on inhaled corticosteroid therapy. It is best to consider the various steps of asthma management guidelines in attempting to integrate these antileukotriene therapies with existing asthma management. Should they be used as first-line treatment for mild intermittent asthma at Step 1 or Step 2 on equal par to the use of low-dose inhaled corticosteroid therapy or sodium cromoglycate and nedocromil sodium? Data showing a reduction in cellular airway infiltration on allergen challenge and an attenuation of the late phase response would indicate that these agents possess antiinflammatory properties disease-modifying effects, although more studies are needed. Finally, there has been no fully-published comparison of these treatments to low-dose inhaled steroids for efficacy in improving lung function and bronchial hyperresponsiveness. It is possible that such clinical studies may help identify groups of patients that may particularly benefit from either one or other first-line therapy. The relative responsiveness of patients to one or other treatment may be important in determining their clinical usage. The recent United States National Heart Lung & Blood Institute Expert Panel Report II guidelines have indicated that leukotriene modifiers may be used as an alternative to low dose inhaled corticosteroids in mild persistent asthma. One advantage of these drugs particularly for its consideration as a Step1/2 therapy, as chronic therapy is its availability as a well-tolerated oral formulation which should promote improved patient compliance and more predictable drug bioavailability compared with inhaled medication, and thus avoid the necessity for teaching and insisting on proper inhaler technique.

Compliance may also be helped by the relatively rapid onset of effect of zafirlukast. A study of twice daily oral zafirlukast showed a compliance of 81% in a group of symptomatic asthmatic patients using an electronic tracking cap device system, which is about twice that of previously-published compliance rates for twice daily inhaled corticosteroid therapy [125]. Another potential area of advantage of the leukotriene inhibitors over inhaled steroid therapy is the combined effect on co-existing allergic rhinitis symptoms. Therefore, much of the basis for the choice would lie in the superior efficacy of inhaled corticosteroids *versus* the likely superior compliance associated with leukotriene inhibitors.

At the more severe level of Step 3 where usually high-dose inhaled corticosteroid therapy is considered, the beneficial effects of leukotriene inhibitors have been demonstrated and these would be recommended as additive therapy to corticosteroids. A combination of low-dose steroids with leukotriene inhibitors may provide better control than high-dose inhaled steroids alone. Certainly, there is an additive effect of leukotriene inhibitors with high-dose inhaled steroid therapy and for more severe asthma patients (Steps 4 and 5), additive therapy to inhaled or oral steroid therapy should be considered.

Neither inhaled nor oral corticosteroid therapy reduce leukotriene production in asthmatic patients as measured by urinary LTE_4 excretion [126, 127]. Comparative studies are now needed regarding the additive effects of leukotriene inhibitors compared to other available agents such as long-acting inhaled β_2-adrenergic agonists and slow-release theophylline at these steps.

Finally, are there any advantages of leukotriene receptor antagonists over 5-lipoxygenase inhibitors and *vice versa* in the treatment of asthma? Zileuton has broader action that the leukotriene receptor antagonists in that it also inhibits the actions of the leukotriene B_4 However, the contribution of LTB_4 to asthma control is not clear and several studies indicate that LTB_4 may not contribute to asthma pathogenesis. There are no direct comparisons of zileuton to the receptors antagonists yet. The need to use zileuton four times a day compared to the once or twice daily dosage for montelukast and zafirlukast respectively may represent a clinical disadvantage. However, currently no firm recommendations can be made on the use of one group *versus* the other.

References

1 Rouzer CA, Matsumoto T, Samuelsson B (1986) Single protein from human leukocytes possesses 5-lipoxygenase and leukotriene A synthase activities. *Proc Natl Acad Sci USA* 83: 857–861

2 Rouzer CA, Samuelsson B (1985) On the nature of the 5-lipoxygenase reaction in human leukocytes: enzyme purification and requirement for multiple stimulatory factors. *Proc Natl Acad Sci USA* 82: 6040–6044

3 Miller DK, Gillard JW, Vickers PJ, Sadowski S (1990) Identification and isolation of a membrane protein necessary for leukotriene production. *Nature* 343: 278–281

4 Haeggstrom JZ, Wetterholm A, Vallee BL, Samuelsson B (1990) Leukotriene A_4 hydrolase: an epoxide hydrolase with peptidase activity. *Biochem Biophys Res Commun* 173: 431–437

5 Lam BK, Penrose JF, Freeman GJ, Austen KF (1994) Expression cloning of a cDNA for human leukotriene C_4 synthase, an integral membrane protein conjugating reduced glutathione to leukotriene A_4. *Proc Natl Acad Sci USA* 91: 7663–7667

6 Sala A, Voelkel N, Maclouf J, Murphy RC (1990) Leukotriene E_4 elimination and metabolism in normal human subjects. *J Biol Chem* 265: 21 771–21 778

7 Maltby NH, Taylor GW, Ritter JM, Moore K, Fuller RW, Dollery CT (1990) Leukotriene C_4 elimination and metabolism in man. *J Allerg Clin Immunol* 85: 3–9

8 Feinmark SJ, Cannon PJ (1986) Endothelial cell leukotriene C_4 synthesis results from intercellular transfer of leukotriene A_4 synthesized by polymorphonuclear leukocytes. *J Biol Chem* 261: 16 466–16 472

9 Bigby TD, Lee DM, Meslier N, Gruenert DC (1989) Leukotriene A_4 hydrolase activity of human airway epithelial cells. *Biochem Biophys Res Commun* 164: 1–7

10 Silberstein DS, Owen WF, Gasson JC, Di Pierso JF, Golde DW, Bina JC, Soberman RJ, Austen KF, David JR (1986) Enhancement of human eosinophil cytotoxicity and leukotriene synthesis by biosynthetic (recombinant) granulocyte-macrophage colony stimulating factor. *J Immunol* 137: 3290–3294

11 Takafuji S, Bischoff SC, De Weck AL, Dahinden CA (1991) IL-3 and IL-5 prime normal human eosinophils to produce leukotriene C_4 in response to soluble agonists. *J Immunol* 147: 3855–3861

12 Dahlén S-E, Hedqvist P, Hammarström S, Samuelsson B (1980) Leukotrienes are potent constrictors of human bronchi. *Nature* 288: 484–486

13 Davidson AB, Lee TH, Scanlon PD, Solway J, McFadden ER, Ingram RH, Corey EJ, Austen KF, Drazen JM (1987) Bronchoconstrictor effects of leukotriene E_4 in normal and asthmatic subjects.

Am Rev Respir Dis 135: 500–504

14 Griffin M, Weiss JW, Leitch AG, McFadden ER, Corey EJ, Austen KF, Drazen JM (1983) Effects of leukotriene D on the airways in asthma. *N Engl J Med* 308: 436–439

15 Arm JP, O'Hickey SP, Hawksworth RJ (1990) Asthmatic airways have a disproportionate hyper-responsiveness to LTE_4 as compared with normal airways, but not to LTC_4, LTD_4, methacholine and histamine. *Am Rev Respir Dis* 142: 1112–1118

16 Bel EH, Van der Veen H, Kramps JA, Dijkman JH, Sterk PJ (1987) Maximal airway narrowing to inhaled leukotriene D_4 in normal subjects. Comparison and interaction with methacholine. *Am Rev Respir Dis* 136: 979–984

17 Arm JP, Spur BW, Lee TH (1988) The effects of inhaled leukotriene E_4 on the airway responsiveness to histamine in subjects with asthma and normal subjects. *J Allerg Clin Immunol* 82: 654–660

18 Sampson SE, Costello JF, Sampson AP (1997) The effect of inhaled leukotriene B_4 in normal and in asthmatic subjects. *Am J Respir Crit Care Med* 155: 1789–1792

19 Woodward DF, Wasserman MA, Weichmann BM (1983) Investigation of leukotriene involvement in the vasopermeability response associated with guinea-pig tracheal anaphylaxis: comparison with cutaneous anaphylaxis. *Eur J Pharmacol* 93: 9–19

20 Hua XY, Dahlen SE, Lundberg JM, Hammerstrom S, Hedqvist P (1985) Leukotrienes C_4 and E_4 cause widespread and extensive plasma extravasation in the guinea-pig. *Naunyn-Schmied Arch Pharmacol* 330: 136–141

21 Hui KP, Lotvall J, Chung KF, Barnes PJ (1991) Attenuation of inhaled allergen-induced airway microvascular leakage and airflow obstruction in guinea-pigs by a 5-lipoxygenase inhibitor (A-63162). *Am Rev Respir Dis* 143: 1015–1019

22 Marom Z, Shelhamer JH, Bach MK, Morton DR, M Kaliner (1982) Slow-reacting substances leukotrienes C_4 and D_4 increase the release of mucus from human airways *in vitro*. *Am Rev Respir Dis* 126: 449–451

23 Coles SJ, Neill KH, Reid LM, Austen KF, Nii Y, Corey EJ, Lewis RA (1983) Effects of leukotrienes C_4 and D_4 on glycoprotein and lysozyme secretion by human bronchial mucosa. *Prostaglandins* 25: 155–170

24 Johnson HG, McNee ML (1983) Secretagogue responses of leukotriene C_4, D_4: comparison of potency in canine trachea *in vivo*. *Prostaglandins* 25: 237–243

25 Bousquet JP, Chanez P, Lacoste JY, Barneon G, Ghavanian N, Enander I, Venge P, Ahlstedt S, Simony-Lafontaine J, Godard P, Michel FB (1990) Eosinophilic inflammation in asthma. *N Engl J Med* 323: 1033–1039

26 Krell RD, Dehaas CJ, Lengel DJ, Kusner EJ, Williams JC, Buckner CK (1994) Preclinical exploration of the potential antiinflammatory properties of the peptide leukotriene antagonist ICI 204,219 (Accolate). *Ann N Y Acad Sci* 744: 289–298

27 Laitinen LA, Laitinen A, Haahtela T, Vilkka V, Spur BW, Lee TH (1993) Leukotriene E_4 and granulocytic infiltration into asthmatic airways. *Lancet* 341: 989–990

28 Panettieri RA, Tan EM, Ciocca V, Luttmann MA, Leonard TB, Hay DW (1998) Effects of LTD_4 on human airway smooth muscle cell proliferation, matrix expression, and contraction *in vitro*: differential sensitivity to cysteinyl leukotriene receptor antagonists. *Am J Respir Cell Mol Biol* 19: 453–461

29 Taylor GW, Taylor IK, Black P, Maltby NH, Turner N, Fuller RW, Dollery CT (1989) Urinary leukotriene E_4 after antigen challenge and in acute asthma and allergic rhinitis. *Lancet* i: 584–587

30 Drazen JM, O'Brien J, Sparrow D, Weiss ST, Martins MA, Israel E, Fanta CH (1992) Recovery of leukotriene E_4 from the urine of patients with airways obstruction. *Am Rev Respir Dis* 146: 104–108

31 Kikawa Y, Miyanomae T, Inoue Y, Saito M, Nakai A, Shigematsu Y, Hosoi S, Sudo M (1992) Urinary leukotriene E_4 after exercise challenge in children with asthma. *J Allerg Clin Immunol* 89: 1111–1119

32 Reiss TF, Hill JB, Harman E, Zhang J, Tanaka WK, Bronsky E, Guerreiro D, Hendeles L (1997) Increased urinary excretion of LTE_4 after exercise and attenuation of exercise-induced bronchospasm by montelukast, a cysteinyl leukotriene receptor antagonist. *Thorax* 52: 1030–1035

33 Taylor IK, Wellings R, Taylor GW, Fuller RW (1992) Urinary leukotriene E_4 excretion in exercise induced asthma. *J Appl Physiol* 73: 743–748

34 Smith LJ, Geller S, Ebright L, Glass M, Thyrum PT (1990) Inhibition of leukotriene D_4-induced

bronchoconstriction in normal subjects by the oral LTD_4 receptor antagonist ICI 204,219. *Am Rev Respir Dis* 141: 988–992

35 Christie PE, Tagari P, Ford-Hutchinson AW (1992) Urinary leukotriene E_4 concentrations increase after aspirin challenge in aspirin-sensitive asthmatic subjects. *Am Rev Respir Dis* 145: 65–69

36 Kumlin M, Dahlen B, Björck T, Zetterstrom O, Granstrom E, Dahlén S-E (1992) Urinary excretion of leukotriene E_4 and 11-dehydro-thromboxane B_2 in response to bronchial provocations with allergen, aspirin, leukotriene D_4 and histamine in asthmatics. *Am Rev Respir Dis* 146: 96–103

37 Wenzel SE, Larsen GL, Johnston G, Voelkel NF, Westcott JY (1990) Elevated levels of leukotriene C_4 in bronchoalveolar lavage fluid from atopic asthmatics after endobronchial allergen challenge. *Am Rev Respir Dis* 142: 112–119

38 Lam S, Chan H, Leriche JC, Chan Yeung M, Salari H (1988) Release of leukotrienes in patients with bronchial asthma. *J Allerg Clin Immunol* 81: 711–717

39 Wardlaw AJ, Hay H, Cromwell O, Collins JV, Kay AB (1989) Leukotrienes, LTC_4 and LTB_4, in bronchoalveolar lavage in bronchial asthma and other respiratory diseases. *J Allerg Clin Immunol* 84: 19–26

40 Crea AEG, Nakhosteen JA, Lee TH (1992) Mediator concentrations in bronchoalveolar lavage fluid of patients with mild asymptotic bronchial asthma. *Eur Respir J* 5: 190–195

41 McMillan RM, Girodeau JM, Foster SJ (1990) Selective chiral inhibitors of 5-lipoxygenase with anti-inflammatory activity. *Br J Pharmacol* 101: 501–503

42 Foster SJ, Bruneau P, Walker ER, McMillan RM (1990) 2-Substituted indazolinones: orally active and selective 5-lipoxygenase inhibitors with anti-inflammatory activity. *Br J Pharmacol* 99: 113–118

43 Carter GW, Young PR, Albert DH, Bouska J, Dyer R, Bell RL, Summers JB, Brooks DW (1991) 5-Lipoxygenase inhibitory activity of zileuton. *J Pharmacol Exp Ther* 256: 929–937

44 Rubin P, Dube L, Braeckman R, Swanson L, Hansen R, Albert D, Carter G (1991) Pharmacokinetics, safety, and ability to diminish leukotriene synthesis by zileuton, an inhibiter of 5-lipoxygenase. *In*: NR Acherman, RJ Bonney, N Doherty (eds): *Progress in inflammation research and therapy.* pp103–112

45 McMillan RM, Spruce KE, Crawley GC, Walker ER, Foster SJ (1992) Pre-clinical pharmacology of ICI D2138, a potent orally-active non-redox inhibitor of 5-lipoxygenase. *Br J Pharmacol* 107: 1042–1047

46 Brideau C, Chan C, Charleson S, Denis D, Evans JF, Ford-Hutchinson AW, Fortin R, Gillard JW, Guay J, Guevremont D et al (1992) Pharmacology of MK-0591 (3-[1-(4-chlorobenzyl)-3-(*t*-butylthio)-5-(quinolin-2-yl-methoxy)-indol-2-yl 2, 2-dimethyl propanoic acid), a potent, orally active leukotriene biosynthesis inhibitor. *Can J Physiol Pharmacol* 70: 799–807

47 Depre M, Friedman B, Tanaka W, Van Hecken A, Buntinx A, DeSchepper PJ (1993) Biochemical activity, pharmacokinetics, and tolerability of MK-886, a leukotriene biosynthesis inhibitor, in humans. *Clin Pharmacol Ther* 53: 602–607

48 Gillard J, Ford-Hutchinson AW, Chan C, Charleson S, Denis D, Foster A, Fortin R, Leger S, McFarlane CS, Morton H et al (1989) L-663, 536 (MK-886) (3-[1-(4-chlorobenzyl)-3-t-butyl-thio-5-isopropylindol-2-yl]-2,2-dimethylpropanoic acid), a novel, orally active leukotriene biosynthesis inhibitor. *Can J Physiol Pharmacol* 67: 456–464

49 Prasit P, Belley M, Blouin M, Brideau C, Chan C, Charleson S, Evans JF, Frenette R, Gauthier JY, Guay J et al (1993) A new class of leukotriene biosynthesis inhibitor: the development of MK-0591. *J Lipid Mediators* 6: 239–244

50 Depre M, Friedman B, Van Hecken A, de Lepeleire I, Tanaka W, Dallob A, Shingo S, Porras A, Lin C, de Schepper PJ (1994) Pharmacokinetics and pharmacodynamics of multiple oral doses of MK-0591, a 5-lipoxygenase-activating protein inhibitor. *Clin Pharmacol Ther* 56: 22–30

51 Grimes D, Sturm RJ, Marinari LR, Carlson RP, Berkenkopf JW, Musser JH, Kreft AF, Weichman BM (1993) WY-50,295 tromethamine, a novel, orally active 5-lipoxygenase inhibitor: biochemical characterization and antiallergic activity. *Eur J Pharmacol* 236: 217–228

52 Evans JF, Leville C, Mancini JA, Prasit P, Therien M, Zamboni R, Fortin R, Charleson P, MacIntyre DE et al (1991) 5-Lipoxygenase-activating protein is the target of a quinoline class of leukotriene synthesis inhibitors. *Mol Pharmacol* 40: 22–27

53 Gorenne I, Labat C, Gascard JP, Norel X, Muller-Peddinghaus R, Mohrs KH, Taylor WA, Gardiner PJ, Brink C (1994) (R)-2-[4-(quinolin-2-yl-methoxy)phenyl]-2-cyclopentyl] acetic acid

(BAY x1005), a potent leukotriene synthesis inhibitor: effects on anti-IgE challenge in human airways. *J Pharmacol Exp Ther* 268: 868–872

54 Israel E, Dermarkarian R, Rosenberg M, Sperling R, Taylor G, Rubin P, Drazen JM (1990) The effects of a 5-lipoxygenase inhibitor on asthma induced by cold, dry air. *N Engl J Med* 323: 1740–1744

55 Meltzer EO, Orgel HA, Ellis EF, Eigen HN, Hemstreet MP (1992) Long-term comparison of three combinations of albuterol, theophylline, and beclomethasone in children with chronic asthma. *J Allerg Clin Immunol* 90: 2–11

56 Israel E, Fischer AR, Rosenberg MA, Lilly CM, Callery JC, Shapiro J, Rubin P, Drazen JM (1993) The pivotal role of 5-lipoxygenase products in the reaction of aspirin-sensitive asthmatics to aspirin. *Am Rev Respir Dis* 148: 1447–1451

57 Shuaib Nasser SM, Bell GS, Hawksworth RJ, Spruce KE, MacMillan R, Williams AJ, Lee TH, Arm JP (1994) Effects of the 5-lipoxygenase inhibitor ZD 2138 on aspirin induced asthma. *Thorax* 49: 749–756

58 Hui KP, Rubin P, Kesterson J, Barnes NC, Barnes PJ (1991) Effect of a 5-lipoxygenase inhibitor on leukotriene generation and airway responses after allergen challenge in asthmatics. *Thorax* 46: 184–189

59 Friedman BS, Bel EH, Buntinx A, Tanaka W, Han YH, Shingo S, Spector R, Sterk P (1993) Oral leukotriene inhibitor (MK-886) blocks allergen-induced airway responses. *Am Rev Respir Dis* 147: 839–844

60 Shuaib Nasser SM, Bell GS, Hawksworth RJ, Spruce KE, MacMillan R, Williams AJ, Lee TH, Arm JP (1994) Effect of the 5-lipoxygenase inhibitor ZD2138 on allergen-induced early and late asthmatic responses. *Thorax* 49: 743–748

61 Diamant Z, Timmers MC, Van der Veen H (1995) The effect of MK-0591, a novel 5-lipoxygenase activating protein (FLAP) inhibiter, on leukotriene biosynthesis and allergen-induced airway responses in asthmatic subjects *in vivo*. *J Allerg Clin Immunol* 95: 42–51

62 Hamilton AL, Watson RM, Wyile G, O'Byrne PM (1997) Attenuation of early and late phase allergen-induced bronchoconstriction in asthmatic subjects by a 5-lipoxygenase activating protein antagonist, BAYx 1005. *Thorax* 52: 348–354

63 Knapp HR (1990) Reduced allergen-induced nasal congestion and leukotriene synthesis with an orally active 5-lipoygenase inhibitor. *N Engl J Med* 323: 1745–1748

64 Kane GC, Pollice M, Kim CJ, Cohn J, Dworski RT, Murray JJ, Sheller JR, Fish JE, Peters SP (1996) A controlled trial of the effect of the 5-lipoxygenase inhibitor, zileuton, on lung inflammation produced by segmental antigen challenge in human beings. *J Allerg Clin Immunol* 97: 646–654

65 Israel E, Rubin P, Kemp JP, Grossman J, Pierson W, Siegel SC, Murray JJ, Busse WW, Segal AT et al (1993) The effect of inhibition of 5-lipoxygenase by zileuton in mild-to-moderate asthma. *Ann Intern Med* 119: 1059–1066

66 Liu MC, Dube LM, Lancaster J (1996) Acute and chronic effects of a 5-lipoxygenase inhibitor in asthma: a 6-month randomized multicenter trial. Zileuton Study Group. *J Allerg Clin Immunol* 98: 859–871

67 Israel E, Cohn J, Dube L, Drazen JM (1996) Effect of treatment with zileuton, a 5-lipoxygenase inhibitor, in patients with asthma. A randomized controlled trial. Zileuton Clinical Trial Group. *JAMA* 275: 931–936

68 Schwartz HJ, Petty T, Dube LM, Swanson LJ, Lancaster JF (1998) A randomized controlled trial comparing zileuton with theophylline in moderate asthma. The Zileuton Study Group. *Arch Intern Med* 158: 141–148

69 Dahlen B, Nizankowska E, Szczeklik A, Zetterstrom O, Bochenek G, Kumlin M, Mastalerz M, Pinis G, Swanson LJ, Boodhoo TI, Wright S, Dube LM, Dahlen S-E (1998) Benefits from adding the 5-lipoxygenase inhibitor zileuton to conventional therapy in aspirin-intolerant asthmatics. *Am J Respir Crit Care Med* 157: 1187–1194

70 Augstein J, Farmer JB, Lee TB, Sheard P, Tattersall ML (1973) Selective inhibitor of slow reacting substance of anaphylaxis. *Nature* 245: 214–217

71 Britton JR, Hanley SP, Tattersfield AE (1987) The effect of an oral leukotriene D_4 antagonist L-649, 923 on the response to inhaled antigen in asthma. *J Allerg Clin Immunol* 79: 811–816

72 Cheng JB (1992) Early efficacy data with a newer generation of LTD_4 antagonists in antiasthma trials: early promise for a single mediator antagonist. *Pulmonary Pharmacol* 5: 77–80

73 Kips JC, Joos GF, De Lepeleire I, Margolskee DJ, Buntinx A, Pauwels RA, Van der Straeten ME

(1991) MK-571: a potent antagonist of LTD_4 induced bronchoconstriction in the human. *Am Rev Respir Dis* 144: 617–621

74 Jones TR, Labelle M, Belley M, Champion E, Charette L, Evans J, Ford-Hutchinson AW, Gauthier JY, Lord A, Masson P et al (1995) Pharmacology of montelukast sodium (Singulair), a potent and selective leukotriene D_4 receptor antagonist *Can J Physiol Pharmacol* 73: 191–201

75 de Lepeleire I, Reiss TF, Rochette F, Botto A, Zhang J, Kundu S, Decramer M (1997) Montelukast causes prolonged, potent leukotriene D_4-receptor antagonism in the airways of patients with asthma. *Clin Pharmacol Ther* 61: 83–92

76 Manning PJ, Watson RM, Margolskee DJ, Williams VC, Schwartz JI, O'Byrne PM (1990) Inhibition of exercise-induced bronchoconstriction by MK-751, a potent leukotriene-D_4 receptor antagonist. *N Engl J Med* 323: 1736–1739

77 Finnerty JP, Wood-Baker R, Thomson H, Holgate ST (1992) Role of leukotrienes in exercise-induced asthma. *Am Rev Respir Dis* 145: 746–749

78 Makker HK, Lau LC, Thomson HW, Binks SM, Holgate ST (1993) The protective effect of inhaled leukotriene D_4 receptor antagonist ICI 204,219 against exercise-induced asthma. *Am Rev Respir Dis* 147: 1413–1418

79 Robuschi M, Riva E, Fuccella LM, Vida E, Barnabe R, Rossi M, Gambaro G, Spagnotto S, Bianco S (1992) Prevention of exercise-induced bronchoconstriction by a new leukotriene antagonist (SKandF) 104,353: A double-blind study *versus* disodium cromoglycate and placebo. *Am Rev Respir Dis* 145: 1285–1288

80 Adelroth E, Inman MD, Summers E, Pace D, Modi M, O'Byrne PM (1997) Prolonged protection against exercise-induced bronchoconstriction by the leukotriene D_4-receptor antagonist cinalukast. *J Allerg Clin Immunol* 99: 210–215

81 Leff JA, Busse WW, Pearlman D, Bronsky EA, Kemp J, Hendeles L, Dockhorn R, Kundu S, Zhang J, Seidenberg BC, Reiss TF (1998) Montelukast, a leukotriene-receptor antagonist, for the treatment of mild asthma and exercise-induced bronchoconstriction *N Engl J Med* 339: 147–152

82 Taylor IK, O'Shaughnessy KM, Fuller RW, Dollery CT (1991) Effect of cysteinyl-leukotriene receptor antagonist ICI 204-219 on allergen-induced bronchoconstriction and airway hyperreactivitiy in atopic subjects. *Lancet* 337: 690–694

83 Findlay SR, Barden JM, Easley CB, Glass M (1992) Effect of the oral leukotriene antagonist ICI 204,219 on the antigen-induced bronchoconstriction in subjects with asthma. *J Allerg Clin Immunol* 89: 1040–1045

84 Rasmussen JB, Eriksson LO, Margolskee DJ, Tagari P, Williams VC (1992) Leukotriene D_4 receptor blockade inhibits the immediate and late bronchoconstrictor responses to inhaled antigen in patients with asthma. *J Allerg Clin Immunol* 90: 193–201

85 Dahlen B, Zetterstrom O, Bjorck T, Dahlen S-E (1994) The leukotriene-antagonist ICI-204,219 inhibits the early airway reaction to cumulative bronchial challenge with allergen in atopic asthmatics. *Eur Respir J* 7: 324–331

86 O'Shaughnessy KM, Taylor IK, O'Connor BJ, O'Connell F, Thomson H, Dollery CT (1993) Potent leukotriene D_4 receptor antagonist ICI 204,219 given by the inhaled route inhibits the early but not the late phase of allergen-induced bronchoconstriction. *Am Rev Respir Dis* 147: 1431–1435

87 Bel EH, Timmers MC, Dijkman JH, Stahl EG, Sterk PJ (1990) The effect of an inhaled leukotriene antagonist, L-648,051, on early and late asthmatic reactions and subsequent increase in airway responsivenss in man. *J Allerg Clin Immunol* 85: 1067–1075

88 Roquet A, Dahlen B, Kumlin M, Ihre E, Anstren G, Binks S, Dahlen SE (1997) Combined antagonism of leukotrienes and histamine produces predominant inhibition of allergen-induced early and late phase airway obstruction in asthmatics. *Am J Respir Crit Care Med* 155: 1856–1863

89 Calhoun WJ, Lavins BJ, Minkwitz MC, Evans R, Gleich GJ, Cohn J (1998) Effect of zafirlukast (Accolate) on cellular mediators of inflammation: bronchoalveolar lavage fluid findings after segmental antigen challenge. *Am J Respir Crit Care Med* 157: 1381–1389

90 Cowburn AS, Sladek K, Soja J, Adamek L, Nizankowska E, Szczeklik A, Lam BK, Penrose JF, Austen KF, Holgate ST, Sampson AP (1998) Over-expression of leukotriene C_4 synthase in bronchial biopsies from patients with aspirin-intolerant asthma. *J Clin Invest* 101: 834–846

91 Sanak M, Simon HU, Szczeklik A (1997) Leukotriene C_4 synthase promoter polymorphism and risk of aspirin-induced asthma. *Lancet* 350: 1599–1600

92 Christie PE, Smith CM, Lee TH (1991) The potent and selective sulfidopeptide leukotriene antagonist, SKandF 104353, inhibits aspirin-induced asthma. *Am Rev Respir Dis* 144: 957–958

93 Dahlen B, Kumlin M, Margolskee DJ, Larsson C, Blomqvist H, Williams VC, Zetterstrom O, Dahlen SE (1993) The leukotriene-receptor antagonist MK-06079 blocks airway obstruction induced by bronchial provocation with lysine-aspirin in aspirin-sensitive asthmatics. *Eur Respir J* 6: 1018–1026

94 Kidney J, Ridge S, Chung KF, Barnes PJ (1993) Inhibition of PAF-induced bronchoconstriction by the oral leukotriene D_4 receptor antagonist, ICI 204,219. *Am Rev Respir Dis* 147: 215–217

95 Spencer DA, Evans JM, Green SE, Piper PJ, Costello JF (1991) Participation of the cysteinyl leukotrienes in the acute bronchoconstrictor response to inhaled platelet activating factor in man. *Thorax* 46: 441–445

96 O'Connor BJ, Uden S, Carty TJ, Eskra JD, Barnes PJ, Chung KF (1994) Inhibitory effects of UK 74505, a potent and specific oral platelet activating factor (PAF) receptor antagonist, on airway and systemic responses to inhaled PAF in man. *Am J Respir Crit Care Med* 150: 35–40

97 Fujimura M, Sakamoto S, Kamio Y, Matsuda T (1993) Effect of a leukotriene antagonist, ONO-1078, on bronchial hyperresponsiveness in patients with asthma. *Respir Med* 87: 133–138

98 Hui KP, Barnes NC (1991) Lung function improvement in asthma with a cystemyl-leukotriene receptor antagonist. *Lancet* 337: 1062–1063

99 Kips JC, Joos GF, Felman EA, Pauwels RA (1993) The effect of inhaled ICI 204,219 on baseline lung function in moderate asthma. *Am Rev Respir Dis* 147: A297 Abstract

100 Joos GF, Kips JC, Pauwels RA, Van Der Straeten ME (1991) The effect of aerosolized SKandF 104353-Z2 on the bronchoconstrictor effect of leukotriene D_4 in asthmatics. *Pulmonary Pharmacol* 4: 37–42

101 Gaddy JN, Margolskee DJ, Bush RK, Williams VC, Busse WW (1992) Bronchodilation with a potent and selective leukotriene D_4 (LTD_4) receptor antagonist (MK-571) in patients with asthma. *Am Rev Respir Dis* 146: 358–363

102 Gaddy J, Bush RK, Margolskee D, Williams VC, Busse WW (1990) The effects of a leukotriene D_4 (LTD_4) antagonist (MK-571) in mild to moderate asthma. *J Allerg Clin Immunol* 85: 197A. Abstract

103 Dahlen B, Margolskee DJ, Zetterstrom O, Dahlen S-E (1993) Effect of leukotriene receptor antagonist MK-0679 on baseline pulmonary function in aspirin-sensitive asthmatic subjects. *Thorax* 48: 1205–1210

104 Cloud ML, Enas GC, Kemp J, Platts-Mills T, Altman LC, Townley R, Tinkelman D, King T, Middleton E, Sheffer AL, McFadden ER, Farlow DS (1989) A specific LTD_4/LTE_4-receptor antagonist improves pulmonary funcion in patients with mild, chronic asthma. *Am Rev Respir Dis* 140: 1336–1339

105 Margolskee DJ (1991) Clinical experience with MK-571. A potent and specific LTD_4 receptor antagonist. *Ann New York Acad Sc* 629: 148–156

106 Reiss TF, Altman LC, Chervinsky P, Bewtra A, Stricker WE, Noonan GP, Kundu S, Zhang J (1996) Effects of montelukast (MK-0476), a new potent cysteinyl leukotriene (LTD_4) receptor antagonist, in patients with chronic asthma. *J Allergy Clin Immunol* 98: 528–534

107 Noonan MJ, Chervinsky P, Brandon M, Zhang J, Kundu S, McBurney J, Reiss TF (1998) Montelukast, a potent leukotriene receptor antagonist, causes dose-related improvements in chronic asthma. Montelukast Asthma Study Group. *Eur Respir J* 11: 1232–1239

108 Spector SL, Smith LJ, Glass M (1994) Effects of six weeks of therapy with oral doses of ICI 204,219, a leukotriene D_4 receptor antagonist, in subjects with bronchial asthma. *Am J Respir Crit Care Med* 150: 618–623

109 Reiss TF, Chervinsky P, Dockhorn RJ, Shingo S, Seidenberg B, Edwards TB (1998) Montelukast, a once-daily leukotriene receptor antagonist, in the treatment of chronic asthma: a multicenter, randomized, double-blind trial. Montelukast Clinical Research Study Group. *Arch Intern Med* 158: 1213–1220

110 Barnes NC, Pujet JC (1997) Pranlukast, a novel leukotriene receptor antagonist: results of the first European, placebo controlled, multicentre clinical study in asthma. *Thorax* 52: 523–527

111 Knorr B, Matz J, Bernstein JA, Nguyen H, Seidenberg BC, Reiss TF, Becker A (1998) Montelukast for chronic asthma in 6- to 14-year-old children: a randomized, double-blind trial. Pediatric Montelukast Study Group. *JAMA* 279: 1181–1186

112 Kemp JP, Dockhorn RJ, Shapiro GG, Nguyen HH, Reiss TF, Seidenberg BC, Knorr B (1998) Montelukast once daily inhibits exercise-induced bronchoconstriction in 6- to 14-year-old children with asthma. *J Pediat* 133: 424–428

113 Tamaoki J, Kondo M, Sakai N, Nakata J, Takemura H, Nagai A, Takizawa T, Konno K (1997)

Leukotriene antagonist prevents exacerbation of asthma during reduction of high-dose inhaled corticosteroid. The Tokyo Joshi-Idai Asthma Research Group. *Am J Respir Crit Care Med* 155: 1235–1240

114 Reiss TF, Chervinsky P, Dockhorn RJ, Shingo S, Seidenberg B, Edwards TB (1998) Montelukast, a once-daily leukotriene receptor antagonist, in the treatment of chronic asthma: a multicenter, randomized, double-blind trial. Montelukast Clinical Research Study Group. *Arch Intern Med* 158: 1213–1220

115 Murray KJ, England PJ, Hallam TJ, Maguire J, Moores K, Reeves ML, Simpson AWM, Rink TJ (1990) The effect of signazodan, a selective phosphodiesterase inhibitor, on human platelet function. *Br J Pharmacol* 99: 612–616

116 Reiss TF, Sorkness CA, Stricker W, Botto A, Busse WW, Kundu S, Zhang J (1997) Effects of montelukast (MK-0476); a potent cysteinyl leukotriene receptor antagonist, on bronchodilation in asthmatic subjects treated with and without inhaled corticosteroids. *Thorax* 52: 45–48

117 Virchow J, Hassall SM, Summerton L (1997) Improved asthma control over 6 weeks with Accolate (zafirlukast) in patients on high dose corticosteroids. *Allergy* 52: 183 Abstract

118 Laitinen LA, Nanya IP, Binks S et al (1997) Comparative efficacy of zafirlukast and low dose steroids on prn β-agonists. *Eur Respir J* 10 (Suppl 25): 419s

119 Malmstrom K, Guerra J, G Rodriguez-Gomez et al (1998) A comparison of montelukast, a leukotriene receptor antagonist, and inhaled beclomethasone in chronic asthma. *Eur Respir J* 12 (Suppl 28): 36s

120 Nakamura Y, Hoshino M, Sin JJ, Ishii K, Hosaka K, Sakamoto T (1998) Effect of leukotriene receptor antagonist pranlukast on cellular infiltration in the bronchial mucosa of patients with asthma. *Thorax* 53: 835–841

121 Leff JA, Pizzichini E, Efthimiadis A et al (1997) Effect of montelukast (MK-0476) on airway eosinophilic inflammation in mildly controlled asthma: a randomised placebo controlled trial. *Am J Respir Crit Care Med* 155: A977

122 Wechsler ME, Garpestad E, Flier SR, Kocher O, Weiland DA, Polito AJ, Klinek MM, Bigby TD, Wong GA, Helmers RA, Drazen JM (1998) Pulmonary infiltrates, eosinophilia, and cardiomyopathy following corticosteroid withdrawal in patients with asthma receiving zafirlukast. *JAMA* 279: 455–457

123 British Thoracic Society (1993) Guidelines on the management of asthma. *Thorax* 48 (Suppl: S1–S24):

124 Global Initiative for Asthma (1995) Global strategy for asthma management and prevention: NHLBI/WHO workshop report. National Institutes of health,

125 Chung KF, Kennelly JC, Summerton L, Harris A (1997) Compliance with an oral asthma treatment: electronic monitoring of twice daily dosing with zafirlukast. *Allergy Clin Immunol Int* 241 Abstract

126 Dworski R, Fitzgerald GA, Oates JASheller JR (1994) Effect of oral prednisone on airway inflammatory mediators in atopic asthma. *Am J Respir Crit Care Med* 149: 953–959

127 O'Shaughnessy KM, Wellings R, Gillies B, Fuller RW (1993) Differential effects of fluticasone propionate on allergen-evoked bronchoconstriction and increased urinary leukotriene E_4 excretion. *Am Rev Respir Dis* 147: 1472–1476

128 Fish JE, Kemp JP, Lockey RF, Glass M, Hanby LA, Bonuccelli CM (1997) Zafirlukast for symptomatic mild-to-moderate asthma: a 13-week multicenter study. The Zafirlukast Trialists Group. *Clin Ther* 19: 675–690

Asthma: Epidemiology, Anti-Inflammatory Therapy and Future Trends
ed. by M. A. Giembycz and B. J. O'Connor
© 2000 Birkhäuser Verlag/Switzerland

CHAPTER 10
Theophylline and New Generation Phosphodiesterase Inhibitors in the Treatment of Asthma

Clive P. Page[1] and John Costello[2]

[1] *Sackler Institute of Pulmonary Pharmacology, Division of Pharmacology & Therapeutics, Guy's, King's & St. Thomas', School of Biomedical Sciences, 5th Floor, Hodgkin Building, Guy's Campus, London SE1 9RT, UK*
[2] *Department of Respiratory Medicine & Allergy, Guy's, King's & St Thomas's School of Medicine, King's College London, Bessemer Road, London SE5,UK*

1. Theophylline in the Treatment of Asthma

Theophylline has been in clinical use for more than a century, although it is only during the last 50 years that this drug has been in regular use for the treatment of asthma. Theophylline was first used in the treatment of asthma in 1937, when it was administered i.v. for the treatment of acute asthma. In 1940, theophylline was first used orally in combination with ephedrine, and there are now many studies in the literature describing the effects of theophylline in the treatment of asthma [1]. Theophylline is now most commonly used in various slow-release formulations to overcome its rapid metabolism. However, over the last decade, the number of prescriptions being written for theophylline has declined, as newer medications have been introduced for the treatment of asthma, and this decline has come about mainly due to concerns about the narrow therapeutic window of theophylline, which has typically been classified as being 10–20 µg/ml in plasma [1].

However, whilst theophylline has traditionally been classified as a bronchodilator drug, it is now apparent that this drug has a range of other effects of potential therapeutic value in the treatment of respiratory diseases [2], that occur independently of the bronchodilator actions, including anti-inflammatory and immunomodulatory actions [3, 4], and increased respiratory drive [5]. These effects often occur at plasma levels below 10 µg/ml, suggesting that lower plasma levels of theophylline than have previously been used to obtain bronchodilation may be of benefit in the treatment of lung diseases, thus reducing the side-effect profile and improving its safety margin.

A number of studies have reported that theophylline can inhibit allergen-induced late onset responses in the airways of allergic asthmatics without significantly affecting acute bronchoconstriction [3, 6–8], although this was not seen in all studies [9]. The late onset response to allergen is known to be accompanied by an influx of inflammatory cells into the airways [10] and this allergen-induced infiltration of activated eosinophils into the airways (assessed as the total number of eosinophils and as an increase in the number of EG_2+ eosinophils in biopsies) was also reduced significantly by 6 weeks of treatment with theophylline [11], an effect that occurred at plasma levels well below the 10–20 µg/ml plasma levels required for bronchodilation. Confirmation that this anti-inflammatory effect of theophylline is not due to its bronchodilator effects has recently been provided by the observation that theophylline will also reduce allergen-induced eosinophil recruitment and activation in allergic rhinitis [12].

The mechanism whereby theophylline inhibits the recruitment of activated eosinophils into the airways is not known, but several mechanisms have been put forward to explain this observation. The first mechanism relates to an immunomodulatory action of theophylline on T-lymphocytes, an action that has been recognized for more than two decades [13–17]. It is now recognized that T-lymphocytes play a central role in the pathogenesis of allergic asthma, in particular the orchestration of eosinophil migration into the airways, *via* the release of cytokines such as IL-5 [18]. Regular treatment with theophylline has also been reported to inhibit allergen-induced recruitment of T-lymphocytes into the airway [19] and to increase the number of suppressor CD8 cells in peripheral blood [3, 17, 20]. Furthermore, withdrawal of theophylline from asthmatics has been shown to unmask a significant increase in asthma symptoms [4, 21], which was associated with an increase in T-lymphocytes in the airways [4], an immunomodulatory effect that again occurred at plasma levels below 10 µg/ml. Regular treatment with theophylline has also been reported to reduce the number of inflammatory cells expressing IL-4 in the airway [22] and to induce the production of IL-10 from peripheral blood mononuclear cells obtained from asthmatics [23], an observation of considerable interest as IL-10 can shorten eosinophil survival [24] and induce tolerance in T-cells [25].

Another suggested mechanism of action of theophylline that occurs at clinically relevant concentrations is its ability to alter eosinophil survival. A number of cytokines, including IL-5 have been shown to prolong eosinophil survival [26]. Theophylline has been shown to inhibit IL-5 mediated survival of human eosinophils and to accelerate apoptosis, again at concentrations below 10 µg/ml [27]. This effect could readily explain the ability of regular treatment with theophylline to reduce the number of eosinophils in the airways at plasma levels lower than 10 µg/ml. Many of the biological effects of theophylline have been suggested to be mediated *via* an inhibitory effect on the phosphodiesterase (PDE) family of enzymes [2, 28]. However, the effect of theophylline on apoptosis of eosinophils was not shared by the selective PDE4 inhibitor rolipram suggesting that this anti-inflammatory effect of theophylline may not be through inhibition of PDE4 [27].

This observation supports other recent work carried out in mononuclear cells obtained from asthmatics where theophylline was able to inhibit mononuclear cell proliferation *via* mechanisms distinct from selective PDE4 inhibitors [29] and recent data with the related xanthine, pentoxyphylline, showing that this drug can inhibit proliferation of fibroblasts *via* a mechanism unrelated to c-AMP generation [30].

Another prominent action of theophylline is the ability to antagonise adenosine receptors [31]. However, for more than a decade this suggestion was questioned as the related drug enprophylline had similar effects to theophylline clinically [6], yet was claimed to lack adenosine receptor antagonism [31]. However, recent studies have reported that enprophylline can act as a selective A2b receptor antagonist on human mast cells [32], a property shared by theophylline and which has been suggested to be of potential importance for the clinical activities of theophylline [33]. Other studies have shown that whilst asthmatics are very sensitive to inhaled adenosine [34], an effect that is blocked by theophylline [35, 36], but there is no evidence to date that this effect is mediated *via* activation of A2b receptors; rather there is evidence from experimental animals that it is the A1 receptor that is upregulated as a result of allergic sensitization [37, 38], an observation supported by the study of Nyce and Metzger [39] that an anti-sense oligonucleotide against A_1 receptors blocks allergen-reduced eosinophilia and allergen-induced bronchial hyperresponsiveness in allergic rabbits.

Recently regular theophylline treatment has been demonstrated to produce anti-inflammatory activity in patients having natural exacerbations of their asthma, in the form of nocturnal asthma. Theophylline treatment significantly improved the overnight deterioration in lung function associated with nocturnal asthma compared with placebo treatment [40], a finding consistent with previous studies using theophylline for the treatment of asthma [41]. Theophylline also inhibited the ability of neutrophils to migrate into the airways of patients undergoing nocturnal attacks of asthma [40], associated with a reduction in the ability of PMNs to release LTB4. This work not only extends the anti-inflammatory actions of theophylline, but also supports earlier work that regular treatment with theophylline can reduce PMN activation [42, 43], in addition to the actions of theophylline on eosinophils and lymphocytes discussed above. Theophylline treatment has also been reported to reduce the slope of methacholine dose-response curves in asthmatics *versus* placebo treatment [44, 45], a change also seen with glucocorticosteroids [46], but not with β_2-agonists [47], which actually steepen the curve.

The clinical relevance of these anti-inflammatory actions of theophylline is now being evaluated and a number of recent clinical studies lend weight to the suggestion that such activities may offer clinical benefit. The combination of low-dose inhaled budesonide plus theophylline, and conventional treatment with high-dose inhaled budesonide produced equivalent clinical efficacy in patients already receiving 800 µg of budesonide and whose asthma was not controlled [48]. These effects occurred at plasma levels below 10 µg/ml and suggest that lower than conventional plasma levels of theophylline may offer real clinical benefit with a reduced risk of side-effects for both drug classes [48]. These results also suggest that theophylline may offer additional benefit to glucocorticosteroids as has been previously suggested from other clinical studies by the use of different types of protocol [4, 49, 50].

Studies in paediatric asthma have shown that there is a clear effect of theophylline in the treatment of asthma that is comparable to low doses of glucocorticosteroids [51]. This observation is of particular interest given that theophylline is an orally active drug and has been shown to have a better compliance rate than inhaled medications [52], which is particularly relevant to the treatment of asthmatic children. With the low cost of theophylline, relative to other anti-asthma medications [53], and the fact that it is still one of the few drugs available for use orally in the treatment of this common disease, the growing body of evidence suggests that theophylline has anti-inflammatory and immunomodulatory properties at lower than conventional plasma levels. It is timely, therefore, to reconsider the wider use of theophylline in the overall management of asthma [28].

2. New Generation Phosphodiesterase (PDE) Inhibitors in the Treatment of Asthma

2.1. Phosphodiesterase Isoenzymes and Inflammatory Cells

Cyclic nucleotide PDEs (EC 3.1.4.17) hydrolyze the phoshpodiester bond of purine cyclic nucleotides (cAMP, cGMP) to the inactive metabolites, 5'-AMP and 5'-GMP, respectively. These metabolites lack the ability to activate cyclic nucleotide-dependent kinases. At least seven isoenzymes families have been identified to date, whose properties include an affinity for cyclic nucleotides. Theophylline is the archetypal non-selective PDE inhibitor. However, a wide range of more selective inhibitors of the various PDE isoenzyme faculties have now been discussed and example selective inhibitors are summarized in Table 1.

It is readily apparent that PDEs are widely distributed throughout the body and regulate the function of many cells. Particular interest has focused on the role of PDE4 and to a lesser extent PDE3 in allergic diseases such as asthma, as these isoenzymes are found in many inflammatory cells.

Table 1. Characteristics of phosphodiesterase isoenzymes

Family	Isoenzyme	Km (μM) cAMP	Km (μM) cGMP	Selective inhibitors	Cell types
1	Ca^{2+} calmodulin-stimulated	1–30	3	Vinpotecine, KS-505a	Brain, testes, trachea
2	cGMP-stimulated	50	50	EHNA	Hear, kindney
3	cGMP-inhibited	0.2	0.3	Siguazodan (SKF 94120) Milrinone Ciclostamide (SKF 95654)	Platelets, smooth muscle
4	cAMP-specific	4	>100	Rolipram, RP 73401 denbufylline, CDP 840, Ro 201724 CP 80633	Inflammatory cells
5	cGMP-specific	150	1	Zaprinast, Sidenefil	Platelets, smooth muscle
6	Phototeceptor	60	>100	Zaprinast, Sidenefil	Retina
7	High-affinity cAMP-specific	0.2	>100	None identified	T-cells

PDE enzymes have been identified in human basophils (PDE3 and PDE4) [54], neutrophils (PDE4) [55]; eosinophils (PDE4), (2) monocytes (PDE4) [56], lymphocytes (PDE3, 4 & 7) [57, 58]. There are now many studies that have demonstrated that such biochemical data are supported by pharmacological studies showing that selective inhibitors of the appropriate PDE isoenzyme families will inhibit a variety of functions of inflammatory cell activation *in vitro* (see [2] for a comprehensive review). In addition PDE3 and PDE4 isoenzyme have been identified in macrophages [59] and vascular endothelial cells [60]. Inhibition of PDE3 and PDE4 by selective inhibitors will also modulate a variety of function of these two cell types (see 2 for review). Furthermore, PDE 1, 3 & 5 have been identified in vascular and airway smooth muscle (see 2 for review) and for studies with selective PDE inhibitors, it would appear that PDE3 plays the dominant role in causing smooth muscle relaxation (see 2 for review).

2.2. Effects of PDE Inhibitors in Experimental Models of the Features of Asthma

2.2.1. Acute Bronchospasm: A variety of selective PDE inhibitors, including rolipram [61–67], RP 73401 [64], CDP 840 [65], and the mixed PDE3/PDE4 inhibitor zardaverine [63], significantly attenuated acute bronchospasm to antigen in the guinea pig. Similary, CDP 840 [68] but not rolipram [69] attenuated allergen-induced bronchoconstriction in the rabbit. In contrast, the PDE3 inhibitor Cl-930 [61], and to a lesser extent siguazodan [63], inhibited the allergen-induced bronchoconstrictor response in the guinea pig, while the PDE5 inhibitor zaprinast was without effect [61].

The effect of PDE4 inhibitors on bronchospasm induced by allergen is most likely due to inhibition of IgE/IgG-dependent mediator release from inflammatory cells rather than functional antagonism of airway smooth muscle shortening, as the predominant PDE isoenzymes in airway smooth muscle in PDE3. Indeed, rolipram significantly attenuated PGD_2 but not histamine release from guinea pig senisitized tracheal preparations *in vitro* [62]. In contrast, rolipram [62–64, 68], RP 73401 [64] and CDP840 [66] were less effective against spasmogen (LTC_4, methacholine, or histamine)-induced bronchoconstriction in the guinea pig, and it is clear that β_2-adrenoceptor agonists are superior to PDE4 inhibitors as functional antagonists.

2.2.2. Recruitment and Activation of Inflammatory Cells: PDE4 inhibitors have been shown to attenuate the ability of various stimuli, including various mediators and allergen to induce the recruitment of inflammatory cells, particularly eosinophils, into the lung.

The mixed PDE 3/4 inhibitor benzafentrine inhibited the pulmonary recruitment of eosinophils induced by the intraperitoneal injection of the cytokines GM-CSF, IL-3, and TNF-α [70]. Similarly, intratracheal instillation of human recombinant IL-5, IL-8, but not IL-3, and RANTES elicited a concentration-dependent increase in eosinophils recovered in BAL fluid that was inhibited by rolipram, and RO-20174, but not by the PDE3 inhibitors milrinone and Siguazodan, or by the PDE5 inhibitor zaprinast [71]. The IL-5-induced pleural eosinophilia in rats was also significantly attenuated by various PDE4 inhibitors, including CDP 840, RP 73401, and rolipram [66].

The PDE4 inhibitor rolipram has also been shown to attenuate allergen-induced pulmonary eosinophilia in the guinea pig whether administered *via* the oral [62, 71] or intraperitoneal route [63, 64, 66, 67, 72, 73] or following direct instillation into the airway [74]. Other PDE4 inhibitors, including Ro 201724 [72], RP 73401 [64, 66], and CDP 840 [66], were effective against eosinophilia induced by allergen. This effect is not a feature peculiar to the guinea pig since rolipram and CDP 840 attenuated the allergen-induced eosinophilia in the allergic rabbit [68, 69], while rolipram [75–77] and RP 73401 [64] inhibited allergen-induced pulmonary eosinophilia in the allergic rat and monkey. In allergic mice, the mixed PDE3/PDE4 inhibitor benzafentrine and the PDE4 inhibitor rolipram attenuated macrophage and eosinophil accumulation in BAL fluid [65]. Moreover, in addition to the ability of rolipram, Ro 201724, and CDP 840 [72, 73, 66] to inhibit pulmonary recruitment of eosinophils induced by allergen challenge, there is some evidence that these inhibitors and CP 80633 [78] also attenuate the activation of eosinophils recruited to the lung, as assessed by measurements of eosinophil peroxidase (EPO) contained in and/or secreted by the eosinophil.

The PDE3 inhibitor siguazodan has been shown to attenuate the ovalbumin-induced pulmonary eosinophilia in guinea pigs [62], although in some studies, siguazodan [72, 73] and milrinone [73, 67] were ineffective. These discrepancies could be attributed to differences in the degree of sensitization and/or dose of allergen employed to challenge the animals. Interestingly, the PDE3 inhibitor milrinone also inhibited pulmonary eosinophilia in allergic rats [77]. The PDE5 inhibitor zaprinast appeared to have no efect on allergen-induced eosinophilia in the rat [77] or the guinea pig [72, 67].

The mixed PDE3/PDE4 inhibitors zardaverine [79, 63, 65] and ORG 20421 [76] inhibited pulmonary eosinophilia in the guinea pig and neutrophilia in the rat, respectively. Furthermore, pulmonary neutrophilia and the attendant increase in elastase and TNF-α in BAL fluid following exposure to LPS in the rat were significantly reduced by zardaverine [80].

Many studies have demonstrated that acute treatment with a PDE4 inhibitor is effective against allergen-induced pulmonary eosinophilia. However, few studies have examined the effect of chronic treatment with PDE4 inhibitors. Seven-day delivery of benzafentrine inhibited eosinophilia induced by PAF [81] and allergen [82] in the guinea pig. Similarly, the intraperitoneal administration of Ro 201724 and zardverine twice daily for 1 week inhibited allergen-induced eosinophilia in the guinea pig [83]. Eosinophilia induced by allergen in allergic monkeys was abrogated following administration of rolipram over a 10-day period [75]. Similarly, the allergen-induced pulmonary recuritment of eosinophils in the allergic rabbit was inhibited following administration of rolipram [69] or CDP 840 [68] over a 3-day period.

In contrast, 7-day treatment with rolipram, benzafentrine, or aminophylline did not inhibit pulmonary eosinophilia to inhaled antigen but did reduce EPO activity in BAL fluid [73]. However, RP 73401 inhibited both eosinophil recruitment and activation [73]. It remains to be established whether chronic treatment with certain PDE4 inhibitors leads to tolerance subsequent to an upregulation of activity and/or expression of PDE4.

2.2.3. Bronchial Hyperresponsiveness: PAF-induced bronchial hyperresponsiveness to various spasmogens was attenuated by the non-selective PDE inhibitor, isbufylline [84], the mixed PDE3/4 inhibitor benzafentrine [70] and the PDE4 inhibitors rolipram [67] and RP73401 [64]. Rolipram [67] also attenuated allergen-induced bronchial hyperresponsiveness. Similarly, inhalation of pollutants such as ozone caused an eight- to 10-fold increase in airway sensitivity to histamine that was significantly attenuated by CDP840 [85]. Rolipram was 100 fold less potent than CDP840, although, RP73401 and aminophylline were found to be ineffective [85]. It is unclear whether differences in the bioavailability of these PDE4 inhibitors can account for the lack of effect of RP73401 on ozone-induced bronchial hyperresponsiveness. The effect of the PDE4 inhibitors on bronchial hyperresponsiveness was unrelated to functional antagonism of airway smooth muscle shortening since these inhibitors failed to attenuate bronchoconstriction induced by various spasmogens.

Both rolipram [69] and CDP840 [68] significantly inhibited allergen-induced bronchial hyperresponsiveness in the rabbit and the mixed PDE3/4 inhibitor zardaverine attenuated LPS-induced bronchial hyperresponsiveness to serotonin in the rat [80].

Few studies have investigated the effect of chronic treatment with PDE4 inhibitors on bronchial hyperresponsiveness. In one study, a 20-fold increase in airways sensitivity to methacholine was observed following repeated antigen challenge of atopic cynomolgus monkeys. This response was abolished by chronic treatment with rolipram [75]. Once again this effect was unlikely to be a consequence of functional antagonism of airway smooth muscle shortening since rolipram failed to attenuate the bronchoconstrictor response to inhaled allergen. In contrast, the mixed PDE 3/4 inhibitor benzafentrine administered over a 7-day period did not attenuate bronchial hyperresponsiveness induced by allergen, despite inhibiting the associated eosinophilia [81].

2.2.4. Phosphodiesterase Inhibitors in Asthma: Very few studies have been published concerning the efficacy of PDE inhibitors in the treatment of asthma. Ibudilast have been reported to significantly improve baseline airways responsiveness to spasmogen by two-fold after 6 months' treatment [86]. We have recently demonstrated that the PDE4 inhibitor CDP840 attenuated the development of the LAR in mild asthmatics with no effect on the acute response [87]. The effect of CDP840 on the LAR was modest, although treatment with this drug was not associated with significant side-effects. This study is the first to document the potential utility of this class of drug in the treatment of asthma, and other more selective orally active compounds are currently under development that are well tolerated in phase 1 studies in man [88]. Furthermore, recent studies with the orally active PDE4 inhibitor SB207499 (Ariflo) have shown that this drug is well tolerated and produces significant clinical benefit in patients with COPD [89] raising the distinct possibility that selective PDE4 inhibitors may well offer a therapeutic benefit in a wider range of respiratory diseases.

References

1 Weinberger M, Hendeles L (1996) Theophylline in asthma. *N Engl J Med* 334: 636–42
2 Spina D, Landells LJ, Page CP (1998) The role of theophylline and phosphodiesterase4 isoenzyme inhibitors as anti-inflammatory drugs. *Clin Exp Allergy* 28: 24–34
3 Ward AJM, McKenniff M, Evans JM, Page CP, Costello JF (1993) Theophylline—an immunomodulatory role in asthma? *Am Rev Respir Dis* 147: 518–523
4 Kidney J, Dominguez M, Taylor PM, Rose M, Chung KF, Barnes PJ (1995) Immunomodulation by theophylline in asthma: demonstration by withdrawal of therapy. *Am J Respir Crit Care Med* 151: 1907–1914
5 Ashutosh K, Sedat M, Fragale-Jackson J (1997) Effect of theophylline on respiratory drive in patients with chronic obstructive pulmonary disease. *J Clin Pharmacol* 37: 1100–1107
6 Pauwels R, Van Renterghem D, Van der Straeten M, Johannesson N, Persson CGA (1985) The effect of theophylline and enprofylline on allergen-induced bronchoconstriction. *J Allerg Clin*

Immunol 76: 583–590

7   Crescioli S, Spinazzi A, Plebani M, Pozzani M, Napp CE, Boschetto P, Fabbri LM (1992) Theophylline inhibits early and late asthmatic reactions induced by allergens in asthmatic subjects. *Ann Allergy* 66: 245–251

8   Hendeles L, Harman E, Huang D, O'Brien R, Blake K, Delafuente J (1995) Theophylline attenuation of airway responses to allergen: comparison with cromolyn metered dose inhaled. *J Allerg Clin Immunol* 95: 505–514

9   Cockcroft DW, Murdock KY, Gore BP, O'Byrne PM, Manning P (1989) Theophylline does not inhibit allergen induced increase in airway responsiveness to methacholine. *J Allerg Clin Immunol* 83(5): 913–920

10 De Monchy JGR, Kauffman HP, Venge P, Koeter GH, Jansen HM, Sluiter HJ, DeVries K (1985) Bronchoalveolar eosinophilia during allergen-induced late asthmatic reactions. *Am Rev Respir Dis* 131: 373–376

11 Sullivan PJ, Bekir S, Jaffar Z, Page C, Jeffery P, Costello J (1994) Anti-inflammatory effects of low-dose oral theophylline in atopic asthma. *Lancet* 343: 1006–1008

12 Aubier M, Neukirch C, Maachi M, Boucara D, Engelstatter R, Steinijans V, Samoyeau R, Dehoux M (1998) Effect of slow-release theophylline on nasal antigen challenge in subjects with allergic rhinitis. *Eur Resp J* 11: 1105–1110

13 Limatibul S, Shore A, Dorsch HM, Gelfard E (1987) Theophylline modulation of E-rosette formation: an indication of T-cell maturation. *Clin Exp Immunol* 33: 503–513

14 Pardi R, Zocchi M, Ferrero E, Cibaldo GF, Inverandi L, Rugarli C (1984) *In vivo* effects of a single infusion of theophylline on human peripheral blood lymphocytes. *Clin Exp Immunol* 57: 722–728

15 Mary D, Aussel C, Ferrua B, Fehlmann M (1987) Regulation of interleukin-2 synthesis by cAMP in human T cells. *J Immunol* 139: 1179–1184

16 Scordamaglia A, Ciprandi G, Ruffoni S, Caria M, Paolieri F, Venuti D, Cannonica GW (1988) Theophylline and the immune response: *in vitro* and *in vivo* effects. *Clin Immunol Immunopathol* 48: 238–246

17 Shohat B, Volovitz B, Varsano I (1983) Induction of suppressor T Cells in asthmatic children by theophylline treatment. *Clin Allergy* 13: 487–493

18 Hamid Q, Azzawi M, Ying S et al (1991) Expression of MRNA for interleukin-5 in mucosal bronchial biopsies from asthma. *J Clin Invest* 87: 1541–1546

19 Jaffar Z, Sullivan PJ, Page CP, Costello JF (1996) Low dose theophylline therapy modulates T-lymphocyte activity in subjects with atopic asthma. *Eur Resp J* 9: 456–463

20 Fink G, Mittelman M, Shohat B, Spitzer SA (1987) Theophylline-induced alterations in cellular immunity in asthmatic patients. *Clin Allergy* 17: 313–316

21 Brenner MR, Berkowitz R, Marshall N, Strunk RC (1988) Need for theophylline in severe steroid-requiring asthmatics. *Clin Allergy* 18: 143–150

22 Finnerty JP, Wilson LS, Madden J, Djukanovic R, Holgate ST (1996) Effects of theophylline on inflammatory cells and cytokines in asthmatic subjects: a placebo-controlled parallel group study. *Eur Respir J* 9: 1672–1677

23 Mascali JJ, Cvietusa P, Negri J, Borish L (1996) Anti-inflammaatory effects of theophylline: modulation of cytokine production. *Ann Allergy Asthma Immunol* 77: 34–38

24 Punnonen J, deWall Malefyt R, van Vlasselaer P (1993) IL-10 and viral IL-10 prevent IL-4 induced IgE synthesis by inhibiting the accessory cell function of monocytes. *J Immunol* 151: 1280–1289

25 Enk AH, Angeloni VL, Udey MC, Katz SI (1993) Inhibition of Langerhans cell antigen-presenting function by IL-10: a role for IL-10 in induction of tolerance. *J Immunol* 151: 2390–2398

26 Yamouguchi Y, Hayashi Y, Sugama Y (1988) Highly purified murine interleukin-5 (IL-5) stimulates eosinophil function and prolonges *in vitro* survival: IL-5 as an eosinophil chemotactic factor. *J Exp Med* 167: 1737–1742

27 Yasui K, Hu B, Nakazawa T, Agematsu K, Komiyama A (1997) Theophylline accelerates human granulocyte apoptosis not via phosphodiesterase inhibition. *J Clin Invest* 7: 1677–1684

28 Barnes PJ, Pauwels RA (1994) Theophylline in the management of asthma: time for reappraisal? *Eur Respir J* 7: 579–591

29 Banner KH, Page CP (1997) Prostaglandins contribute to the anti-proliferative effect of isoenzyme selective phosphodiesterase 4 inhibitors but not theophylline in human mononuclear cells. *Br J Pharmacol* 120: 11P

30 Peterson TC, Slysz G, Isbrucker R (1998) The inhibitory effect of ursodeoxycholic acid and pentoxifylline on platelet derived growth factor-stimulated proliferation is distinctive from an effect by cyclic AMP. *Immunopharmacology* 39: 181–191

31 Persson CGA, Pauwels R (1989) Pharmacology of Anti-Asthma Xanthines. *In*: CP Page, PJ Barnes (eds): *Pharmacology of Asthma*. Academic Press London 7: 207–225

32 Feoktistov I, Biaggioni I (1995) A2b Receptors evoke interleukin-8 secretion in human mast cells. An eroprofylline-sensitive mechanism with implications for asthma. *J Clin Invest* 96: 1979–1986

33 Feoktistov I, Polosa R, Holgate ST, Baggioni I (1998) Adenosine A2b receptors: novel therapeutic target in asthma? *Trends Pharmacol Sci* 19: 148–153

34 Cushley MJ, Tattersfield AE, Holgate ST (1983) Inhaled adenosine and guanosine on airway resistance in normal and asthmatic subjects. *Br J Clin Pharmacol* 15: 161–165

35 Mann JS, Holgate ST (1985) Specific antagonism of adenosine-induced broncocosntriction in asthma by oral theophylline. *Br J Clin Pharmacol* 19: 685–692

36 Cushley MJ, Tattersfield AE, Holgate ST (1984) Adenosine-induced bronchoconstriction in asthma. Antagonism by inhaled theophylline. *Am Rev Respir Dis* 129: 380–384

37 El-Hashim A, D'Agostino B, Matera MG, Page CP (1996) Characterization of adenosine receptors involved in adenosine-induced bronchoconstriction in allergic rabbits. *Br J Pharmacol* 119: 1262–1268

38 Ali S, Mustafa SJ, Metzger WJ (1994) Adenosine receptor-mediated bronchoconstriction and bronchial hyperresponsiveness in an allergic rabbit model. *Am J Physiol* 266: L271–L277

39 Nyce JW, Metzger WJ (1997) An anti-sense oligonucleotide against A_1 receptors inhibits allergen-induced airway responsiveness in allergic rabbits. *Nature* 97: 721–725

40 Kraft M, Torvik JA, Trudeau JB, Wenzel SE, Martin RJ (1996) Theophylline: potential antiinflammatory effects in nocturnal asthma. *J Allerg Clin Immunol* 97: 1242–1246

41 D'Alonzo G, Smolensky M, Feldman S (1990) Twenty-four hour lung function in adult patients with asthma. *Am Rev Respir Dis* 142: 84–90

42 Nielson CP, Crowley JJ, Cusak BJ, Vestal RE (1986) Therapeutic concentrations of theophylline and enprofylline potentiate catecholamine effects and inhibit leukocyte activation. *J Allerg Clin Immunol* 76: 660–667

43 Nielson CP, Crawley JJ, Morgan ME, Vestal RE (1988) Polymorphonuclear leukocyte inhibition by therapeutic concentrations of theophylline is mediated by cyclic 3', 5' adenosine monophosphate. *Am Rev Respir Dis* 137: 25–30

44 Page CP, Cotter T, Kilfeather S, Sullivan P, Spina D, Costello JF (1998) The effect of chronic theophylline treatment on position and shape of the methacholine dose-response curve in allergic asthmatic subjects. *Eur Resp J* 12: 24–29

45 Magnussen H, Reuss G, Jorres R (1987) Theophylline has a dose-related effect on the airway response to inhaled histamine and methacholine in asthmatics. *Am Rev Respir Dis* 136: 1163–1167

46 Bel EH, Timmers MC, Zwinderman AH, Dijkman JH, Sterk PJ (1991) The productive effect of inhaled corticosteroid on the maximal degree of airway narrowing to methacholine in asthmatic subjects. *Am Rev Respir Dis* 43: 109–113

47 Bel EH, Zwinderman AH, Timmers MC, Dijkman JH, Sterk PJ (1991) The protective effect of a beta 2 against excessive airway narrowing in response to bronchoconstrictor stimuli in asthma and chronic obstructive lung disease. *Thorax* 46: 9–14

48 Evans DJ, Talor DA, Zetterstrom O, Chung KF, O'Connor BJ, Barnes PJ (1997) A comparison of low-dose inhaled budesonide plus theophylline and high-dose budesonide for moderate asthma. *N Eng J. Med* 337: 1412–1418

49 Rivington RN, Boulet L-P, Cote J et al (1995) Efficacy of uniphyl, salbutamol, and their combination in asthmatic patients on high-dose inhaled steroids. *Am J Respir Crit Care Med* 151: 325–332

50 Ukena D, Harnest U, Sakalauskas R, Magyar P, Vetter N, Steffen H, Leichtl S, Rathgeb F, Keller A, Steinijans VW (1997) Comparison of addition of theophylline to inhaled steroid with doubling of the dose of inhaled steroid in asthma *Eur Respir J* 10: 2754–2760

51 Tinkelman DG, Reed CE, Nelson HS, Offord KP et al (1993) Aerosol beclomethasone dipropionate compared with theophylline as primary treatment of chronic, mild to moderately severe asthma in children. *Paediatrics* 92(1): 64–77

52 Kellaway JS, Wyatt RA, Addis SA (1994) Comparison of patients compliance with prescribed

oral and inhaled asthma medications. *Arch Intern Med* 154: 1349–1354
53 Barnes PJ, Jonsson B, Klim JP (1996) The cost of asthma. *Eur Resp J* 9: 636–642
54 Peachell PT, Undem BJ, Schleimer RP, MacGlashan DWJr Lichtenstein LM, Cielinski LB, Torphy TJ (1992) Preliminary identification and role of phosphodiesterase isoenzymes in human basophils *J Immunol* 148: 2503–2510
55 Muller T, Engels P, Fozard JR (1996) Subtypes of the type 4 cAMP phosphodiesterases: structure, regulation and selective inhibition. *Trends Pharmacol Sci* 17: 294–298
56 Sounes JE, Griffin M, Maslen C, Ebsworth K, Scott LC, Pollock K, Palfreyman MN, Karlsson JA (1996) Evidence that cyclic AMP phosphodiesterase inhibitors suppress TNFα generation from human monocytes by interacting with a 'low-affinity' phosphodiesterase 4 conformer *Br J Pharmacol* 118: 649–658
57 Tenor H, Staniciu L, Schudt C, Hatzelmann A, Wendel A, Djukanovic R, Church MK, Shute JK (1995). Cyclic nucleotide phosphodiesterases from purified human CD4$^+$ and CD8$^+$ T lymphocytes. *Clin Exp Allergy* 25: 616–624
58 Giembycz MA, Corrigan CJ, Seybold J, Newton R, Barnes PJ (1996) Identification of cyclic AMP phosphodiesterase 3,4 and 7 in human CD4$^+$ and CD8$^+$ T-lymphocytes: role in regulating proliferation and the biosynthesis of interleukin-2. *Br J Pharmacol* 118: 1945–1958
59 Schudt C, Tenor H, Hatzelmann A (1995) PDE isoenzymes as targets for anti-asthma drugs *Eur Respir J* 8: 1179–1183
60 Souness JE, Diocee BK, Martin W, Moodie SA (1990) Pig aortic endothelial-cell cyclic nucleotide phosphodiesterases. Use of phosphodiesterase inhibitors to evaluate their roles in regulating cyclic nucleotide levels in intact cells. *Biochem J* 266: 127–132
61 Howell RE, Sickels BD, Woeppel SL (1993) Pulmonary antiallergic and bronchodilator effects of isozyme-selective phosphodiesterase inhibitors in guinea pigs. *J Pharmacol Exp Ther* 264: 609–615
62 Underwood DC, Osborn RR, Novak LB, Matthews JK, Newsholme SJ, Undem BJ, Hand JM, Torphy TJ (1993) Inhibition of antigen-induced bronchoconstriction and eosinophil infiltration in the guinea pig by the cyclic AMP-specific phosphodiesterase inhibitor, rolipram. *J Pharmacol Exp Ther* 266: 306–313
63 Underwood DC, Kotzer CJ, Bochnowicz S, Osborn RR, Luttmann MA, Hay DW, Torphy TJ (1994) Comparison of phosphodiesterase III, IV and dual III/IV inhibitors on bronchospasm and pulmonary eosinophil influx in guinea pigs. *J Pharmacol Exp Ther* 270: 250–259
64 Raeburn D, Underwood SL, Lewis SA, Woodman VR, Battram CH, Tomkinson A, Sharma S, Jordan R, Souness JE, Webber SE, et al (1994) Anti-inflammatory and bronchodilator properties of RP 73401, a novel and selective phosphodiesterase type IV inhibitor. *Br J Pharmacol* 113: 1423–1431
65 Nagai H, Takeda H, Iwama T, Yamaguchi S, Mori H (1995) Studies on anti-allergic action of AH 21-132, a novel isozyme-selective phosphodiesterase inhibitor in airways. *Jpn J Pharmacol* 67: 149–156
66 Hughes B, Howat D, Lisle H, Holbrook M, Tames T, Gozzard N, Blease K, Hughes P, Kingaby R, Warrellow G et al (1996) The inhibition of antigen-induced eosinophilia and bronchoconstriction by CDP840, a novel stereo-selective inhibitor of phosphodiesterase type 4. *Br J Pharmacol* 118: 1183–1191
67 Ortiz JL, Valles JM, MartiCabrera M, Cortijo J, Morcillo EJ (1996) Effects of selective phosphodiesterase inhibitors on platelet-activating factor- and antigen-induced airway hyperreactivity, eosinophil accumulation, and microvascular leakage in guinea pigs. *Naunyn-Schmied Arch Pharmacol* 353: 200–206
68 Gozzard N, El-Hashim A, Herd CM, Blake SM, Holbrook M, Hughes B, Higgs GA, Page CP (1996a). Effect of the glucocorticosteroid budesonide and a novel phosphodiesterase type 4 inhibitor CDP840 on antigen-induced airway responses in neonatally immunised rabbits. *Br J Pharmacol* 118: 1201–1208
69 Gozzard N, Herd CM, Blake SM, Holbrook M, Hughes B, Higgs GA, Page CP (1996b). Effects of theophylline and rolipram on antigen-induced airway responses in neonatally immunized rabbits. *Br J Pharmacol* 117: 1405–1412
70 Kings MA, Chapman I, Kristersson A, Sanjar S, Morley J (1990) Human recombinant lymphokines and cytokines induce pulmonary eosinophilia in the guinea pig which is inhibited by ketotifen and AH 21-132. *Int Arch Allergy Appl Immunol* 91: 354–361
71 Lagente V, Pruniaux MP, Junien JL, Moodley I (1995) Modulation of cytokine-induced

eosinophil infiltration by phosphodiesterase inhibitors. *Am J Respir Crit Care Med* 151: 1720–1724

72 Lagente V, Moodley I, Perrin S, Mottin G, Junien JL (1994) Effects of isozyme-selective phosphodiesterase inhibitors on eosinophil infiltration in the guinea-pig lung. *Eur J Pharmacol* 255: 253–256

73 Banner KH, Marchini F, Buschi A, Moriggi E, Semeraro C, Page CP (1995) The effect of selective phosphodiesteraseinhibitors in comparison with other anti-asthma drugs on allergen-induced eosinophilia in guinea-pig airways. *Pulm Pharmacol* 8: 37–42

74 Raeburn D, Souness JE, Tomkinson A, Karlsson JA (1993) Isozyme-selective cyclic nucleotide phosphodiesterase inhibitors: biochemistry, pharmacology and therapeutic potential in asthma. *Prog Drug Res* 40: 9–32

75 Turner CR, Andresen CJ, Smith WB, Watson JW (1994) Effects of rolipram on responses to acute and chronic antigen exposure in monkeys. *Am J Respir Crit Care Med* 149: 1153–1159

76 Elwood W, Sun J, Barnes PJ, Giembycz MA, Chung KF (1995) Inhibition of allergen-induced lung eosinophilia by type-III and combined type III- and IV-selective phosphodiesterase inhibitors in brown-Norway rats. *Inflamm Res* 44: 83–86

77 Howell RE, Jenkins LP, Fielding LE, Grimes D (1995) Inhibition of antigen-induced pulmonary eosinophilia and neutrophilia by selective inhibitors of phosphodiesterase types 3 or 4 in Brown Norway rats. *Pulm Pharmacol* 8: 83–89

78 Turner CR, Cohan VL, Cheng JB, Showell HJ, Pazoles CJ, Watson JW (1996) The *in vivo* pharmacology of CP-80,633, a selective inhibitor of phosphodiesterase 4. *J Pharmacol Exp Ther* 278: 1349–1355

79 Schudt C, Winder S, Eltze M, Kilian U, Beume R (1991b). Zardaverine: a cyclic AMP specific PDE III/IV inhibitor. *Agents Actions Suppl* 34: 379–402

80 Kips JC, Joos GF, Peleman RA, Pauwels RA (1993) The effect of zardaverine, an inhibitor of phosphodiesterase isoenzymes III and IV, on endotoxin-induced airway changes in rats. *Clin Exp Allergy* 23: 518–523

81 Sanjar S, Aoki S, Boubekeur K, Chapman ID, Smith D, Kings MA, Morley J (1990a). Eosinophil accumulation in pulmonary airways of guinea-pigs induced by exposure to an aerosol of platelet-activating factor: effect of anti-asthma drugs. *Br J Pharmacol* 99: 267–272

82 Sanjar S, Aoki S, Kristersson A, Smith D, Morley J (1990b). Antigen challenge induces pulmonary airway eosinophil accumulation and airway hyperreactivity in sensitized guinea-pigs: the effect of anti-asthma drugs. *Br J Pharmacol* 99: 679–686

83 Banner KH, Page CP (1995) Acute *versus* chronic administration of phosphodiesterase inhibitors on allergen-induced pulmonary cell influx in sensitized guinea-pigs. *Br J Pharmacol* 114: 93–98

84 Manzini S, Perretti F, Abelli L, Evangelista S, Seeds EA, Page CP (1993) Isbufylline, a new xanthine derivative, inhibits airway hyperresponsiveness and airway inflammation in guinea pigs. *Eur J Pharmacol* 249: 251–257

85 Holbrook M, Gozzard N, James T, Higgs G, Hughes B (1996) Inhibition of bronchospasm and ozone-induced airway hyperresponsiveness in the guinea-pig by CDP840, a novel phosphodiesterase type 4 inhibitor. *Br J Pharmacol* 118: 1192–1200

86 Kawasaki A, Hoshino K, Osaki R, Mizushima Y, Yano S (1992) Effect of ibudilast: a novel anti-asthmatic agent, on airway hypersensitivity in bronchial asthma. *J Asthma* 29: 245–252

87 Harbinson PL, MacLeod D, Hawksworth R, O'Toole S, Sullivan PJ, Heath P, Kilfeather S, Page CP, Costello J, Holgate ST, Lee TH (1997) The effect of a novel orally active selective PDE4 isoenzyme inhibitor CDP840 on allergen-induced responses in asthmatic subjects. *Eur Respir J* 10: 1008–1914

88 Landells LJ, Jensen MW, Spina D, Donigi Gale D, Miller AJ, Nichols T, Smith K, Rotshetyn Y, Burch RM, Page CP, O'Connor BJ (1998) Oral adminsitration of the phosphodiesterase (PDE) 4 inhibitor, V11294A inhibits *ex vivo* agonist-induced cell activation. *Eur Respir J* 12: 362

89 Torphy TJ, Murduch RD, Nieman R, Compton CH (1998) Ariflo (SB 207499), a second generation PDE4 inhibitor for the treatment of asthma and COPD. *In: Proceedings of New Drug for Asthma IV*, Official Satellite of the XIII IUPHAR Symposium, Konstanz, July 23–25, 1998

Index